KU-722-746

Acknowledgements

The principal author of this report was Mat Kinton of the MHAC Policy Unit.

The Commission is grateful to all persons who acted in a consultative capacity in the preparation of this report, many of whom offered their valuable time to discuss issues with us and suggest means of expression.

We are particularly grateful to our "experts panel" who agreed to act as readers and many of whom kindly gave a day of their time to meet with us to discuss our shared ideas and concerns: Christian Dingwall, Prof Nigel Eastman, Catherine Grimshaw, David Hewitt, Camilla Parker, Andrew Parsons, Robert Robinson, Oliver Thorold, June Tweedie and Prof K W M (Bill) Fulford. All responsibility for the content of this report rests, of course, with the Commission itself, and what follows cannot be assumed to reflect the individual views of those listed above.

It is not practicable to name all the members and secretariat of the Commission who have contributed to this report but we thank them collectively.

We are grateful to Kevin Towers of West London Mental Health NHS Trust for data used at Figure 53 and to Barbara Hatfield of the University of Manchester Mental Health Social Work Unit for data used at Chapter 8.71. We have also taken from Commission-based research, particularly that of Steve Klein and Hazelanne Lewis. Margaret Burn, Lynda Crofts, Fran Mente, Melissa Meritt and Tracey Whittingham have provided information and occasional comment on our ideas from the Department of Health, whilst scrupulously avoiding seeking to influence what we choose to say.

The Commission wishes, finally, to express its gratitude to the managers and staff of hospitals and other authorities responsible for operating the 1983 Act, who have been so willing to co-operate with our work over past years.

This report is dedicated to all patients who have been detained under the 1983 Act.

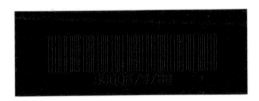

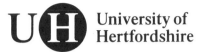

University of Hertfordshire

College Lane, Hatfield, Herts. AL10 9AB

Learning and Information Services

For renewal of Standard and One Week Loans,
please visit the web site **http://www.voyager.herts.ac.uk**

This item must be returned or the loan renewed by the due date.
The University reserves the right to recall items from loan at any time.
A fine will be charged for the late return of items.

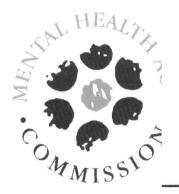

psychiatric compulsion

Tenth Biennial Report
2001–2003

London: **TSO**

Published by TSO (The Stationery Office) and available from:

Online
www.tso.co.uk/bookshop

Mail, Telephone, Fax & E-mail
TSO
PO Box 29, Norwich, NR3 1GN
Telephone orders/General enquiries: 0870 600 5522
Fax orders: 0870 600 5533
E-mail: book.orders@tso.co.uk
Textphone 0870 240 3701

TSO Shops
123 Kingsway, London, WC2B 6PQ
020 7242 6393 Fax 020 7242 6394
68-69 Bull Street, Birmingham B4 6AD
0121 236 9696 Fax 0121 236 9699
9-21 Princess Street, Manchester M60 8AS
0161 834 7201 Fax 0161 833 0634
16 Arthur Street, Belfast BT1 4GD
028 9023 8451 Fax 028 9023 5401
18-19 High Street, Cardiff CF10 1PT
029 2039 5548 Fax 029 2038 4347
71 Lothian Road, Edinburgh EH3 9AZ
0870 606 5566 Fax 0870 606 5588

TSO Accredited Agents
(see Yellow Pages)

and through good booksellers

First published 2003

ISBN 0 11 322652 7

Mental Health Act Commission,
Maid Marian House,
56 Hounds Gate,
Nottingham,
NG1 6BG

Tel: 0115 943 7100

Email: chief.executive@mhac.trent.nhs.uk

Printed in the United Kingdom for The Stationery Office

Contents

Part Two
Issues arising from the application of the MHA 1983

Part Three
Forensic and secure mental health services

Part Six
The work of the Commission and its successor bodies

Chairman's Foreword

Placed Amongst Strangers

The Mental Health Act Commission's Tenth Biennial Report

This Tenth Biennial Report is something of a watershed. Looking back, it signals twenty years of significant focused activity reviewing the lawfulness of detention of detained patients, monitoring the operation of the Mental Health Act, and ensuring that as far as possible the quality of care for patients and service users is of a good and continually improving standard. Looking forward, this may be the last biennial report of the Commission, although at the time of writing it is possible that there will be an eleventh!

The Government has understandably and sensibly decided to streamline monitoring inspection and regulation of health services. Subject to legislation setting up the Commission for Healthcare Audit and Inspection (CHAI), and the proposed Mental Health Bill (which will replace the Mental Health Act 1983), it is proposed that the Mental Health Act Commission will merge with three other Commissions to form CHAI. The Commission has welcomed this change as an opportunity to improve the monitoring of the operation of the Act and to obtain the resources and sanctions required to ensure that any necessary changes are implemented.

This report covers the period 2001 – 2003. During that time there have been significant changes in case law, largely though not exclusively as a result of the Human Rights Act 1998, which came into force in 2000. A number of high profile cases have dealt with issues that have for many years been a concern of the Commission. Seclusion is one of those. Shortly before we completed preparation of this report the *Munjaz* case was heard in the Appeal Court, leading to a landmark judgement which ruled unlawful the seclusion policy at Ashworth Hospital largely on the grounds that it did not accord with the Code of Practice. Such developments are important but create wider uncertainty amongst patients and their advocates about the legal framework within which they are detained. The proposed Bill may clarify some matters, but perhaps will lead to different uncertainties as the new Act, once passed, settles down and as case law emerges.

This report focuses very heavily on the implications of the Human Rights Act 1998, considers a number of critical issues about which the Commission has felt concerned for some time (such as the needs of women and young people), emphasises concerns such as seclusion, and draws powerful attention to the needs of Black and minority ethnic patients. Following the second National Visit in 1999, the Commission has recently published with NIMHE and the University of Central Lancashire Centre for Ethnicity and Health a further paper ('Engaging and Changing') to promote good practice in the provision of care for Black and minority ethnic groups based on the findings of that National Visit. The Commission will continue to give a high priority to diversity issues and will continue to give particular prominence to all those who have extra vulnerability in addition to their mental disorder.

This report makes 70 recommendations, most of which are directed to Government and Parliament. In our Ninth Biennial Report we focused many of our recommendations at service providers. In this report we unambiguously return to addressing the lawfulness of detention of patients. In turn, this leads us to make a number of proposals for improvements in the present law and in the way that the patients are treated which we hope will be incorporated into any new legislation.

I am grateful to many people for assisting the Commission in putting together this report especially the 216 Commissioners named in Appendix B, whose visits to detained patients in hospital have provided the evidential base for that which follows. In particular I wish to pay tribute to Mat Kinton who wrote the report and who worked unstintingly for six months to ensure that the report engages deeply with the issues and is at the same time eminently readable.

Professor Kamlesh Patel OBE
Chairman, Mental Health Act Commission

Summary of this Report

In the English, Gujarati, Hindi, Urdu, Somali and Welsh languages

Summary of this report

The Mental Health Act Commission is charged with monitoring the implementation of powers and discharge of duties arising from the detention and treatment of patients under the Mental Health Act 1983. This report is based upon the experience of the Commission in visiting all psychiatric facilities that detain patients. The report specifically covers the financial years 2001/02 and 2002/03, but draws upon the work of the Commission over the two decades of its existence and looks to the future application and monitoring of compulsion in mental health services.

A central theme of the report is the need for Government to take a lead in policy-level guidance and intervention on the use and impact of mental health law. We see this as particularly important in the current climate for the following reasons.

* Human rights based challenges are reshaping existing mental health law. Whilst this creates welcome improvements to practice, it also generates great uncertainty amongst practitioners as the law changes from month to month.

* Wider uncertainties exist because of proposals for fundamental changes in mental health law, particularly where it is felt that such changes are in response to requirements of human rights legislation.

* The increasing development of less institutional and more diverse inpatient units, whilst welcome in many respects, risks creating small-scale, fragmented services without uniformity or transparency in the application of legal powers of coercion.

The report also suggests that the development of a truly human rights based approach to mental health services involving compulsion will require:

* new legislation to be based upon explicit principles, similar to those provided in the Mental Health Act Code of Practice;

* particular attention given to ensuring that mental health services are provided equitably and without discrimination according to gender, sexual orientation ethnicity, religion, or social class;

* statutory regulation of specific areas of compulsion, such as those dealing with, control and discipline (including seclusion), to ensure uniform good practice;

* the active promotion across all areas of Government of anti-stigma and anti-discriminatory measures in relation to mentally disordered people, with particular focus on those made subject to powers of compulsion; and

* effective and focussed monitoring of the use of legal powers and the care of patients subject to such powers.

We welcome and support the National Institute for Mental Health's commitment to Values-Based Practice. Practice founded on respect for human rights must develop genuine user and carer-involvement, even when State powers of coercion are invoked.

The Commission continues to have many concerns about the care and treatment of patients under compulsion. Our report notes the vulnerability of children and minors admitted to adult facilities; and of women patients, especially those admitted to largely male environments, or affected by transfers within the High Secure Hospital sector. We highlight the problems of access to therapeutic and recreational activities on many wards, environmental problems in hospitals and the broad uncertainties existing over the extent of powers of control and discipline, especially the way seclusion is practiced in some hospitals. We note the continuing over-representation amongst detained patients from Black and minority ethnic groups, and we are particularly concerned about racial harassment of patients. The Commission continues to press for as little detriment to patients' clinical care as possible in the implementation of the Government's Security Directions for High Security Hospitals.

We hope that the Mental Health Bill as presented to Parliament in the coming session or thereafter will have been considerably amended from the draft of 2002, especially in relation to the criteria for and purpose of compulsory interventions in mental health care. We believe that any plan to extend powers of compulsory treatment into prison under such legislation to be premature, given the infrastructure of prison-based healthcare and the lack of effective monitoring of prison mental health provision at present.

We believe there is and will be a continuing need for a visitorial body charged specifically with monitoring the application of powers and discharge of duties created by mental health legislation for the compulsory treatment of patients. This function is necessary to discharge duties placed upon Government to know about those it detains. Arrangements under new legislation should preserve this function, however it is administered.

સંક્ષિપ્ત હેવાલ

મેન્ટલ હેલ્થ (માનસિક આરોગ્ય) એક્ટ 1983 હેઠળ દરદીઓને રોકી રાખવા અને એમના ઉપચાર કરવાની સત્તાની અને ફરજોની તપાસ રાખવાની જવાબદારી, મેન્ટલ હેલ્થ એક્ટ કમિશનની છે. આ રિપોર્ટ (હેવાલ), બધી સાયકાઅટ્રિક (મનોરોગ ચિકિત્સા) સુવિધાઓ, જ્યાં રોગીઓને રોકી રાખવામાં આવે છે, ત્યાંની કમિશનની બધી મુલાકાતોના અનુભવો પર આધારિત છે. વિશિષ્ટ રીતે હેવાલ 2001/02થી 2002/03ના નાણાંકીય વર્ષોને આવરી લે છે, પરંતુ છેલ્લા બે દસકાઓમાં થયેલી કમિશનની કામગીરી પણ બતાવે છે, તથા ભવિષ્યમાં લાગુ પડતી બાબતોને અને માનસિક આરોગ્ય સેવાઓમાં (મેન્ટલ હેલ્થ સર્વિસિસ) જબરદસ્તીના વલણ માટે તપાસ થવી જોઈએ, એની પણ માહિતી આપે છે.

હેવાલનો મુખ્ય વિષય છે, ગવર્મેંટ કાર્યપદ્ધતિ સ્તર પર યોગ્ય માર્ગદર્શન આપવું જોઈએ અને માનસિક આરોગ્ય કાયદાના ઉપયોગ અને અસર પર દરમ્યાનગીરી કરવી જોઈએ. અત્યારના સમયમાં આનું વિશિષ્ટ મહત્વ નીચેના કારણોસર છે.

- માનવીય અધિકારો પર આધાર રાખતી કસોટીઓના કારણે અત્યારનો માનસિક આરોગ્યનો કાયદો બદલાઈ રહ્યો છે. એક રીતે આ આવકારદાયક રહે છે, પરંતુ એ જ સમયે પ્રેક્ટિશનરોમાં ખૂબ જ અનિશ્ચિતતા પેદા કરે છે, કારણકે કાયદો એક મોઢેથી બીજા મોઢે બદલાતો રહે છે.

- માનસિક આરોગ્યના કાયદામાં પાયારૂપી ફેરફારોની દરખાસ્તો છે, જેને કારણે વિસ્તૃત અનિશ્ચિતતા રહે છે. ખાસ કરીને જ્યારે એમ લાગે છે કે, આવા ફેરફારો માનવીય અધિકારોના કાયદાઓની જરૂરતની પ્રતિક્રિયાના રૂપમાં છે.

- ઓછા ઈન્સ્ટિટ્યૂશનલ હોય એવા અને વિભિન્ન ઈનપેશંટ યુનિટોનો વિકાસ થવાથી નાના-પાયાની, છૂટીછવાઈ સેવાઓ ઉત્પન્ન થવાનું જોખમ રહે છે, જે કાયદાના સત્તાઈના અધિકારને લાગુ કરવામાં એકસરખી કે પારદર્શક નથી હોતી.

રિપોર્ટ એ પણ સૂચવે છે કે, ચોક્કસ રીતે માનવીય અધિકારો પર આધારિત માનસિક આરોગ્ય સેવાઓનો વિકાસ, જેમાં જબરદસ્તીનો સમાવેશ થાય છે, એવા વિકાસ માટે નીચે જણાવેલી બાબતો આવશ્યક રહેશે :

- સ્પષ્ટ સિદ્ધાંતો પર આધારિત નવા કાયદાઓ મેન્ટલ હેલ્થ એક્ટ કોડ ઓફ પ્રેક્ટિસમાં અપાયેલા કાયદાઓ સમાન હોય;

- ખાસ ધ્યાન અપાયું હોય કે, માનસિક આરોગ્ય સેવાઓ સમાન રીતે અપાય છે અને એ માટે લિંગ, જાતિય મૂળ, ધર્મ અથવા સામાજિક વર્ગના આધાર પર ભેદભાવ કરવામાં નથી આવતો;

- વિશિષ્ટ જબરદસ્તીના ક્ષેત્રોનું કાયદા પ્રમાણે ખાસ નિયંત્રણ; ક્ષેત્રો જેવા કે નિયંત્રણ અને શિસ્ત (એકાંતનો સમાવેશ કરીને) સાથે વહેવાર કરતા હોય. આનાથી એક સરખી ઉત્તમ પદ્ધતિની ખાતરી રહેશે;

- ગવર્મેંટના બધા ક્ષેત્રોમાં માનસિક વિકૃતિવાળા લોકો માટે લાંછન વગરની અને ભેદભાવ વગરની પદ્ધતિ માટે સક્રિય પ્રોત્સાહન, ખાસ કરીને જેમના પર જબરદસ્તીના અધિકારો લાગુ પડી શકતા હોય; અને

- કાયદાના અધિકારોના ઉપયોગની અસરકારક અને કેન્દ્રિય તપાસ, તથા આવા અધિકારો હેઠળ આવતા રોગીઓની દેખભાળ.

અમે નૅશનલ ઈન્સ્ટિટ્યૂટ ફોર મેન્ટલ હેલ્થની વૅલ્યુ- બેઝ્ડ પ્રેક્ટિસ માટેની જવાબદારીને આવકાર આપી ટેકો આપીએ છીએ. જે પ્રેક્ટિસ માનવીય અધિકારો માટેના આદર પર આધારિત હોય એણે સાચા વાપરનાર અને દેખરેખ રાખનારની સમાવિષ્ટતા વધારવી જોઈએ, રાજ્યના સત્તાઈના અધિકારનું આવાહ્ન થાય ત્યારે પણ.

જબરદસ્તી હેઠળના રોગીઓની દેખભાળ અને ઉપચાર વિષે કમિશનને ઘણી ચિંતાઓ રહે છે. અમારો રિપોર્ટ, બાળકો અને સગીર વયની વ્યક્તિઓની પુખ્તવયની સુવિધાઓમાં દાખલા માટેની હુમલાપાત્રતા; સ્ત્રી રોગીઓ, જેમને પુરુષોના વાતાવરણમાં રાખવામાં આવતી હોય તથા સ્ત્રીઓ જેમના પર હાઈ સિક્યુર હૉસ્પિટલ વિભાગની અંદર જ બદલી થતી હોય, એ બધી બાબતોને નોંધી રહ્યા છીએ. ઘણા બધા વૉર્ડોમાં રોગનિવારક અને મનોરંજનની પ્રવૃત્તિઓ મેળવવાની સમસ્યાઓ, હૉસ્પિટલના વાતાવરણની સમસ્યાઓ અને નિયંત્રણના તથા શિસ્તના અધિકારોની અનિશ્ચિતતા,ખાસ કરીને જે રીતે કેટલીક હૉસ્પિટલોમાં એકાંતમાં રાખવામાં આવે છે, આ બધી બાબતોનું મહત્વ અમે જણાવી રહ્યા છીએ. બ્લૅક અને લઘુમતિ જાતિના ગ્રૂપોના રોકી રાખેલા રોગીઓની લગાતાર વધારે પડતી રજૂઆતોને અમે જોઈ રહ્યા છીએ. અમે ખાસ કરીને રોગીઓ માટેની વંશવાદી પજવણીથી ચિંતિત રહીએ છીએ. ગવર્મેંટના સિક્યુરિટી ડાયરેકશન્સ ફોર હાઈ સિક્યુરિટી હૉસ્પિટલ્સના કાયદાઓનો અમલ કરવામાં, કમિશન, રોગીઓની ચિકિત્સાની સારસંભાળ ઓછી ન થઈ જાય એનું ખૂબ જ ધ્યાન રાખે છે.

અમે આશા રાખીએ છીએ કે, મેન્ટલ હેલ્થ બિલ, જેને આગળ આવતી પાર્લિઆમેન્ટ બેઠકમાં રજૂ કરવામાં આવે અથવા ત્યારપછી રજૂ કરવામાં આવે, એને પૂરી રીતે 2002ના ડ્રાફ્ટથી સુધારેલું હોય; ખાસ કરીને માનસિક આરોગ્યની દેખભાળ માટે જબરદસ્તીની દરમ્યાનગીરીના હેતુ સંબંધિત બદલેલું હોય. અમે માનીએ છીએ કે જેલમાં જબરદસ્તીના ઉપચાર માટેના અધિકારો વધારવાની કોઈપણ યોજના, જે આવા કાયદાઓ હેઠળ હોય, એ પૂરી રીતે પરિપક્વ થઈ નથી, કારણકે અત્યારે જેલમાં માનસિક આરોગ્યને અસરકારક રીતે તપાસવા માટે કોઈ જોગવાઈ નથી.

અમે માનીએ છીએ કે, રોગીઓ માટે જબરદસ્તીના ઉપચારના અધિકારોને અમલમાં લાવવા માટે મુલાકાતીઓની સંસ્થા દ્વારા લગાતાર તપાસની જરૂર રહે છે. માનસિક આરોગ્યના કાયદાઓએ ઘડેલી ફરજો નિભાઈ રહી છે કે નહિ, એની તપાસની પણ લગાતાર આવશ્યકતા રહે છે. ગવર્મેંટની ફરજોને નિભાવવા, જે ફરજો હેઠળ રોગીઓને રોકી રાખવામાં આવે છે, એમના વિષે જાણકારી મેળવવાની ગવર્મેંટને જરૂર રહે છે. નવા કાયદાઓ હેઠળની ગોઠવણોએ કોઈપણ વહીવટની રીતથી કાર્યને જાળવી રાખવું જોઈએ.

इस रिपोर्ट का सार

मानसिक स्वास्थ्य अधिनियम (मैंटल हैल्थ ऐक्ट) कमीशन का काम मानसिक स्वास्थ्य अधिनियम 1983 के अंतर्गत रोगीयों को नज़रबंद करने और उनका इलाज करने संबंधी अधिकार और कर्तव्य का मॉनीटरन करना है। यह रिपोर्ट उस अनुभव पर आधारित है जो रोगियों को नज़रबंद करने वाली मनोरोग चिकित्सा संस्थाओं में जाकर कमीशन को प्राप्त हुआ। यह रिपोर्ट विशेष करके 2001/02 से 2002/03 वित्तीय वर्षों से संबंधित है परंतु कमीशन के पिछले दो दशकों के काम को भी ध्यान में रखती है और मनोरोग चिकित्सा सेवाओं की भावी ज़िम्मेवारियों के प्रसंग और मॉनीटरन को भी नज़र में रखती है।

इस रिपोर्ट का मूल विषय सरकार की वह अगुआई प्रदान करने की ज़िम्मेवारी है जो मानसिक स्वास्थ्य क़ानून के उपयोग और प्रभाव क्षेत्र में उसकी ओर से नीति स्तर पर मार्गदर्शन और दखल देने की बनती है। हम इसे वर्तमान स्थिति में निम्नलिखित कारणों से विशेष महत्त्वपूर्ण मानते हैं।

- मानव अधिकार चुनौतियां वर्तमान के मानसिक स्वास्थ्य क़ानून में परिवर्तन ला रही हैं। ये पद्धति में स्वागत योग्य सुधार लाती तो हैं, परंतु साथ ही ये क़ानून में माह दर माह परिवर्तन लाने के कारण चिकित्सकों में भारी अनिश्चितता भी पैदा करती हैं।
- मानसिक स्वास्थ्य क़ानून में बुनियादी परिवर्तन लाने के प्रस्तावों के कारण व्यापक अनिश्चितताएं पैदा हुई हैं विशेष करके जब यह महसूस होता है कि ये परिवर्तन मानव अधिकार विधान की शर्तों को पूरा करने के लिए लाए जा रहे हैं।
- अंतरंग रोगियों के लिए कम संस्थागत और अधिक नानाविध सुविधाओं के विकास में बढ़ौतरी किन्ही मामलों में स्वागत योग्य होते हुए भी छोटी-छोटी, टुकड़ों में बंटी हुई ऐसी सेवाओं को जन्म देने का जोखिम उठाती है जिन में अनिवार्यता के वैधानिक अधिकारों का उपयोग असमान और अपारदर्शी हैं।

रिपोर्ट यह भी सुझाव देती है कि मानव अधिकारों पर सचमुच आधारित मानसिक स्वास्थ्य की अनिवार्यता वाली सेवाओं का विकास करते समय निम्नलिखित की भी आवश्यकता पड़ेगी:

- मानसिक स्वास्थ्य अधिनियम की पद्धति संहिता की तरह स्पष्ट सिद्धांतों पर आधारित एक नया विधान;
- यह सुनिश्चित करने के लिए विशेष ध्यान देना कि मानसिक स्वास्थ्य सेवाएं लिंग, लैंगिक रूझान, मानव जातीय मूल, धर्म या सामाजिक वर्ग के आधार पर भेदभाव किए बिना प्रदान की जाती हैं;
- नियंत्रण और अनुशासन (अलग रखने समेत) से संबंधित अनिवार्यता के विशेष अंगों में समान और सुचारू पद्धति की स्थापना को सुनिश्चित करने के लिए क़ानूनी विनियम;
- मनोविकृत लोगों, विशेष करके उनके तई जिन्हें अनिवार्यता के अधिकारों के अधीन लाया जाता है, कलंक और भेदभाव विरोधी संस्कार को सरकार के सभी क्षेत्रों में सक्रिय बढ़ावा देना; और

- कानूनी अधिकारों के उपयोग का और इन अधिकारों के अधीन आने वाले रोगियों की देख-भाल का प्रभावकारी और केंद्रित मॉनीटरन।

हम राष्ट्रीय मानसिक स्वास्थ्य संस्थान (नैशनल इंस्टीट्यूट फ़ॉर मैंटल हैल्थ) की मान्यता आधारित पद्धति के लिए वचनबद्धता का स्वागत और समर्थन करते हैं। जो पद्धति मानव अधिकारों के लिए सम्मान पर आधारित होगी वह, भले ही अनिवार्यता के क़ानूनी अधिकारों को लागू किया जाए, सच्चे अधिकार को काम में लाने वाला और देख-भाल कर्ता की भागीदारी का विकास अवश्य करेगी।

जो अनिवार्यता के अधीन हैं, उन रोगियों की देख-भाल और उनके इलाज के बारे में कमीशन की लगातार कई चिंताएं है। वयस्कों के लिए बनी संस्थाओं में दाखिल बच्चों और नाबालिगों की नाज़ुक स्थिति की ओर हमारी रिपोर्ट ने ध्यान दिया है; और उन स्त्री रोगियों की ओर भी जो मुख्यत: आदमियों के क्षेत्र में दाखिल हैं और उन स्त्रीयों की ओर भी जो अस्पतालों में उच्च-सुरक्षा के क्षेत्रों में रखे जाने से प्रभावित हैं। हम ने कई वार्डों में चिकित्सा और मनोरंजन संबंधी गतिविधियों तक पहुंच पाने की समस्याओं को, अस्पतालों में वातावरण संबंधी समस्याओं को और नियंत्रण व अनुशासन (विशेष कर कुछ अस्पतालों में जिस प्रकार रोगियों को अकेला रखा जाने का चलन है) की सीमा में व्यापक अनिश्चितता को भी उजागर किया है। हम ने नज़रबंद रोगियों में काले और अल्प-संख्यक लोगों का लगातार बाहुल्य देखा है और रोगियों को नस्ली मूल के कारण परेशान किए जाने पर हमें विशेष चिंता है। उच्च-सुरक्षा के अस्पतालों के लिए सरकारी सुरक्षा निर्देशों के लागू करने के कारण रोगियों की उपचार संबंधी देख-भाल में यथा संभव न्यूनतम कमी लाने के लिए कमीशन ने अपना दबाव बनाए रखा है।

हम आशा करते हैं कि संसद के अगले या बाद के सत्र में पेश किए विधेयक में 2002 के मसौदे के मुक़ाबले में, विशेष करके मानसिक स्वास्थ्य देख-भाल के लिए अनिवार्य हस्तक्षेप के औचित्य और प्रयोग के मानदंडों में काफी संशोधन किया गया होगा। हमें विश्वास है कि जेलों में उपलब्ध स्वास्थ्य देख-भाल की सुविधाओं की आज की स्थिति और मानसिक स्वास्थ्य की सुविधाओं के प्रभावी मॉनीटरन की वर्तमान की कमी को देखते हुए किसी भी क़ानून में जेलों के अंदर अनिवार्य उपचार के अधिकारों का विस्तार करने की योजना अधूरी और कच्ची होगी।

हमें यक़ीन है कि मानसिक स्वास्थ्य क़ानून के अंतर्गत रोगियों के अनिवार्य उपचार के लिए प्रदत्त अधिकारों के उपयोग और कर्तव्यों के पालन के मॉनीटरन के लिए एक अधिकृत निरीक्षण समिति की लगातार आवश्यकता है और सदा रहेगी। यह सरकार की अपनी ज़िम्मेवारी को निभाने के लिए आवश्यक है कि उसे उनके बारे में जानकारी हो जिन्हें उसने नज़रबंद किया है। भले ही इस पर किसी प्रकार की कार्रवाई हो, नए क़ानून में इस ज़िम्मेवारी को निभाने के लिए व्यवस्था होनी ही चाहिए।

اس رپورٹ کا خلاصہ

مینٹل ہیلتھ کمیشن پر مینٹل ہیلتھ ایکٹ 1983 کے تحت مریضوں کو اسپتال وغیرہ میں رکھے اور ان کے علاج سے متعلق اختیارات اور فرائض کا جائزہ لینے کی ذمہ داری عائد کی گئی ہے۔ اس رپورٹ کی بنیاد کمیشن کی طرف سے ان تمام ''سائیکائٹرک'' (نفسیاتی) سہولیات (اداروں) کے دوروں سے حاصل ہونے والے تجربے پر ہے جو مریضوں کو رکھتے (داخل کرتے) ہیں۔ یہ رپورٹ خاص طور پر 2001/02 سے 2002/03 کے مالی سالوں کے بارے میں ہے 'لیکن اس میں کمیشن کے دو دھائیوں کے دوران کام کے وجود اور اس کا استعمال کیا گیا ہے اور اس میں دماغی صحت سے متعلق سروسز میں جبر اور زبردستی کے اطلاق اور اس کے جائزے پر بھی غور کیا گیا ہے۔

رپورٹ کا مرکزی موضوع یہ ہے کہ حکومت کو پالیسی کے لیول پر رہنمائی اور دماغی صحت سے متعلق قانون کے استعمال اور اس کے اثرات میں مداخلت کرنے کی ضرورت ہے۔ ہم درج ذیل وجوہات کی بنا پر موجودہ صورت حال اسے خاص اہمیت سے دیکھتے ہیں۔

- انسانی حقوق کی بنیاد پر رونما ہونے والے مبارزات دماغی صحت کے موجودہ قانون کو تبدیل کررہے ہیں۔ اگر چہ اس کے نتیجے میں کارکردگی میں بہتر تبدیلیاں پیدا ہورہی ہیں 'لیکن جیسے جیسے ایک ماہ سے دوسرے ماہ قانون تبدیل ہوتا ہے 'یہ تبدیلیاں کارکنوں کے درمیان غیر یقینی کی سی کیفیت بھی پیدا کرتی ہیں۔

- دماغی صحت سے متعلق قانون میں بڑی تبدیلیوں کے لیے بڑی سے وسیع تر غیر یقینی کیفیتیں موجود ہیں خاص طور پر جہاں یہ محسوس کیا جاتا ہے کہ اس قسم کی تبدیلیاں انسانی حقوق سے متعلق قانون کے ردعمل میں پیدا ہوئی ہیں۔

- کم دستوری اور زیادہ گوناگوں مریضوں کو رکھنے والے یونٹس کی تشکیل میں اضافہ اگر چہ کئی لحاظ سے یہ ایک اچھی چیز ہے 'لیکن جبر زبردستی کے قانونی اختیارات کے استعمال کے دوران بنا کیسانیت اور ناقابل فہم چھوٹی چھوٹی سروسز کی تشکیل کا خطرہ بھی پیدا ہو جائے گا۔

رپورٹ میں اس بات کا ذکر بھی کیا گیا ہے کہ جبر کی حامل دماغی صحت کی سروسز کی طرف سے انسانی حقوق کی بنیاد پر ایک سچار جحان پیدا کرنے کے لیے درج ذیل کی ضرورت بھی ہوگی؛

- نئے قانون کی بنیاد واضح اصولوں پر ہو بالکل ویسے ہی اصول جو دماغی صحت سے متعلق قانون کے ضابطہ عمل جیسے ہوں؛

- اس بات کا اطمینان کرنے کے لیے خاص توجہ دینا کہ صحت سے متعلق سروسز منصفانہ طور پر اور لوگوں کی صنف 'جنسی جحان 'نسلی تعلق 'مذہب یا ساجی طبقے کے مطابق کسی قسم کے تعصب کے بغیر فراہم کی جائیں؛

- جبر (زبردستی) کے خاص پہلوؤں سے متعلق قانونی اصول و ضوابط 'جیسے کہ وہ جو کنٹرول اور نظم و ضبط (بشمول علیحدگی) سے نپٹتے ہیں 'تا کہ ایسا اچھی کارکردگی کا اطمینان کیا جا سکے۔

- حکومت کے تمام پہلوؤں میں دماغی خلل میں مبتلا افراد کے لیے منفی خیالات کے خلاف اور تعصب کے تحت اقدامات کو سرگرمی کے ساتھ فروغ دینا' اور ان لوگوں پر خاص طور پر توجہ مرکوز کرنا جنہیں جبری اختیارات (طاقتوں) کا شکار بنایا جاتا ہے؛ اور

- قانونی طاقتوں کے استعمال اور ایسی طاقتوں کے شکار مریضوں کی دیکھ بھال کا موثر اور مرکز جائزہ لینا۔

ہم قدر شناسی کی بنیاد پر کارکردگی کے لیے نیشنل انسٹی ٹیوٹ فار مینٹل ہیلتھ کی پابندی کا خیر مقدم اور ان کی حمایت کرتے ہیں 'انسانی حقوق کے احترام میں کی جانے والی کارکردگی میں حقیقی طور پر سروس استعمال کرنے والے اور اس کی دیکھ بھال کرنے والے فرد کی شمولیت ہونی چاہیے جہاں قانونی طور پر جبری اختیارات کو استعمال بھی کیا جائے۔

کمیشن کو جبر (زبردستی) کے تحت مریضوں کی دیکھ بھال اور علاج سے متعلق مسلسل بہت سی تشویشات لاحق ہیں۔ ہماری رپورٹ میں بالغ افراد کے لیے فراہم کی جانے والی سہولیات میں بچوں اور نوجوانوں کے داخلے کے بارے میں بھی ذکر کیا گیا ہے 'اور مریض خواتین' خاص طور پر وہ جنہیں زیادہ تر مردوں کے ماحول میں رکھا جاتا ہے اور وہ خواتین جو اسپتال کے انتہائی محفوظ شعبے سے منتقلی سے متاثر ہوتی ہیں۔ ہم نے بہت سے وارڈز میں معالجاتی اور تفریحی سرگرمیوں تک رسائی میں پیش آنے والے مسائل 'اسپتالوں میں ماحولیاتی مسائل اور کنٹرول اور نظم و ضبط کے اختیارات کی وجہ سے پیدا ہونے والی غیر یقینی کیفیتوں کا ذکر کیا ہے' خاص طور پر جس طرح سے بعض اسپتالوں میں مریضوں کو علیحدہ علیحدہ رکھا جاتا ہے۔ ہم نے سیاہ فام اور اقلیتی نسلی گروپس سے تعلق رکھنے والے مریضوں کی نسبتاً زیادہ تعداد کو زیر نگرانی داخل رکھنے کے بارے میں بھی ذکر کیا ہے اور ہمیں خاص طور پر مریضوں کے ساتھ نسلی ہراسانی کے بارے میں فکر ہے۔ کمیشن اس بات کے لیے زور دار تیار ہوگا کہ نہایت محفوظ اسپتالوں میں حکومت کی طرف سے حفاظتی ہدایات کے اطلاق سے مریضوں کی طبی دیکھ بھال میں خلل کو کم سے کم رکھا جا سکے۔

ہم امید کرتے ہیں کہ اگلے سیشن اور اس کے بعد آنے والے سیشنز میں پارلیمنٹ کے سامنے پیش کیے جانے والے مینٹل ہیلتھ بل میں 2002 کے مسودے کافی حد تک ترمیم کی جائے گی' خاص طور پر دماغی صحت سے متعلق دیکھ بھال میں لازمی مداخلت اور مقصد کے معاملات میں۔ ہمارے خیال میں اس قسم کے قانون کے تحت زبردستی علاج کے اختیار کو جیل میں وسعت دینے کے لیے کسی بھی قسم کی منصوبہ بندی کرنا نہایت جلد بازی ہو گی' جس کی وجہ جیل میں فراہم کی جانے والی دیکھ بھال اور فی الوقت جیل میں دماغی صحت کی سہولیات کے موثر جائزے میں کمی ہے۔

ہم اس بات پر یقین رکھتے ہیں کہ اس وقت اور مستقبل میں بھی کسی ایسے ادارے کی طرف سے مسلسل دوروں کی ضرورت رہے گی جن پر خاص طور پر مریضوں پر دماغی صحت سے متعلق قانون کی طرف سے پیدا کیے گئے اختیارات کے اطلاق اور فرائض کا جائزہ لینے کی ذمہ داری عائد کی جاتی ہے۔ حکومت پر عائد کیے جانے والے فرائض کو پورا کرنے کے لیے ضروری ہے 'تا کہ ان مریضوں کے بارے میں مکمل طور پر خبر رہے جنہیں زیر نگرانی رکھا جا رہا ہے۔ نئے قانون کے انتظامات کے تحت اس عمل کو جاری رکھا جائے گا' جیسا جا رہا ہے 'اس پر جس طریقے سے بھی عمل کیا جائے۔

18

Qodobada ugu muhiimsan Warbixintan

Guddiga Shuruucda Caafimaadka Maskaxda - The Mental Health Act Commission – waxa uu mas'uul ka yahay kormeerka xarigga iyo daryeelka bukaanka maskaxda ka jirran iyadoo la cuskanayo Shuruucda Caafimaadka Maskada ee soo baxay 1983. Warbixintani waxay ku salaysantahay khibradda ay guddigani heleen intii ay kormeerayeen adeegga iyo dhammaan goobaha lagu hayo dadka maskaxda ka jirran. Gaar ahaan waxay warbixintani khusaysaa sannadaha 2001/02 ilaa 2002/03, inkastoo guud ahaan warbixintu ay saamaynayso waxqabadka Guddiga ee labaatanka sano ee uu dhisnaa iyo sidii mustaqbalka lagama maarmaan looga dhigi lahaa joogtaynta adeegyada dhinaca caafimaadka maskaxda khuseeya.

Laf dhabar waxaa u ah qoraalkan baahida loo qabo inay dawladdu ay qaaddo tallaabo siyaasadeed oo mas'uulnimo ku dheehantahay oo hoggaamin ka bixinaysa dhaqangelinta ku shaqaynta shuruucda caafimaadka maskaxda ka degsan. Sababta aan arrintaas muhiim ugu aragno marka la fiiriyo xaaladda haatan lagu jiro waxa weeye.

- Qodobada ka degsan dhinaca Xuquuqda Aadanaha ayaa ay tahay in la waafajiyo sharciyada adeegga maskaxda. Inkastoo arrintaan hawsheeda la bilaabay haddana sharciyada waxaa la beddelaa bil kasta.
- Waxaa kale oo aan iyana laysla meel dhigin xaddiga ay yeelanayaan isbeddelada lagu samaynayo shuruuxda caafimaadka maskaxda markii la tixgelinayo dhinaca xuquuqda aadanaha.
- Waxaa iyana jirta inay sii badanayaan dhismaha hay'ado aan qaynuun adag ku salaysnayn oo lagu hayo dadka jirran, oo inkastoo ay dhinac ka wanaagsantahay, hadana la mid ah machadyo kala qoqoban oo aan lahayn xiriir adag oo isku xiran marka ay timaaddo hirgelinta shuruucda.

Warbixintu waxay kaloo ku talinaysaa in dhismaha qaynuun dhab ah oo ku salaysan bani'aadminimo oo lagu waajaho adeegga caafimaadka maskaxda ay u baahanayso:

- sharci-dejin cusub oo ku salaysan xeerar qeexan, oo la mid ah kuwa ku jira Sharciga Caafimaadka Maskaxda Qodobkiisa ku Shaqaynta;
- in si gaar ah loola socdo in adeegyadan lagu bixiyo hab aan ku dhisnayn midab kala-faquuq jinsi, farac, diin, nolosha gaarka ah iyo dabaqadda bulsho;
- in la xoojiyo qaynuunada gaarka ah sida kuwa, qaabilsan dhinaca, maamulka iyo anshaxa (oo ay ku jiraan kuwa asturnaanta qofka), si loo xaqiijiyo shaqo loo simanyahay;

- in dhammaan qaybaha kala duwan ee dawladda laga sameeyo abaabul looga horjeedo in bartimaameed ama midab kala sooc lala beegsado dadka maskaxda ka jirran, gaar ahaan kuwa loo adeegsado awoodaha qasabka; iyo
- kormeerista iyo xaqiijinta in adeegsada awoodaha qasabka iyo daryeelka bukaanka ay isku dheellitiran yihiin.

Waxaan soo dhoweynaynaa shaqada uu hayo Machadka Qaranka ee Caafimaadka Maskaxda ee ku salaysan Habka-Qiimaynta Shaqada - Values-Based Practice. Shaqada waa inay noqotaa mid a ay ka muuqato ixtiraam badan oo loo hayo xuquuqda aadanaha, xataa marka ay awoodaha dawladda ee qasabka la adeegsado.

Guddigu waxay weli ka walaacsanyihiin daryeelka iyo adeegsiga awoodaha qasabka. Warbixintu waxay taabanaysaa saamaynta ay taasi ku yeelan karto carruurta iyo dadka tabarta daran eel ala xiro dadka ka tabarta roon; haweenka bukaanka ah, gaar ahaan kuwa lala xiro dad rag u badan ama haweenka laysku kala beddelo Qaybta Ammaanku Sarreeyo ee Cisbitaalka. Waxaan farta ku fiiqnay dhibaatooyinka ka jira helitaanka adeegyada maskax-dejinta iyo firfircooni gelinta bukaanka, sixada caafimaadka ee cisbitaallada qaar iyo qodobada khuseeya awoodaha maamulka iyo anshaxa gaar ahaan sida loo qiimeeyo asturnaanta bukaanka cisbitaalada qaar. Waxaan taabanay tirada badan ee ka xiran bulshada Madow iyo kuwa laga tiro badanyahay, gaara ahaan waxaan ka walaacnay cabsi gelin dhinaca midabka ku dhisan. Guddigu waxa uu daba taaganyahay yaraynta xad-gudub lagu sameeyo daawada bukaanka marka la hirgelinayo qorshaha dawladda ee Cisbitaallada Ammaankoodu Sarreeyo.

Waxaan rajaynaynaa in Sharciga Caafimaadka Maskaxda ee baarlamaanka la hordhigayo fadhiga soo socda laga beddelo qoraalkiisii sannadka 2002, gaar ahaan qorshaha faragelinta qasabka iyo daryeelka caafimadka maskaxda. Waxan qabna inay degdegtahay go'aan lagu sii ballaarinayo awoodda qasabka, marka la tixgeliyo xaaladda kormeerka iyo adeegga caafimaad ee xabsiga gudihiisa.

Waxaan aaminsannahay inay jiri doonaan guddi kormeera hirgelinta awoodaha qasabka iyo adeegga caafimaadka maskaxda ee bukaanka. Shaqadani waa u muhiim yaraynta awoodda dawladda ee bukaanka xiran. Qodobadan waa in lagu daraa sharci-dejinta cusub si kasta oo lagu maamuloba.

Crynodeb o'r Adroddiad hwn

Comisiwn y Ddeddf Iechyd Meddwl sydd â'r cyfrifoldeb o fonitro'r pwerau a'r dyletswyddau sy'n deillio o gadw a thrin cleifion dan Ddeddf Iechyd Meddwl 1983. Seiliwyd yr adroddiad hwn ar brofiad y Comisiwn o ymweld â'r holl gyfleusterau seiciatrig sy'n cadw cleifion. Mae'r adroddiad yn benodol yn ymdrin â'r blynyddoedd ariannol 2001/02 hyd 2002/03, ond mae'n tynnu ar waith y Comisiwn dros y ddau ddegawd y bu mewn bodolaeth ac yn edrych tua'r dyfodol o ran defnyddio a monitro gorfodaeth mewn gwasanaethau iechyd meddwl.

Un o themâu canolog yr adroddiad yw'r angen i'r Llywodraeth roi arweiniad, o ran cyfarwyddyd ac ymyrraeth ar lefel polisi, ar y defnydd o gyfraith iechyd meddwl a'i heffaith. Gwelwn hyn yn arbennig o bwysig yn yr hinsawdd gyfredol am y rhesymau canlynol.

- Mae sialensiau ar sail iawnderau dynol yn ailffurfio'r gyfraith iechyd meddwl sy'n bodoli. Tra bod hyn yn creu gwelliannau a groesawir, mae hefyd yn creu ansicrwydd mawr ymhlith yr ymarferwyr wrth i'r gyfraith newid o fis i fis.
- Mae ansicrwydd ehangach yn bodoli oherwydd yr argymhellion ar gyfer newidiadau sylfaenol i gyfraith iechyd meddwl, yn arbennig pan deimlir bod y newidiadau hynny yn ymateb i ofynion deddfwriaeth iawnderau dynol.
- Mae'r cynnydd yn y datblygu ar unedau cleifion mewnol llai sefydliadol a mwy amrywiol, tra'n cael ei groesawu ar lawer ystyr, yn debygol o greu gwasanaethau bratiog, ar raddfa fechan, heb unffurfiaeth na thryloywder wrth weithredu pwerau cyfreithiol gorfodaeth.

Mae'r adroddiad hefyd yn awgrymu y bydd datblygu ymagwedd sy'n wironeddol seiliedig ar iawnderau dynol tuag at wasanaethau iechyd meddwl sy'n cynnwys gorfodaeth yn gofyn am:

- ddeddfwriaeth newydd yn seiliedig ar egwyddorion clir, tebyg i'r rhai a ddarperir yng Nghôd Ymarfer y Ddeddf Iechyd Meddwl;
- roi sylw arbennig i sicrhau bod gwasanaethau iechyd meddwl yn cael eu darparu'n deg a heb gamwahaniaethu yn ôl rhyw, tuedd rywiol, ethnigrwydd, crefydd na dosbarth cymdeithasol;
- reolaeth statudol ar feysydd penodol mewn gorfodaeth, fel y rhai yn ymdrin â rheolaeth a disgyblaeth (gan gynnwys neilltuaeth), i sicrhau ymarfer da unffurf;
- hyrwyddo gweithredol ar draws pob adran o Lywodraeth ar gamau gwrth-stigma a gwrth-gam wahaniaethu yng nghyswllt pobl gydag

anhwylderau meddwl, gyda phwyslais arbennig ar y rhai sy'n ddarostyngedig i bwerau gorfodi; a

- monitro effeithiol ac wedi eu ffocysu ar y defnydd o bwerau cyfreithiol a gofal i gleifion sy'n ddarostyngedig i bwerau o'r fath.

Rydym yn croesawu ac yn cefnogi ymrwymiad y Sefydliad Cenedlaethol dros Iechyd Meddwl i Ymarfer ar Sail Gwerthoedd. Rhaid i ymarfer a seilir ar barch i iawnderau dynol ddatblygu cyfranogiad gwirioneddol i'r defnyddwyr a'r cynhalwyr, hyd yn oed pan ddefnyddir pwerau gorfodi'r wladwriaeth.

Pery'r comisiwn i goleddu nifer o bryderon am ofal a thriniaeth cleifion dan orfodaeth. Mae ein hadroddiad yn nodi pa mor hawdd eu niweidio yw plant a phobl ifanc a dderbynnir i gyfleusterau oedolion; a chleifion o fenywod, yn arbennig y rhai a dderbynnir i amgylchedd gwrywaidd yn bennaf, a menywod y mae trosglwyddiadau yn effeithio arnynt o fewn y sector Ysbyty Diogel Iawn. Rydym yn tanlinellu'r problemau parthed mynediad at weithgareddau therapiwtig a hamdden ar nifer o wardiau, problemau amgylcheddol mewn ysbytai a'r ansicrwydd sy'n bodoli parthed graddfa'r pwerau rheoli a disgyblu, yn arbennig y ffordd y mae neilltuaeth yn cael ei weithredu mewn rhai ysbytai. Nodwn y ffaith bod cleifion duon ac o leiafrifoedd ethnig yn dal i gael eu gor-gynrychioli, ac rydym yn bryderus iawn am aflonyddu hiliol ar gleifion. Mae'r Comisiwn yn parhau i bwyso am cyn lleied o niwed â phosibl i ofal clinigol cleifion wrth weithredu Cyfarwyddiadau Diogelwch y Llywodraeth i Ysbytai Diogel Iawn.

Gobeithiwn y bydd y Mesur Iechyd Meddwl fel y'i cyflwynir i'r Senedd yn y sesiwn nesaf neu'n ddiweddarach wedi cael ei ddiwygio'n sylweddol ers y drafft yn 2002, yn arbennig o ran y meini prawf ar gyfer ymyrraeth orfodol a'i diben mewn gofal iechyd meddwl. Credwn fod unrhyw fwriad i ymestyn pwerau triniaeth orfodol i'r carchar dan ddeddfwriaeth o'r fath yn gynamserol, o ystyried yr isadeiledd gofal iechyd yn y carchardai a'r diffyg monitro effeithiol ar y ddarpariaeth iechyd meddwl mewn carchardai ar hyn o bryd.

Credwn y bydd angen parhaus am gorff ymweld gyda chyfrifoldeb penodol am fonitro'r modd y gweithredir pwerau a'r modd y gweithredir y dyletswyddau a grëir gan ddeddfwriaeth iechyd meddwl ar gyfer triniaeth orfodol ar gleifion. Mae'r swyddogaeth hon yn angenrheidiol i gyflawni'r dyletswyddau a osodwyd ar y Llywodraeth i wybod am y rhai sydd yn y ddalfa ganddi. Dylai'r trefniadau dan y ddeddfwriaeth newydd gadw'r swyddogaeth hon, pa fodd bynnag y bydd yn cael ei gweinyddu.

Instead of my understanding being addressed and enlightened, and my path being made as clear and plain as possible, in consideration of my confusion, I was committed … to unknown and untried hands; and I was placed amongst strangers, without introduction, explanation or exhortation. Instead of great scrupulousness being observed in depriving me of my liberty or privilege, and of the exercise of so much choice and judgment as might be conceded to me with safety – on the just ground, that for the safety of society my most valuable rights were already taken away – on every occasion, in every dispute, in every argument, the assumed premise immediately acted upon was that I was to yield, my desires were to be set aside, my few remaining privileges to be infringed upon for the convenience of others. Yet I was in a state of mind not likely to acknowledge even the justice of my confinement … and jealous of any further invasion of my natural and social rights; but this was a matter that never entered into their consideration.

John Perceval (1840)

A Narrative of the Treatment Experienced by a Gentleman,
During a State of Mental Derangement[1]

---

[1] Perceval J (1840) *A Narrative of the Treatment Experienced by a Gentleman, During a State of Mental Derangement; Designed to Explain the Causes and the Nature of Insanity, and to Expose the Injudicious Conduct Pursued Towards Many Unfortunate Sufferers Under That Calamity.* Extracts reprinted in Peterson D [ed] (1982) *A Mad People's History of Madness,* University of Pittsburgh 1982 p96-107.

Introduction –
Placed amongst strangers

1.1 This Tenth Biennial Report of the Mental Health Act Commission may be our last. Proposed changes in mental health legislation and the framework of health service inspection and regulation look set to dissolve the MHAC into a wider Commission for Healthcare Audit and Inspection, perhaps within the next two years.

1.2 Although the Mental Health Act Commission has had a lifespan so far of just over twenty years, its roots lie much deeper in the history of mental health reforms. On the facing page we have reproduced the words of John Perceval, an early service-user voice, who had been detained in two of the most prestigious English asylums for about 18 months during the 1830s[2]. His book was instrumental in the reform movement that led to the Lunacy Act of 1845, ('not inaptly called "the Magna Charta of the Liberties of the insane"'[3]) and the permanent establishment of the Lunacy Commission, the ancestor of the Mental Health Act Commission. Perceval's complaints – that his natural rights had been invaded beyond that which was necessary for his treatment, that he was denied respect as an autonomous individual, and that he was not given sufficient information about his circumstances to understand them or to make choices about his care – are strikingly contemporary. Indeed, these themes still feature in patients' accounts on our visits to them; in our concerns from our general observations on visits; and as the backbone of this report.

1.3 We have taken the title of this report – *Placed Amongst Strangers* – from Perceval's account of his detention. For all that psychiatric care may have developed between Perceval's time and our own, the experience that every patient who has been detained under one of the Mental Health Acts of the last half century will have had in common with Perceval is precisely that of being taken from his or her usual environment and 'committed to unknown and untried hands': of being 'placed amongst strangers'. The removal of a mentally disordered person who is in crisis from their situation to a place of care and treatment is no doubt frequently necessary, and often the most beneficent act possible, but it is nevertheless the most serious interference with human rights available to the State under civil powers.

---

[2]   Ticehurst House and Brislington House: the description of these as 'prestigious' is from Porter, R (ed) (1991) *The Faber Book of Madness*, p23. John Perceval (1803-1876) was a son of the assassinated Prime Minister, Spencer Perceval (d.1812). He was a founder member of the Alleged Lunatic's Friend Society (from 1845) and described himself, whilst giving evidence to an 1860 Parliamentary Committee, as "the attorney general of all Her Majesty's madmen". See also Peterson D [ed] (1982) *A Mad People's History of Madness*, p92-6.

[3]   Hodder E (1890) *The Life and Work of the Seventh Earl of Shaftesbury K G.* Cassell & Co, 1890 ed. p332

1.4   There remains much to do to bring about a truly humane psychiatric service. That persons are still compelled to reside on wards that are acknowledged by those responsible for them to be substandard, frightening and even dangerous is a resounding indictment of the current infra-structure of mental health services[4]. For this reason the Commission welcomes the stated policy intention of Government to make mental health care 'a little less institutional and a little more diverse' through the provision of smaller inpatient units with closer links to the community[5]. We also note that recent case law appears to have anticipated proposed changes in mental health law that would sever the link between compulsory treatment and continued detention in hospital[6].

1.5   The move towards community-based settings and less formal approaches towards providing care is, in some senses, a continuation of an existing policy trend. The idea that a modern mental health service should be built upon the dismantling of large institutional establishments into clusters of small units that are, wherever possible, absorbed into communities has, despite its many political vicissitudes, remained relatively constant from at least the 1950s[7]. However, a large-scale extension of formal powers of psychiatric compulsion out of the confines of recognisable 'hospital' environments will mark a departure for much of the mental health service. Whilst, even under proposed new legislation, 'in-patient' units will continue to form the core of services at least at the initial assessment stages of compulsion, it seems likely that these units may, eventually, also be small in scale and relatively specialized and scattered.

1.6   The Commission fully supports the development of community-based care as an important step in reducing social exclusion of people with mental health problems. There are, however, particular and perhaps obvious risks inherent in having physically decentralised structures of smaller inpatient units operating powers of compulsion on behalf of the State. One such risk, which we discuss in more detail at Chapters 10.32 and 11.23 below, is the spreading of available medical and other expertise too thinly, so that no inpatient units can realistically have immediate access to a doctor when emergencies arise. Where patients are detained for their own safety, such a lack creates an ethical dilemma, if not a legal one. Similar issues relating to economies of scale pose other challenges. Staff who are given powers of coercion (and the responsibilities that go with such powers, from using them appropriately to being held accountable when things go wrong) must of course be allowed appropriate resources, human and otherwise, to carry them out effectively. For example, Mental Health NHS Trusts and large independent hospitals usually now employ a Mental Health Act adminis-trator to ensure that legal powers and duties of compulsion are operated and documented correctly. Where such employees establish an effective foothold within their organisation, their work can have marked benefits for the treatment and safety of patients. Although it is perhaps likely that some shared managerial structures, such as the increasingly large NHS Trusts of today, will allow for such posts to continue, isolated units may not have sufficient resources.

---

[4]   see Chapter 8.81 below, but also Mental Health Act Commission (2001) *Ninth Biennial Report, 1999-2001* London: Stationery Office. Chapters 3 and 4.

[5]   Professor Louis Appleby (National Director for Mental Health) giving evidence to the David Bennett inquiry [2003]. Inquiry transcript II.6-650.

[6]   see Chapter 9.47 below.

1.7 A less obvious risk of decentralised structures, and indeed the potential converse of positive attempts to make the provision of mental health services 'patient-centred', is what a "less institutional" framework could mean for the practice of compulsion. The danger of emphasising the need for less formal structures of care is that these may disguise or detract from underlying realities of coercion. At Chapter 8.1 *et seq* below we discuss our concerns over patients who, under current mental health legislation, are "*de facto*" detained in hospitals with none of the protections of the law or the oversight of this body. We have similar concerns that, under envisaged structures of mental health care, and in the absence of sufficient central guidance and monitoring, laudable aims of less formality with greater immediacy of response and availability of appropriate care could lead, in practice, to the casual and unregulated application of powers of coercion. It is obvious that not all coercion in mental health care takes place within a recognised framework of established legal powers (see Chapter 11.6 *et seq* below). It may not be reasonable to expect either Tribunal systems established to provide a check on the use of formal powers, or general inspectorates charged with monitoring healthcare outcomes, to provide any safeguard against abuses of patients' rights under such a system. In the Commission's view, Government must therefore provide for specific guidance and monitoring to ensure that any necessary deinstitutionalisation of mental health wards does not create twenty-first century equivalent of workhouse "casual wards", providing relatively open access to those in need but at the cost of much civil liberty.

1.8 As mental health services are reshaped by the severance of the link between detention and compulsion, community-based treatment of those subject to compulsion could end the isolation of seriously mentally disordered people from the community. However, this change alone will do nothing to prevent isolation caused by other factors, such as social exclusion, discrimination and the stresses placed upon families and carers of severely mentally ill persons. There is a great deal of work to be done if psychiatric patients are to receive appropriate support and opportunity whilst being treated outside hospital environments.

1.9 There are no reasons why the concerns expressed above should be insurmountable. We highlight these concerns not to argue against the direction of Government policy, but to highlight those matters which, if attended to with sufficient care and resources, could ensure that such policies are not deemed to have failed in the coming years.

1.10 We started this introduction on a historical note, and will end it on another. Ninety years ago the final Lunacy Commission Report[8] looked back over the history of its work, and forward to the work of its successor body, the Board of Control. The Lunacy Commissioners believed the history of their times "as regards the care and treatment of the insane, a record of uninterrupted progress"[9]. We would not make such an extravagant claim, although we have no doubt of the Mental Health Act Commission's positive effect in supporting better practice in mental health compulsion. However, both then and now the major anxiety over

---

[7] see Bennett, D (1991) 'The drive towards the community' in Berrios G.E. & Freeman H (eds) (1991) *150 years of British Psychiatry 1841-1991*, Gaskell, p321-332

[8] Lunacy Commission (1914) *The Sixty-Eighth Report of the Commissioners in Lunacy*, Part I. His Majesty's Stationery Office, 1914.

[9] *ibid*, p3

the change process has been whether a proper system of visits to patients will survive into the new organisations:

> 'The Commissioners trust that the policy which has been so successfully carried out over the last seventy years will be adhered to by the Board of Control. They are confident that any relaxation of personal interest and attention of the Commissioners would react most unfavourably on the patients'[10].

We end our report at Chapter 20 with a discussion of how patients might be assured of the continued protection of a visiting body charged with monitoring the use of psychiatric compulsion.

---

[10]   *ibid*, p4

Part 1

Human Rights, Human Values:

The Structure of Mental Health Law

2

Developing a culture of respect for human rights

2.1 The Human Rights Act 1998, which came into force in October 2000, established a duty on public authorities[11] to act in accordance with the European Convention of Human Rights (ECHR) within the scope permitted by primary legislation. This, as a part of the legislation's general aim of introducing elements from the European Convention to domestic law, was intended by the Government to "bring rights home" and establish a human rights culture within the UK[12].

2.2 This year, the Parliamentary Joint Committee on Human Rights (JCHR) recognised only limited progress towards the above aim, and feared that "the highwater mark has been passed". "Too often", according to the JCHR, "human rights are looked upon as something from which the State needs to defend itself, rather than to promote as its core ethical values…human rights should provide a framework within which people who need to can negotiate with public authorities for better conditions and treatment, both in individual cases and in wider contexts" [13].

2.3 The Joint Committee on Human Rights recognised that bodies such as the Mental Health Act Commission, whose concern is with the State in its coercive rather than enabling role, demonstrate an awareness of "human rights as important grounding principles to the legislative framework or standards of good practice"[14] within which we work. The Commission was reported by the JCHR to view "the promotion of a human rights culture in the mental health field, and the provision of advice on human rights issues, [as] a core element in its work"[15].

2.4 Despite the apparent understanding and good intentions of the Mental Health Act Commission and bodies like it, the JCHR nevertheless concluded that "human rights have not taken root in the wider public sector [specifically local and health authorities], other than as a compliance issue for the lawyers, because public authorities are not being encouraged or enabled to act in this area"[16].

---

[11] on the identification of 'public authorities', see Chapter 3.20 below.

[12] *Rights Brought Home: the Human Rights Bill.* Cm.3782 (1997).

[13] Joint Committee on Human Rights (2003) *The Case for a Human Rights Commission: Sixth Report of Session 2002-03*, Volume 1. HL Paper 67-I, HC 489-I. London, The Stationery Office, March 2003. Pages 6 - 7.

[14] *ibid.* para 54

[15] *ibid.* para 55

[16] *ibid.* para 61

2.5   In our experience, health and social services authorities that have powers and duties under the Mental Health Act 1983 are alive to their responsibilities under the Human Rights Act 1998. Unfortunately, such awareness as exists may not always reach down to front-line staff where it is most needed, and many authorities do undoubtedly adopt a primarily defensive approach to human rights issues. Concerns about breaches of human rights have raised anxiety over the less regulated aspects of care under compulsion and, in some cases, have led to unnecessary constraints in the care of patients. For example, the Commission has been involved with one complaint where a patient's movements to and from the open ward where he was detained were unrestricted by hospital staff, despite the warnings of his family that he was putting himself at serious risk, because the Human Rights Act "wouldn't allow" them to interfere. Our observations echo the findings of the British Institute of Human Rights, whose December 2002 report, *Something for Everyone*, suggested that much human rights awareness in public services focused on defensive, anti-litigation measures, and suggested that lack of awareness had led to the Human Rights Act being cited as a barrier to providing appropriate services on the grounds of non-interference with a persons' rights[17].

2.6   We recognise the thrust of Government policy to be that health and social authorities should become more locally accountable, and that this implies a lessening of prescriptive guidance from central government. We agree that nursing and other professional leadership is needed to effect changes and improvements to services. Indeed, in this way grassroots pioneers of local services can be encouraged to revitalise the notion of human rights as positive entitlements that are considered on a day-to-day level in service development. But such an approach will not, by itself, work in the context of psychiatric compulsion.

2.7   Practitioners who use the Mental Health Act 1983 and who will use subsequent mental health legislation face the difficulty that they act primarily on behalf of the State in its coercive rather than enabling role. They take decisions that are *prima facie* interference with patients' human rights, even though they may feel that they may be thanked for doing so (or held accountable for not doing so) after the event. For such practitioners to attain the confidence to move beyond a defensive approach to human rights they must have the support of adequate and authoritative guidance on legal and practice issues. Whilst general service development may not be led from central government, the same may not be true of the use of compulsion. We discuss this further at Chapter 6.9 below.

2.8   We believe it to be the task of Government to provide authoritative guidance on the law and requirements of good practice relating to the compulsion of psychiatric patients. Whilst this report was being written, the Court of Appeal has similarly stated that the State has a duty towards those who are detained under its powers[18]. We therefore welcome the Government's intention to restate in new legislation a duty to provide a Code of Practice similar to that imposed by the 1983 Act. We trust that this duty will be established by primary legislation

---

[17]   British Institute for Human Rights (2002) *Something for Everyone: The impact of the Human Rights Act and the need for a Human Rights Commission*, British Institute for Human Rights, researched and written by Jenny Watson, pages 10, 31. (available from 020-7401 2712 or www.bihr.org). See also Brown, M. *Shameful Act*, Guardian Society, 23 July 2003.

[18]   *R (on the application of Colonel Munjaz) v Mersey Care NHS Trust and (i) Secretary of State for Health and (ii) MIND; S v Airedale NHS Trust (i) the and Secretary of State for Health and (ii) MIND* [2003]. Cases cited are listed in full at Appendix A of this report

and thus be indivisible from the powers that such a Code seeks to advise upon. We discuss the debate over the status and legal force of the present Code, which the Court of Appeal has now hopefully resolved, at Chapter 3.2 *et seq* below. As well as pressing Government to establish and maintain a robust Code of Practice, we also continue to argue that Government should seize the opportunity of new legislation to regulate a number of areas of compulsory care and treatment, such as seclusion, control and restraint and certain forms of treatment (such as the naso-gastric feeding of anorectic patients): these matters are further discussed at Chapters 11.24, 11.27 and 10.54 respectively.

2.9   We urge the Department of Health to remain vigilant over its own role in promoting human rights. In some cases Government must be applauded for its actions in this respect: there have been a number of examples where Department of Health officials have taken up a proactive role in giving guidance or establishing legal positions (see, for example, Chapter 3.27 below). We are also confident that the Department of Health is receptive to concerns raised by the Commission and other bodies. Nevertheless, there remains a danger that the passing of the Human Rights Act 1998 may yet have a paradoxical effect on the way in which the state recognises and fulfils its duties in promoting human rights. Because the Human Rights Act has brought the ECHR into domestic law and charged all public authorities with a duty to uphold human rights principles in their actions, executive agencies of government may appear to divest themselves *as government* of day-to-day human rights responsibility on matters of detail. This gives the appearance of delegating powers *and responsibilities* regarding human rights to the authorities operating on behalf of the State. For example, the submission made by Department of Health officials on behalf of the Secretary of State to the Court of Appeal in *Munjaz* [2003] argued that, even if a "special hospital" secludes patients in such a way as to possibly breach their human rights,

> "the State has nevertheless discharged its positive obligations to provide protection against breaches of human rights because …[the hospital]… is under an obligation … to act compatibly with …[the HRA]…[and] …any alleged failure or threatened failure to comply with …[the HRA]… can be brought before a court, which must itself, as a public authority, act to protect the appellant's …[ECHR]… rights"[19]

We take the view that, particularly in relation to the restriction of fundamental human rights as a health or safety measure on the authority of the State, any divestiture of responsibility by Government is inappropriate, both in legal terms and in a wider ethical sense. We are therefore pleased that the Court of Appeal took a similar view in the *Munjaz* case, which underlined the State's general responsibility for the treatment of those whom it has deprived of their liberty. We discuss this in relation to the status of the Code of Practice at Chapter 6.17 *et seq* below, and examine the 2003 *Munjaz* judgment itself at Chapter 3.2 *et seq* below.

2.10   We urge Government to re-affirm its commitment towards and responsibility for discharging positive responsibilities in the promotion of a human rights culture. The decentralisation of the NHS must not be allowed to create a vacuum of policy-level advice on the implementation of mental health law. We are heartened by the energy of the Welsh Assembly Government and NHS Wales in this respect (see Chapter 18.18 *et seq* below). We

---

[19]   Court of Appeal Respondent Notice issued by the Secretary of State in *Munjaz*, para 1.2

look with renewed optimism upon the emerging role of the National Institute of Mental Health for England (NIMHE) as the policy-arm of the Department of Health in England. We are pleased to see NIMHE's recent publications recognise this need for active Government intervention:

> "It is interesting to reflect that the ideas enshrined in the National Service Framework for Mental Health (DOH 1999) and other recent Mental Health policy guidance were rehearsed in a way 25 years ago, highlighting the importance of active Government leadership and facilitating change"[20]

We hope that this report will play a role in fostering such leadership.

---

[20] Department of Health (2003) *Cases for Change: Policy Context.* National Institute for Mental Health in England (NIMHE). p3

3

The effect of human rights challenges to the MHA 1983

3.1 Early in our reporting period, two Mental Health Act Commissioners published an article in the *Nursing Standard* suggesting the likely effects on mental health care of the introduction of the ECHR into domestic law[21]. Persaud and Hewitt's forecast that "a relatively small number of cases will transform clinical services in the UK" seems to have been vindicated by the cases of the last two years: their suggestion that such cases should be seen as an opportunity rather than a threat by mental health professionals is discussed specifically at Chapter 5.1. Some of the more significant human rights based cases are outlined below.

Seclusion and the status of the Code of Practice

3.2 This reporting period has seen two major legal challenges in relation to seclusion practice which culminated in a single Court of Appeal ruling in July 2003[22]. Although the power to seclude patients has long been considered to be implied by powers of detention, neither the 1983 Act nor its subsidiary legislation mentions seclusion (see Chapter 11.13 below on the legal basis for seclusion under the Act). The Code of Practice (chapters 19.16-23) provides guidance on the definition and use of seclusion. As an element of both legal challenges was that seclusion practices in both cases had departed from the Code's guidance, the courts had to determine what legal weight should be attached to such a departure. The determination therefore extended beyond the specific issue of seclusion to encompass the proper status of the Code of Practice itself.

3.3 The facts of the cases may be summarised very briefly. The first case (*Munjaz*) involved a patient at Ashworth Hospital who had been secluded on four occasions for between four and 20 days at a time. He challenged the lawfulness of the hospital's seclusion policy, which followed neither the Code of Practice guidance nor a previous judgment that found against the hospital's seclusion procedures[23]. The second case (*S v Airedale NHS Trust*) involved the seclusion of a patient for nearly a fortnight, albeit only at night for the last few days, in a general mental health services hospital while awaiting transfer to a secure bed. The patient

---

[21] Persaud A and Hewitt D (2001) *European Convention on Human Rights: effects on psychiatric care* Nursing Standard, 15, 44, 33-37

[22] *R (on the application of Colonel Munjaz) v Mersey Care NHS Trust and (i) Secretary of State for Health and (ii) MIND; S v Airedale NHS Trust (i) the and Secretary of State for Health and (ii) MIND* [2003]

[23] *R v Ashworth Hospital Trust, ex parte Munjaz* [2000]

challenged the lawfulness of this seclusion on the grounds that it too departed from the Code's guidance, both in purpose (in that there was no incident of current aggression to justify its duration) and in other practical details[24]. Both cases specifically challenged the lack of regular medical reviews as required by the Code. Both claimants argued that their cases raised issues under the European Convention.

3.4   The Commission was joined as an interested party in the first-instance *Munjaz* hearing[25]. We argued to the court that it should not be acceptable to depart from the guidance of the Code of Practice except where an individual patient's circumstances dictate that the Code cannot be followed, and that such departures should be recorded in the patient's medical record. We were surprised that our approach was not supported at that time by the Department of Health, whose submissions appeared to accept Ashworth Hospital's view that it could be legitimate to determine at policy level not to follow Code of Practice guidance. In the *Munjaz* judgment of 2002, the view held on this issue by the hospital, apparently with Government sanction, prevailed[26]. This judgment was upheld by the first instance decision in *S v Airedale NHS Trust* [2002]. The claims of both patients were therefore dismissed at first instance, with the respective judgments agreeing that authority to seclude where it was necessary to so could be implied from the 1983 Act, and that authorities had only to regard the Code as a guide to which they should refer when drafting policies, but from which they might depart where they had sensible reason to do so[27].

3.5   In our evidence to the Appeal Court hearing, we maintained the position regarding the proper weight to be attached to the Code of Practice that we had held in the first instance *Munjaz* hearing. We also disclosed a letter that we had addressed to the Department of Health in December 2002, in which we had expressed concern at the Department's apparent expectations of authorities in relation to the Code and had sought clarification of its position.

3.6   On the 16 July 2003 the Court of Appeal upheld both patients' appeals against the first-instance dismissal of their cases. The court accepted the Commission's suggested approach to the Code of Practice, which was that the Code's guidance should be observed by all hospitals unless they have a good reason for departing from it in relation to an individual patient[28]. The court ruled that hospitals' policies or actions can be unlawfully in breach of the Code of Practice[29]. It declared Ashworth Hospital's seclusion policy and the seclusion of *S* by Airedale General Hospital to have been unlawful. The detail of the judgment in relation to seclusion practice is set out at Figure 2 below.

3.7   The court made an important qualification to its determination that the Code's guidance should be observed by all hospitals unless they have a good reason for departing from it in relation to an individual patient. The court also allowed that hospitals may identify good

---

[24]   *S v Airedale NHS Trust* [2002]

[25]   *R (on the application of Munjaz) v Ashworth Hospital Authority* [2002]

[26]   *ibid*, para 105

[27]   Hewitt D, *A room of one's own – seclusion is at last lawful.* The Times, 26 November 2002

[28]   *R (on the application of Colonel Munjaz) v Mersey Care NHS Trust & Another; S v Airedale NHS Trust* [2003] para 76

[29]   *ibid*, para 77

reasons for particular departures from the Code's guidance in relation to groups of patients who share particular well-defined characteristics, so that if a patient falls within that category there will be good reason for departing from the Code in his or her case. The Commission suggests that this does not absolve services from the necessity of basing such departures upon the individual assessment of patients, even if such assessment is primarily to determine whether the patient falls within a category recognised in hospital policies as justifying practice not in accordance with the Code's guidance.

3.8 The Commission is pleased that the Department of Health agreed to issue a short statement on the status of the Code of Practice following the judgment. At Figure 1 below we reproduce the Department's statement, which was issued in its Chief Executive's Bulletin, issue 187, September 2003. We reproduce it here for promulgation amongst services and authorities without access to that bulletin.

Department of Health statement on the status of the Code of Practice

"In its recent judgment in *R (Munjaz) v. Mersey Care NHS Trust*, the Court of Appeal has confirmed that the Code of Practice should be observed by all to whom it is addressed unless they have good reason for departing from it in relation to an individual patient. The Court has also made clear that good reasons for particular departures may be identified in relation to relation to an individual or groups of patients who share particular well-defined character-istics, so that if a patient falls within that category there will be good reason for departing from the Code in his or her case. The Department considers it best practice for the reasons for any departure to be recorded. Further, it should be noted that the Mental Health Act Commission's policy is to treat unsubstantiated departures from the Code to be *prima facie* evidence of poor practice".

Fig 1: Department of Health statement on the status of the Code of Practice after *Munjaz* [2003]

Seclusion, the ECHR and the Code of Practice following *R (on the application of Colonel Munjaz) v Mersey Care NHS Trust and others; & S v Airedale NHS Trust and others* [2003]

1 Seclusion itself is not a violation of a patient's rights to protection from inhuman or degrading treatment under ECHR Article 3, although used improperly or with little regard to the patient's welfare, it could become so. [para 53-55]

2 Seclusion, by denying association and placing a patient under close surveillance, is necessarily an interference with the right to respect for private life, but one that may be justifiable under ECHR Article 8(2). To be so justified it must be operated predictably and transparently within limits set by domestic law. [65]

3 The State is under an obligation:

(i) "to know enough about its ...patient to provide effective protection..." [58]; and

(ii) to ensure that other public authorities act compatibly with the ECHR [59].

4   The Code of Practice is one essential means by which the State undertakes its duty at 3(ii) above in respect of detention and treatment of patients under the MHA 1983. The Code of Practice:

   (i) can provide transparency and predictability where ECHR compliance requires this but the law is insufficiently defined [65, 74]; and

   (ii) should be afforded a status consistent with its purpose [60, 71-6].

   The Code should therefore be observed by all hospitals unless there is a good reason for particular departures in relation to individual patients. It is not acceptable to depart from the Code as a matter of policy, although policies may identify circumstances when such departures might be considered on a case-by-case basis [76]

5   Seclusion that is not practiced in accordance with the Code's definition and requirements, unless it can be justified as necessary in an individual patient's case, will not meet the requirement of legality set by the ECHR. Policies that depart from the Code's guidance on an arbitrary basis may be similarly unlawful [74, 76-7].

6   Whilst seclusion of a patient who is already detained does not engage ECHR rights to liberty under Article 5, the process of detention itself clearly does so. Where the Code deals with the processes of detention, adherence to its guidance is similarly an ECHR requirement for the hospital's policy or actions to be lawful, unless a departure from the Code's guidance can be shown to have been necessary in a particular case [70,74].

7   It is therefore possible for a hospital's actions or policies to be in unlawful breach of the Mental Health Act Code of Practice on issues that engage ECHR issues [77]

Fig 2 : Seclusion, the ECHR and the Code of Practice after *Munjaz* [2003]

Burden of proof in Mental Health Review Tribunal hearings

3.9   In April 2001 the Court of Appeal issued a formal Declaration of Incompatibility in relation to the burden of proof in Mental Health Review Tribunal hearings and Articles 5(1) and 5(4) of the ECHR[30]. The court held that, rather than patients being required to establish their suitability for discharge, the Tribunal must be positively satisfied that the criteria for detention continue to be met before refusing to discharge a patient. A Remedial Order was laid before Parliament on the 26 November 2001 amending sections 72 and 73 of the Mental Health Act 1983 to effect this change.

3.10   The Government has offered compensation on an *ex gratia* basis for anyone who can demonstrate to its satisfaction that he or she was subject to unlawful detention as a result of the incompatibility of sections 72(1) and 73(1) of the Act prior to its amendment[31].

---

[30]   *R (on the application of H v Mental Health Review Tribunal North & East London Region (Secretary of State for Health Intervening)*[2001]. The declaration of incompatibility was given on the 4 April 2001.

[31]   Applications for compensation should be addressed to Mrs Melissa Merritt, Mental Health Branch, Department of Health, Room 309, Wellington House, 133-155 Waterloo Road, London SE1 8UG, setting out reasons why the patient believes he or she would have been discharged but for the incompatibility.

3.11 We pointed to this potential conflict with the ECHR in 1999, recommending that the burden be changed in new legislation[32]. We therefore see this change as both welcome and inevitable. It will be interesting to see whether it leads to an increase in discharges by the Tribunal. We are aware of views that the practical effect of the change may be to raise the threshold for detention, by restricting practitioners' discretion to use the Act in 'borderline' cases or where cases where diagnoses remains uncertain after a period of inpatient treatment. We can see no reason *in law* why this should be the case. In making the declaration of incompatibility, the Appeal Court stressed that the thresholds for detention set by ECHR Article 5 are less stringent than those set by section 3 of the 1983 Act[33]. A Tribunal is not, therefore, bound by Article 5 to discharge a mentally disordered patient if it cannot be shown on a balance of probabilities that medical treatment will alleviate or prevent a deterioration of that mental disorder, nor is it bound by Article 5 to discharge a patient from detention if it cannot be convincingly shown that such detention the only means of providing treatment. The 1983 Act only requires Tribunals to "have regard" to these issues in respect of patients detained for treatment, and none of the changes in law over this reporting period have narrowed this wide region of discretion.

Dual role of Tribunal medical member

3.12 The courts have determined that the role of Tribunal medical members as both fact finder, in examining patients prior to a hearing, and decision maker, as a member of the Tribunal panel taking the final decision, was not incompatible with Article 5(4) requirements (*R v MHRT and Department of Health, ex parte S*, [2002]). However, medical members of the Tribunal must regard their pre-hearing assessment of the patient only to result in a provisional view before the case is formally heard, and must ensure that any pre-hearing communication with other panel members makes this clear. The proposals for the next Mental Health Act address this concern by establishing a requirement that Tribunals appoint at least one medical expert from a panel (presumably much as Second Opinion Appointed Doctors are appointed under the 1983 Act) to perform the fact finder role in the Tribunal's deliberations[34]. Under new legislative proposals, the patient will also have a right to appoint his or her own medical expert.

Patients' access to Tribunals

Tribunal delays

3.13 It was established in *R (on the application of C) v MHRT London South & SW Region* [2001] that the policy of listing Tribunal hearings eight weeks from the date that a section 3 patient appeals detention failed the requirement under Article 5(4) for a speedy determination of the lawfulness of detention. In *R (on the application of KB & six others) v MHRT and Secretary of State for Health* [2002], the court confirmed that seven patients whose Tribunal hearings had been delayed for longer than this period by repeated adjournments had been denied their rights under Article 5(4). The court laid the responsibility for this on

---

[32] Mental Health Act Commission (1999) *Mental Health Act Commission Submission to the Mental Health Legislation Review Team.* MHAC, Nottingham. page 27

[33] *R (on the application of H v Mental Health Review Tribunal North & East London Region* [2001], para 32-3

[34] *Draft Mental Health Bill* 2002 Cm 5538-I. Clause 48

Government for failing to provide adequate Tribunal resources. In February 2003 the High Court awarded damages of between £750 and £4,000 to six of the patients as compensation for deprivation of liberty and, in some cases, consequent frustration and distress. Other case law (*B v MHRT and Secretary of State for the Home Department* [2002]) confirms that even patients who are not discharged from detention by their delayed Tribunals may still be able to make successful compensation claims.

Tribunal access for extended section 2 detentions

3.14   In 1997 the Commission highlighted that patients whose detention under section 2 is extended whilst an application for the displacement of their Nearest Relative is pending had no right of access to the Tribunal during that extension. The extension of section 2 by a further 50 days has been recorded under these circumstances. The Commission suggested an amendment to the law to provide a right of appeal in such circumstances[35]. In this reporting period, a patient whose detention was being extended in these circumstances requested the Secretary of State to exercise his discretionary power to refer a case to the Tribunal under section 67(1), and was initially refused. The patient's challenge that this refusal was in breach of Article 5(4) was settled out of court, although it appears that initial approaches regarding a policy for the operation of this discretionary power have now been withdrawn on the grounds that the Secretary of State's discretion cannot be fettered.

3.15   The Commission regrets that, at the time of writing, the procedures for Tribunal access under circumstances described above may still fail ECHR requirements of transparency and predictability. It is in relation to matters such as this that Government could set an example of promoting a human rights culture in mental health services.

> **Recommendation 1:** Government should provide a clear framework within which patients whose section 2 detentions are extended may be assured of their right to challenge their detention in accordance with ECHR requirements.

Extending the role of the Tribunal in conditional discharge arrangements

3.16   In *R (on the application of IH) v Secretary of State for the Home Department and the Secretary of State for Health* [2002], the Court of Appeal held that whilst it was not for the Tribunal to enforce conditions of a patient's discharge, its lack of powers to monitor the implementation of its decision or review that decision denied patients their Article 5 rights. The court therefore held that section 73 should be interpreted so as to allow the Tribunal to make a provisional decision to discharge subject to specified conditions, but to defer its final decision whilst it monitors the implementation of those conditions. If the conditions are not or cannot be met, then the Tribunal may make a further order modifying the conditions or determine that the patient should remain in hospital. We understand that it is now

---

[35]   Mental Health Act Commission (1997) *Seventh Biennial Report 1995-7*, London: Stationery Office. p190

standard practice for Mental Health Review Tribunals to fix a date for a further consideration of any deferred discharge decision made. This nascent monitoring role for Tribunals anticipates, to a limited extent, the proposed role of the Tribunal under the next Act. It is already the case that healthcare professionals or Home Office officials may be summoned before the Tribunal to account for delays in implementing discharge plans. The court underlined the Secretary of State's responsibility to respond to recommendations by the Tribunal or requests from RMOs, and not to obstruct or cause unreasonable delay in the implementation of a Tribunal decision in *R (on the application of R A) v Secretary of State for the Home Department* [2002].

3.17 What might constitute an "unreasonable delay" is, of course, not ascertainable in any general sense, although the Department of Health wrote to all health and social services authorities subsequent to *Johnson v United Kingdom* [1997], asking them to "give priority to ensuring that cases of deferred conditional discharge are implemented within six months of the MHRT's decision". In our view, six months is too long a time for patients to remain in conditions that are no longer appropriate for their clinical requirements.

3.18 Delays in patients' discharge under conditions are likely to be caused by difficulties in identifying appropriate community resources. The courts have considered whether this implies a duty on authorities to provide such resources in a number of recent cases. In September 2001 a European Court ruling suggested a limited recognition of a duty of care similar to that accepted in US law (see Chapter 4.14 *et seq* below). The court acknowledged that "the assumption of responsibilities by the authorities of a Contracting State for the health of the individual may in certain defined contexts engage their liability under the Convention with respect to that individual" (*Clunis v UK* [2001]).

3.19 So far, UK judgments have concluded that neither Strasbourg jurisprudence nor the implications of ECHR Article 5 indicate that a Member State owes a duty under the Convention to put in place facilities for the treatment in the community of patients who would otherwise be detained in hospital[36]. However, where a Member State's own law requires such resources for the express purpose of obviating the need for detention, or where such resources are available but are not utilised, Article 5 might be engaged[37]. In February 2003 the High Court determined that it was sufficient for authorities charged under section 117 of the MHA 1983 with providing aftercare services to make their 'best endeavours' to secure arrangements required for a patient's conditional discharge into the community. The failure of such arrangements would not result in the patient being falsely imprisoned[38]. The courts have also repeatedly found, following *Ashingdane v UK* [1985], that Article 5(1) is not engaged where a patient is detained in inappropriate conditions due to a lack of facilities.[39] However, at the time of writing, at least one of the above judgments is subject to appeal (and is further discussed at 3.21 below).

---

[36] In particular, *Ashingdane v UK [1985]; R (on the application of IH) v the Secretary of State for the Home Department and the Secretary of State for Health* [2002], para 87; *R v Camden and Islington Health Authority, ex parte K* [2001], para 33; *MP v Nottinghamshire NHS Trust* [2003], paras 9-22.

[37] *R (on the application of IH)* [2002], para 87

[38] *R v Doncaster Metropolitan Borough Council ex parte W* [2003].

[39] see *MP v Nottinghamshire NHS Trust* [2003], paras 9-22

Identification of a public authority

3.20 *R (on the application of A and others) v Partnerships in Care Ltd* [2002] determined that Independent Hospitals are public authorities when carrying out the powers and duties of the 1983 Act in the detention and treatment of patients. Thus any health and social services authority and any NHS Trust or independent hospital's Board may be held to account as a public authority in relation to the Human Rights Act 1998.

3.21 A much more difficult question arises in relation to the extent to which employees of such authorities may themselves be held to account as public authorities under the HRA 1998. It is clear that any person exercising "functions of a public nature" is a public authority for the purposes of section 6(3)(b) of the 1998 Act. In certain circumstances, the Mental Health Act 1983 places duties specifically on a job-holder (such as an Approved Social Worker at section 13(1)) rather than their employing authority, and therefore that individual bears the public authority responsibility. However, not all duties imposed or implied by the 1983 Act are so clearly determined. At the time of writing, a case is pending appeal that raises the question of the extent of doctors' public authority responsibilities in relation to the 1983 Act[40]. The Royal College of Psychiatrists has sought to become an interested party to the action, arguing that the claim made on doctor's public authority status by the applicant would, if successful, seriously compromise doctors' autonomy and ability to meet their duty of care. The claim by *IH* is that a community-based doctor, in declining to accept a patient whose discharge from detention was conditional upon such a community-based placement, was in breach of public authority duties to provide suitable arrangements for the patient's care.

3.22 Doctors acting in roles assigned specifically to them as *doctors* by the 1983 Act are acting in a public authority role, just as is the case with social workers acting in an ASW capacity. In such roles, there are limitations on doctors' autonomy as *doctors*, in that both hospital managers and Mental Health Review Tribunals can discharge a patient from a doctor's care under detention against that doctor's advice. However, in such circumstances there is nothing to prevent the doctor from satisfying his or her own duty of care by, for example, offering the patient arrangements for continuing care on an informal basis. The doctor would not have failed his or her duty of care if the patient declined such an offer, as all patients who are not subject to compulsion have a right to do.

3.23 Although doctors' powers are limited by the 1983 Act, the Act does not at present create any general powers or duties that compromise a doctors' autonomy to make positive clinical decisions: a doctor cannot be compelled to provide treatment under civil powers against his or her wishes[41]. The concern expressed by the Royal College of Psychiatrists and others about the judicial review application discussed here is that, if successful, it could reverse this position. The doctor's ability to reject a patient's placement within his or her care for clinical reasons (i.e. because the services provided by that doctor are, in the doctor's opinion, unsuitable for the patient in question) might be fettered if such a rejection creates a failure

---

[40] Application for appeal of *R (on the application of IH)* [2002]. See paragraph 3.16 above for general discussion of the issues in the first instance judgment)

[41] It could be argued that certain aspects of Part III of the 1983 Act – such as the ability of the Secretary of State to bar the discharge of a restricted patient – compromise doctors' autonomy in just such a sense. See also Chapter 13.14 below for a case involving the Criminal Procedures (Insanity) acts that raises these issues.

of a public authority duty to provide sufficient treatment facilities to avoid compulsion[42]. Whilst we are sympathetic to this concern, doctors operating powers and discharging duties under the 1983 Act (which may, perhaps, extend to those doctors responsible for post-discharge aftercare arrangements) *do* have some responsibilities as public authorities. A judgment that doctors do not have such duties could mean that no tribunal, court or service provider could require a doctor to perform any specific duty. Conversely, a judgment that doctors must follow unquestioningly the direction of a tribunal, court or other body in performing any specific medical function, regardless of whether that doctor had the necessary skills, training or resources, would severely compromise the doctor's clinical role and have serious implications for the professional autonomy of all clinicians operating public law duties. We hope that the court, which may reach a judgment whilst this report is in press, will be able to achieve a balance in their determination that does not impose unreasonable responsibilities on clinicians or absolve them of public authority responsibilities where these are warranted.

Double jeopardy of life prisoners subject to hospital orders

3.24   The High Court made a formal declaration of incompatibility over the case of *R v Home Secretary, ex parte D* [2002], concerning a discretionary life prisoner who had been transferred to hospital under section 47/49 and who had served the penal element of his sentence. The court found that the requirement on *D* to appeal for discharge both to the Tribunal and for the Home Secretary's consent to go before the Parole Board was a contravention of his Article 5(4) right to take proceedings to determine the lawfulness of his detention. Two points were argued by *D* to be in breach of Article 5(4). First, that because the referral to the Parole Board is made at the discretion of the Home Secretary, this is inconsistent with the detained person's entitlement to an effective review. Second, that because the application to the MHRT and the referral to the Parole Board are made consecutively, there will not in practice be a "speedy" hearing. The Judge accepted both arguments and found that the current regime breaches Article 5. This was only the fourth such order passed by the UK courts, three of which have been mental health cases. At the time of writing, further legal action is ongoing which may provide a resolution to this matter.

Identification of gay and lesbian partners as Nearest Relatives

3.25   In 1999 we highlighted our existing concern that the statutory protocol for identifying Nearest Relatives under the 1983 Act was discriminatory against same-sex couples[43]. This was the subject of a legal challenge in 2002, where a patient whose lesbian partner had been discounted as Nearest Relative claimed a violation of her right to family life under ECHR Article 8.

3.26   A Court Order finalised on the 7 November 2002 declared that, to avoid incompatibility with the HRA 1998, and provided that the two have cohabited for at least six months, the homosexual partner of a patient can be treated as falling within the phrase "living with the

---

[42]   This case therefore also raises an argument claiming positive rights to treatment under human rights principles. See Chapter 4.17 *et seq* below.

[43]   Mental Health Act Commission (1999) *Submission to the Mental Health Legislation Review Team*. MHAC, Jan 1999, p9

patient as the patient's husband or wife as the case may be" in section 26(6) of the 1983 Act and accordingly as their Nearest Relative within section 26(1) of the Act[44].

3.27 In 2002 we identified a number of local authorities that had refused to recognise the court order as binding law. We approached the Department of Health about this and were pleased to help the Department in promulgating a clarificatory statement on the legal import of the judgment. We entered into discussions with the authorities concerned, who have now all recognised the change in law and advised their practitioners accordingly that, in the words of the Department of Health guidance, the consent order "can and should be followed by decision makers: local authorities can and should regard same sex partners as within the extended definition of husband and wife under section 26".

3.28 The current legal position is an improvement on the previous situation, but it may not prevent further human rights challenges. Some commentators remain dissatisfied that the Act continues to discriminate against unmarried couples, in that the latter (whether homosexual or heterosexual) must have cohabited for six months to be recognised.

Automatic appointment of Nearest Relatives and ECHR Article 8

3.29 In 1997 we first highlighted problems caused by the statutory requirements for consultation with Nearest Relatives[45]. A patient has no say in or veto over the appointment of their Nearest Relative, who is identified according to the statutory scheme set out at section 26 of the 1983 Act, even if the patient has been abused by or is estranged from that person. This is a clear breach of the right to respect for family life under ECHR Article 8. In our Ninth Biennial Report we welcomed the Government's undertaking to amend the Act so as to enable a detained patient to apply to the court "to have the Nearest Relative replaced where the patient reasonably objected to a certain person acting in that capacity", as a part of its friendly settlement of the challenge to this part of the law in *JT v UK* [2000].

3.30 We regret that no action has been taken on this undertaking at the time of writing (October 2003), despite a formal declaration of incompatibility in June 2003 following a further legal challenge[46]. In this case, the patient alleged that she had been sexually abused in childhood by her adoptive father, who was her Nearest Relative under the Act. As a consequence, there was no relationship of trust between her and her adoptive father and she did not wish to see or communicate with him again. But she had no right under the 1983 Act to have him replaced by someone who would be acceptable to her. Mr Justice Maurice Kay found that the automatic appointment of the adoptive father as Nearest Relative and the statutory consequences that result from that appointment constituted a continuous interference with the patient's private life which was not justified under Article 8(2). Further, he found that it was not possible to construe sections 26 and 29 of the 1983 Act compatibly with Article 8. Accordingly, he granted a declaration to that effect.

---

[44] *R on the application of SSG and Liverpool City Council and Secretary of State for Health.* Website address: www.doh.gov.uk/consentorder.doc. See also www.doh.gsi.gov.uk/mhact1983.htm

[45] Mental Health Act Commission (1997) *Seventh Biennial Report 1995-7*. London: Stationery Office. p 119

[46] *R (on the application of M) v Secretary of State for Health* [2003]

3.31 We can see no reason for this matter to have not been attended to before now and very much regret that the situation remains uncertain as we go to press. We trust that remedial legislative action will be introduced as soon as possible.

> **Recommendation 2:** Government should take action to rectify the incompatibility of sections 26 and 29 of the Mental Health Act 1983 with human rights principles by means of a Remedial Order under section 10 of the Human Rights Act 1998.

Challenging Second Opinion authorisations

The *Wilkinson* case

3.32 The Court of Appeal judgement in *Wilkinson* (October 2001) has been subject of much debate and speculation over this period[47]. The case has been frequently misunderstood to limit the authority of the current Act in respect of detained patients with mental capacity who refuse consent, because of a passage in the judgment of Simon Brown LJ that was, and was acknowledged to be, *obiter*[48]. We discuss this aspect of the case at Chapter 4.2 below. In fact, at the time of its hearing in 2002 the court was faced with a single issue on an interlocutory appeal. This was whether medical experts should be required to attend for cross-examination in judicial reviews of Second Opinion Appointed Doctor (SOAD) decisions to authorise treatment.

3.33 The case began in 2000 with a successful application for judicial review of and injunction against the administration of depot medication for mental disorder which had been authorised by a SOAD. By the time of the final Appeal Court hearing, eighteen months later, the authorisation in question had been withdrawn and so the court determined points of principle only. It noted that the human rights implications of enforced treatment on the authorisation of a SOAD may include alleged fundamental Convention breaches (in this case, in relation to ECHR Articles 2 or 3), or such as obviously raise questions of medical necessity and proportionality (in this case Articles 8 and 14). The question of a patient's mental capacity would be relevant, certainly to questions of proportionality. It was determined that any court considering alleged Convention breaches of this kind inevitably would have to reach its own view on these matters. Where, as in this case, there were conflicting medical opinions before the court, it would be necessary for the court to require the attendance and cross examination of medical experts.

3.34 The court recognised the burden that such hearings could place on services and hoped that challenges of this nature would be rare and arise only in the most exceptional circumstances. In our reporting period (financial years 2001 to 2003), only one case has gone to a

---

[47] *R (on the application of Wilkinson) v the Responsible Medical Office, Broadmoor Hospital, the Mental Health Act Commission Second Opinion Appointed Doctor and the Secretary of State for Health* [2001]. For an account of the misunderstandings and a corrective view see also Hewitt, D *An end to compulsory psychiatric treatment?* (2002) <u>New Law Journal</u>, 8 Feb 2002, p194-5.

[48] i.e. *Obiter Dictum* – a judge's remark made in passing in arguing point or giving judgment, but not essential to the decision and therefore without binding legal authority.

full hearing with cross-examinations of witnesses (the *N* case, discussed at 3.35 below). A further such case was concluded as went to press.

3.35 In *R (on the application of N) v Doctor M and others* [2002], the final determination revolved around the question of whether, in the face of opposing medical evidence, a SOAD, RMO or a court could justify the imposition of medical treatment as a "necessary" curtailment of a patient's human rights. The applicant argued to the Court of Appeal that the existence of dissenting medical opinion proved that a treatment was not "considered necessary by a responsible body of opinion" and did not therefore meet the *Bolam* test[49]. This "reverse *Bolam* test" was rejected by the court, which held that the question could be whether the treatment was the best of a number of available options, all of which might pass the *Bolam* test, with the choice between involving issues wider than the medical. In other words, the test was simply whether the proposed treatment had been convincingly shown to be a medical necessity[50]. The existence of dissenting medical views was a matter to take into account in determining this, but was not a decisive factor.

3.36 The *N* judgment suggested that *Wilkinson* should not be regarded as a charter for routine applications to the court for oral evidence in human rights cases, and that courts were entitled to reach decisions on written evidence if they felt able to do so. The court emphasised Hale LJ's qualification in *Wilkinson* that cross-examination should be ordered "if necessary"[51].

3.37 It may therefore be the case that the courts will be slow to grant cross-examination in such cases in future. Nevertheless, we are concerned at the administrative and resource burden that such cases could put on psychiatric services generally, and on our own functions in administering the SOAD system. However, it may be that, under the next Mental Health Act, other appeal mechanisms than judicial can be found when a Tribunal doctor authorises compulsory treatment for mental disorder. The grounding of the "SOAD" role within the Tribunal system may itself, perhaps, provide such a mechanism. We advise Government to consider this matter carefully in the formulation of the next Act.

> **Recommendation 3:** We advise Government to consider how appeals against decisions relating to the authority for patients' care plans might be heard within the framework of new mental health legislation.

---

[49] see *Bolam v Friern Hospital Management Committee* [1957]; *Bolito v City and Hackney Health Authority* [1998]. The 'Bolam test' is a measure of whether a doctor will be deemed to have acted in a patient's best interests and be immune from liability in trespass. The test is whether the doctor acted in accordance with practice accepted as proper at that time by a body of medical opinion skilled in the treatment in question.

[50] see *Herczegfalvy v Austria* [1992]: "the established principles of medicine are admittedly in principle decisive in such cases; as a general rule, a method which is a therapeutic necessity cannot be regarded as inhuman or degrading. The court must nevertheless satisfy itself that the medical necessity has been convincingly shown to exist" (para 82).

[51] *Wilkinson*, para 62 (see also *R (on the application of N) v Doctor M and others* [2002] paras 34-37)

The duty to give reasons for Second Opinion determinations

3.38 *R (on the application of Wooder) v Feggetter and the Mental Health Act Commission* [2002] was heavily influenced by the approach taken in *Wilkinson*. The Court of Appeal held that "with the coming into force of the Human Rights Act 1998 the time has come...to declare that fairness requires that a decision by a SOAD which sanctions the violation of the autonomy of a competent adult patient should also be accompanied by reasons". The common law implied such a duty. The patient was entitled to know a SOAD's reasons for authorising treatment, unless the patient's doctor justified withholding such information on clinical grounds. Reasons should be stated in writing by the SOAD and communicated to the patient by his Responsible Medical Officer (RMO).

3.39 Guidance issued by the Mental Health Act Commission following this decision is available on the Commission's website[52]. The Commission has advised SOADs to provide reasons in respect of any authorisation that they provide, whether or not a patient has mental capacity in their view. A patient may be determined to lack mental capacity to give a competent refusal of consent to treatment and yet still wish to know why his or her stated wishes are being overridden. It is for such patients' RMOs to determine whether to release the information provided by the SOAD.

The Limits of Compulsory Treatment

3.40 In *R (on the application of B) v Ashworth Hospital Authority* [2003], a patient challenged his placement in a personality disorder ward, despite only having the Mental Health Act "classi-fication" of mental illness on his detention documentation. Although the hospital suggested that the patient suffered from a personality disorder alongside the mental illness, it had not sought to reclassify the patient accordingly. Indeed, some doubt remained as to whether the personality disorder was of such a nature and degree alone to warrant the use of the Act. The hospital argued, successfully in the first instance, that section 63 allowed them wide powers to provide care and treatment appropriate to the patient's mental disorder regardless of classification.

3.41 The Appeal Court disagreed, deciding that the phrase "medical treatment...for the mental disorder from which [the patient] is suffering" at section 63 must be read in the wider context of the Act. As such it only permits treatment as is appropriate for the mental disorder(s) that the patient is classified as suffering from under the Act.

3.42 The court made two important caveats in its judgment:

* re-classification under sections 16, 20 or 72(5) was an available tool for RMOs and Tribunals to ensure that the necessary authority to treat is provided;

* even where a secondary mental disorder could not be re-classified, in that its nature or degree would not meet the criteria of the 1983 Act, it is possible that it nevertheless aggravates or prevents the treatment of the disorder for which the patient *is* detained for treatment. Following *B v Croydon* [1995], the treatment of the unclassified mental disorder may in these circumstances be ancillary to, and therefore a necessary part of, the treatment of the classified mental disorder.

---

[52] www.mhac.trent.nhs.uk. For contact details of the Mental Health Act Commission, see appendix F

3.43   Simon Brown LJ noted that following this case "the question of re-classifying patients to include other disorders will assume a far greater importance than hitherto it has had". The court ruled that, unless and until B was reclassified as suffering also from a psychopathic disorder it would be unlawful to continue treating him without consent for that condition.

3.44   This case, although it did not rely directly on any ECHR based challenge, continues the line of judgments where the courts have sought to interpret the Mental Health Act 1983 as limited by extraneous "residual freedoms". It is notable, however, that, contrary to his remarks in *Wilkinson* (see 3.32 above and Chapter 4.2 below), Simon Brown LJ accepted in *B* that a detained patient may be compelled to accept medical treatment for mental disorder even if, being capable, he objects to it. This approach was also taken by the Hon. Mr Justice Silber in *R (on the application of PS) v Dr G & Dr W* [2003], a judgment given as we go to press, which allowed that the administration of medication under section 58 in the face of a patient's capacitated opposition did not infringe ECHR rights where such treatment is in a patient's best interests.

4

Human rights and mental health: future directions

Concern for patient autonomy

4.1   Some general patterns emerge from the cases discussed in Chapter 3 above. Foremost amongst these is the judicial concern with the "canon of construction that Parliament is presumed not to have enacted legislation that interferes with the liberty of the subject without making it clear that this was its intention"[53]. Cases such as *Wilkinson* and *B v Ashworth* (see Chapter 3.32 & 3.40 above) reinforce the fact that a patient who is subject to specific forms of compulsion retains residual freedoms, even if detained in hospital, although the precise limits of such freedoms are far from established. The courts have consistently rejected legal arguments suggesting a 'paternalistic' approach to health issues in general, emphasising instead the rights of patients as autonomous individuals[54]

The role of mental capacity

4.2   There is a considerable body of opinion that would prefer mental health legislation replacing the 1983 Act to draw a clearer distinction between the mentally capable and the mentally incapable when determining the limits of compulsion. At Chapter 3.32 above we noted that the *Wilkinson* case has occasionally been misconstrued as limiting the authority of the current law in relation to capable patients. More often, the case is considered as an example or harbinger of the judiciary's pull on the law towards capacity-based thresholds of compulsion. This is because of a remark made in passing by Lord Justice Simon Brown, one of the Appeal Judges in the case. Drawing on ECHR principles, his Lordship stated that if the appellant against compulsory treatment had genuine capacity to refuse consent, "it is difficult to suppose that he should nevertheless be forcibly subjected to it". It is important to note the qualification that followed this statement, which acknowledged its *obiter* status[55], and then acknowledged that it was "quite inappropriate on such an appeal for this court to try to resolve at this stage all the many questions which [may] arise for decision under the Convention". The *obiter* remark of Simon Brown LJ was opposed by another of the judges in this case, Lady Justice Hale, who stated that she did not take the view that detained patients

---

[53]   *R v Hallstrom ex p W (No 2)*; *R v Gardner ex p L* [1986], per McCullough, J. The subsequent effective overturning of the Hallstrom ruling over renewal of patients' detention on leave (see Chapter 9.47 below) does not, in our view, negate this general point, although it does demonstrate the breadth of potential judicial interpretation of ambiguities in statute law.

[54]   see, for example, *Re B (Adult: Refusal of Medical Treatment)* [2002]

[55]   see note 48 above on the meaning of *obiter*.

with capacity to decide for themselves can never be treated against their will. Lady Justice Hale's remarks were cited in *R (on the application of PS) v Drs G & W* [2003], which confirmed as we go to press that treatment under the 1983 Act in the face of capacited refusal may be consistent with ECHR rights. We also note that neither the Government's Expert Committee, led by Professor Richardson in 1999, nor the Government itself has countenanced a law that would guarantee psychiatric patients a right of competent refusal of treatment where questions of the safety of other persons arise[56].

4.3   We recognise that there is a considerable body of opinion, including within our own membership, that considers the review of current legislation to have missed an important opportunity to refocus the criteria for psychiatric compulsion around issues of mental capacity. Yet we continue to have concerns over whether the concept of mental capacity can, in fact, provide the panacea of natural justice that its supporters seem to suggest. These concerns focus on the indeterminate nature of the concept of mental capacity itself. Mental capacity, like consent, is usually viewed as a point on a sliding scale dependent not only on the patient's mental state but also by the circumstances in which a decision is being made. In the current legal framework, this tends to be interpreted as though the threshold for mental capacity rises according to the invasiveness or seriousness of the intervention for which consent is sought. This is, perhaps, as it should be: a patient probably should be subject to a "higher" capacity threshold if they are to consent to neurosurgery than if they are to consent to a tranquilliser tablet. But the danger of making such capacity, or its absence, the fundamental criterion for giving a treatment, is that no-one with a mental disorder who refuses consent to treatment that a doctor feels to be necessary would ever be judged by that doctor to have made a 'capable' decision. It is the case, perhaps, that such difficulties in defining or determining capacity could be addressed in future medico-legal practice. One safeguard could be that someone other than the treating doctor makes the assessment, although this could lead to a cumbersome and bureaucratic system.

4.4   A second aspect of the indeterminancy of capacity is the wide variety of definitions adopted by different authorities for different purposes and in different jurisdictions. The British Medical Association's helpful 5-point test[57], for example, although directly referring to the standard legal test of capacity set out in *Re C (Adult: Refusal of Treatment)* [1994], differs from it both by addition (eg the BMA test includes the ability to "make a free choice", i.e. one that is "free from pressure") and by subtraction (the BMA test excludes the *Re C* elements of believing the relevant information and of weighing it in the balance in arriving at a choice). The draft Mental Incapacity Bill also excludes the element of belief; and although the Explanatory Notes talk of weighing the information, the Bill itself employs the quite different notion of the ability "to use the information" in coming to a decision[58]. Again, the

---

[56]   Department of Health (1999) *Report of the Expert Committee Review of the Mental Health Act 1983.* London, Department of Health para 7.12-14

[57]   The test is set out in British Medical Association and The Law Society (1995). *Assessment of Mental Capacity: Guidance for Doctors and Lawyers.* London: British Medical Association (page 66), and reproduced in British Medical Association. (2001) *Consent Toolkit.* London: BMA (pages 13-14)

[58]   see Department of Constitutional Affairs (2003) *Draft Mental Incapacity Bill* Cm 5859-1. London: The Stationery Office, Part 1, clause 2.1; the reference to weighing the information comes in Part 1 para 19 of Department of Constitutional Affairs (2003) *Draft Mental Incapacity Bill. Commentary and Explanatory Notes.* Vol 2. London: Stationery Office.

MacCAT-T, a well-validated measure of capacity widely used in both research and medico-legal practice in North America, includes a further element, of "appreciation", which is absent from all three of the above tests[59]. These differences between proposed tests of capacity are more than mere differences of drafting: the ability to "weigh" information is central to the assessment of capacity in a wide range of mental disorders (such as anorexia nervosa, for example[60]); and "appreciation", in the MacCAT-T, equates centrally with the particular kind of loss of insight which is characteristic of the group of disorders that are most likely to be treated on an involuntary basis[61], namely the functional psychotic disorders, such as schizophrenia, hypomania and major depression.

4.5   There is of course considerable scope for debate among experts – clinical, legal and philosophical[62] – about which of the many different ways of understanding capacity is the more appropriate in different contexts and for different purposes. But that is our point. In the absence of a consensus view, the premature adoption in statute of any particular candidate definition of capacity could exclude certain patients from treatment and place mental health professionals in an untenable position. This is a particular problem in relation to two types of patient. Professionals could be prevented from intervening in the care of patients with deteriorating conditions until the point of loss of capacity had been reached, or prevented from effective intervention in the care of patients who may be a danger to others, even when they might still be held responsible for treatment outcomes or patients' actions. The Richardson Committee's attempts at addressing these problems led it to compromise the capacity-based model that it proposed to Government in 1999, and admit that the question of intervention in the case of patients posing a risk to others was a "political decision"[63]. The Richardson Committee's capacity-based approach was not, of course, adopted by the draft Mental Health Bill of 2002, and so this particular dilemma is unlikely to be put before Parliament in relation to England and Wales in the immediate future.

4.6   The Commission's detailed discussions of its concerns in relation to mental incapacity as the key determinant for compulsion were expressed in our submissions to the Expert Committee appointed by Government to report in 1999, and to Government itself in our responses to its

---

[59] Grisso, T., and Appelbaum, P.S. (1998) *Assessing Competence to Consent to Treatment: A Guide for Physicians and other Health Professionals.* Oxford: Oxford University Press, chapter 3: abilities related to competence, pages 31-60.

[60] Tan, J. (forthcoming) *The discrepancy between the legal definition of capacity and the British Medical Association's guidelines.* Journal of Medical Ethics.

[61] see, for an example of empirical research in showing the importance of functional psychotic disorders in relation to compulsion, Sensky, T., Hughes, T., and Hirsch, S., (1991) *Compulsory Psychiatric Treatment in the Community, Part 1. A Controlled Study of Compulsory Community Treatment with Extended Leave under the Mental Health Act: Special Characteristics of Patients Treated and Impact of Treatment.* British Journal of Psychiatry 158:792, and for an example of conceptual and legal analysis Fulford, K.W.M. (1993) *Value, Action, Mental Illness and the Law.* p279-310 in Shute S., Gardner J, and Horder, J., eds. *Action and Value in Criminal Law.* Oxford: Oxford University Press).

[62] see Szmukler, G and Holloway F, *Mental Health Legislation is Now a Harmful Anachronism*, in Psychiatric Bulletin, 1998 22 p. 662-5, with commentaries by Fulford, K.W.M., (1998) *Replacing the Mental Health Act 1983? How to change the game without losing the baby with the bath water or shooting ourselves in the foot*, p666-8, Sayce, L, *Transcending Mental Health Law*, p669-70.

[63] Department of Health (1999) *Report of the Expert Committee Review of the Mental Health Act* 1983. London, Department of Health para 7.12-14

[64] Scottish Executive (2001) *New Directions: Report of the Review of the Mental Health (Scotland) Act 1984.* Edinburgh, The Stationery Office. Chapter 5. www.scotland.gov.uk/millan.

Green Paper and draft Mental Health Bill of 2002. Many of these concerns are echoed in the Millan Committee's report on the review of the Mental Health (Scotland) Act 1984[64].

4.7   The Millan Report states that the issue of incapacity was one of the most difficult that the Committee faced. The report acknowledged that there are powerful arguments in favour of the introduction of a capacity test, including:

∗ The claim that it provides a specific and ethically justifiable reason for overruling a person's autonomy, in that such autonomy has already been usurped as a consequence of the mental disorder.

∗ That it would bring mental healthcare into line with other forms of health intervention, and thus be non-discriminatory.

∗ That consistency between and eventual amalgamation of mental health and mental incapacity legislation is desirable.

∗ That it received strong support from the Law Society, the Scottish Association for Mental Health and many health and social work interests.

4.8   The Millan Committee nevertheless rejected the concept of mental incapacity as a key determinant for compulsion, setting out its concerns which we have summarised at Figure 3 below. The Millan Committee proposed the concept of 'impaired judgment' in place of 'mental incapacity' as the basic criterion for compulsion. The Committee described 'impaired judgment' as "a broadly similar concept to incapacity, but…less legalistic… and one which may be easier to apply in practice. It may also be a term which is easier for service users to accept than the term 'incapable'". It is not clear to the Commission, however, how the concept of impaired judgment can be freed from the circularity discussed at 4.3 above, although its lack of precise definition does at least avoid some of the difficulties that we have suggested in relation to use of thresholds determined by more narrowly defined concepts of mental incapacity.

4.9   The Commission will be taking a keen and constructive interest in the continuing debates over concepts of incapacity that may be applied in relation to the thresholds for compulsory care. We hope that further work can be undertaken to arrive at fully conceived concepts of incapacity specific to the context of compulsion in a range of mental health interventions, for the further consideration of how mental incapacity might operate as a threshold to such compulsion.

4.10   The *Wilkinson* case has raised the profile of mental capacity as a key determinant in considering whether compulsion is warranted. We discuss this in relation to statutory Second Opinion Appointed Doctors' authorisation of such treatment at Chapter 10.38 below.

Difficulties with a capacity test
(summary of arguments set down by the Millan committee report, Chapter 5.29-38)

i)   a capacity test could be difficult to apply in a range of situations, including patients with mood disorders, obsessive compulsive disorders and eating disorders, where patients retain legal capacity but be at such risk to justify intervention;

ii) in relation to forensic patients, the issue is not so much capacity as whether placement is more appropriate in a health care or penal setting;

iii) incapacity was a concept difficult to measure and apply, especially for GPs or doctors in, for example, A&E Departments and might lead to reluctance to use the Act even where it was proper to do so;

iv) people experiencing acute mental distress often present to clinicians in an ambiguous state of mind, ostensibly resisting treatment but perhaps doing so in the hope that someone will intervene;

v) there could be difficulties in defining a threshold at which a patient becomes incapable, particularly with patients whose judgement is affected to some degree by their disorder but who retain some decision-making capability;

vi) it would seem impractical for compulsion to start and stop with the rapid fluctuations in capacity experienced by some mentally ill patients;

vii) although it is true that psychiatrists will have to assess capacity under mental incapacity legislation, and have to do so in relation to specific treatments under the Mental Health Act, in relation to long-term detention under mental health law to allow a range of treatment interventions it may be difficult to identify precisely what it is that the patient must be incapable of making a decision over; and

viii) the practical effect of introducing an incapacity test may discourage early intervention, or prevent a person from receiving help when they might bring severe harm to themselves on the basis of a judgment that they retained mental capacity in their choice of action.

Fig 3: Summary of concerns over mental incapacity as the basis for compulsion as set out in the Millan report

Human rights concerns with the current Mental Health Act

4.11   Elsewhere in this report we discuss the following issues that give cause for concerns specifically related to human rights:

* The '*de facto*' detention of patients without due process or protection may conflict with ECHR Articles 5 (right to liberty and security), 6 (right to a fair trial) and 8 (right to respect for family and private life); (see Chapter 8.1 – 8.11)

* The limitations of patients' access to Tribunals, particularly through administrative difficulties, may conflict with ECHR Articles 5 (right to liberty and security) and 6 (right to a fair trial); (see Chapter 3.13 – 3.15)

* The lack of clarity around explicit and implicit powers of compulsion may give rise to further challenges under ECHR Articles 3 (prohibition of torture); (see Chapter 11.1– 11.12)

* The continued differentiation between married, unmarried and same-sex couples in determining Nearest Relative may conflict with ECHR Articles 8 (right to respect for family and private life) and 14 (prohibition of discrimination); (see Chapter 3.25 – 3.28)

* the automatic appointment of Nearest Relatives regardless of the wishes of the patient conflicts with ECHR Articles 8 (right to respect for family and private life) (see Chapter 3.28 – 3.31)

Human rights concerns with the draft Mental Health Bill of 2002

4.12 Human rights concerns over the implications of the draft Mental Health Bill of 2002 have been widely discussed elsewhere, and have been raised particularly by the Joint Committee on Human Rights (JCHR)[65], to whom we submitted evidence in 2002[66]. We recognise that work will be undertaken on the redrafting of the Bill to meet the concerns raised by the JCHR and other bodies, and therefore confine our comments in this section to the general. However, the JCHR welcomed aspects of the draft Mental Health Bill proposals of 2002, particularly as these related to plans to address the lack of safeguards for 'de facto' detained patients and the extended role of the Tribunal.

4.13 Aspects of the draft Mental Health Bill of 2002 which have been raised as human rights issues by the JCHR and other bodies cover the following general areas:

* the broad criteria for compulsion;

* the relative weakness of the Code of Practice as a regulatory tool[67];

* the possibility of "preventive detention", particularly in relation to personality disordered patients;

* review and termination criteria for compulsion in the community;

* reduced powers of relatives in the initiation and termination of compulsion;

* plans to extend compulsory medical treatment to prisoners (see chapter 14 below); and

* plans to pass the Commission's monitoring role regarding compulsion to a wider, generic healthcare inspectorate (see Chapter 20 below).

The longer term: the example of America

4.14 It may be that the USA, with its constitutionally based culture of concern for individual rights and legal process, provides a useful model in predicting future directions of mental health law, particularly in relation to the likely legal challenges based upon human rights principles. Peay (2003) notes that US jurisprudence has recently begun to be invoked in Human Rights Act submissions to UK courts[68].

4.15 Following a number of federal court judgments in the early 1970s, almost all states in the US enacted "patients' Bills of Rights"[69] underlining the fact that persons resident in psychiatric

---

[65] Joint Committee on Human Rights (2002) *Draft Mental Health Bill: Twenty-fifth report of Session 2001-02.* HL Paper 181, HC 1294. London, Stationery Office

[66] Mental Health Act Commission submission available at www.mhac.trent.nhs.uk

[67] This concern was expressed prior to the *Munjaz* [2003] judgment discussed at Chapter 3.2 *et seq* above, which has strengthened the legal 'weight' of the Code. However, even subsequent to this ruling it is questionable whether a new legislative framework for the compulsory treatment of psychiatric patients should have key elements determined at the level of practice guidance.

[68] Peay, J (2003) *Decisions and Dilemmas: working with mental health law.* Oxford, Hart Publishing. p163

[69] Perlin, M *The United States* in Payne, A (1993) *Sexual activity among psychiatric inpatients: international perspectives.* Journal of Forensic Psychiatry, Vol 4 No 1 109-129.

hospitals retain a broad range of civil rights predicated on the US constitution. Such federal laws have, in turn, provided impetus to Congress to pass rights-based mental health legislation, although judicial action has remained a crucial instigator of change. In this way, the US Bill of Rights is similar, in both content and operation, to the European Convention in UK law since the passing of Human Rights Act 1998. It is the case, of course, that the recognition of certain "civil rights" under US law does not prevent various State practices that cause great ethical concern to patient and professional groups in the US, such as the use of mechanical restraint, and also does not preclude many individual States from assuming powers that reach far beyond those that would be allowed under UK jurisdiction[70]. The formal recognition of concepts of human rights by the State is clearly not an automatic protection against State practices that can be considered abusive.

4.16   One aspect of the US attention to human rights has been the increasing focus on anti-discrimination legislation, culminating so far in the Americans with Disabilities Act 1991. This prohibits specifically forms of discrimination that exclude disabled people from services, programs or activities; or leads to their treatment being unequal to that provided to other persons, or different to that provided to others without good reason. Authorities are further required to provide services in the most integrated settings appropriate to the needs of the disabled individual.[71]

4.17   But the influence of human rights on US law has not been limited to the so-called negative rights of non-discrimination. As early as 1974 (*Wyatt v Stickney*), the courts established positive rights to treatment for persons committed to psychiatric institutions by requiring treatment as a justification for detention with due process of law. *Johnson v Solomon* (1979) established a right to treatment in the least restrictive environment, which has been extended by subsequent judgments to an obligation on authorities to provide adequate community based services and support. In *Youngberg v Romeo* (1982) the Supreme Court ruled that due process also required reasonably safe conditions of confinement, freedom from unreasonable bodily restraint and minimally adequate rehabilitation, with courts giving due deference to professional opinion on what is "reasonable". That US citizens have a right to freedom from harm under the Eighth Amendment has also been successfully argued as a basis for legal action against poor hospital environments and repressive regimes (*New York Association for Retarded Children v Rockerfeller* 1973). The right to freedom from harm is also interpreted as a positive obligation on authorities to protect those citizens to whom it has a "special relationship" (*Martinez v California* 1980). A special relationship clearly exists where a person is detained by the State or subject to community-based powers of coercion, but "government control or custody is not a prerequisite for municipal liability" (*Estate of Bailey v County of York* 1985). A special relationship is therefore established between the State and those who meet program or service guidelines (*Board of Regents v*

---

[70] The American Psychiatric Association has, for example, recently been debating the ethical dilemmas relating to the psychiatric treatment of prisoners condemned to the death penalty.

[71] Marty, D A and Chapin, R (2000) *Ethics in Community Health Care: The legislative tenets of clients' right to treatment in the least restrictive environment and freedom from harm: Implications for community providers.* In Community Mental Health Journal Vol.36, No.6 December 2000, p545-556.

Roth 1972)[72]. US jurisprudence has also provided a relatively narrow definition of 'dangerousness', which must be based upon a finding of evidence, which we discuss at Chapter 7.26 below.

4.18   In summary, over the last quarter century the above cases have established within US law:

* a right to psychiatric treatment, which must also be in the least restrictive environment; and

* a duty of care (with subsequent liabilities for failures) that probably extends to all patients, but certainly extends to any patient whose liberties are curtailed by the State, whether they are detained in hospital or receiving treatment in the community.

It seems likely that issues relating to the State's positive obligations to treat and protect psychiatric patients will arise in future legal challenges to UK mental health law. The extending of compulsory powers into the community will perhaps throw these issues into sharper relief, given the inherent difficulties of managing or protecting non-resident patients.

---

[72]   *ibid.*, p551

5.

Values in Mental Health Services

…the primary concern of the Human Rights Act is not so much rights in the ordinary common law sense, but values.

Lord Woolf, Lord Chief Justice, 15 October 2002[73]

5.1   The coming into force of the Human Rights Act 1998 has been described as a unique opportunity for professionals to influence the debate on future healthcare law far more directly than has ever previously been possible, primarily because judges must now interpret the law in accordance with the "living instrument" of the European Convention on Human Rights, which suggests that judicial weight will have to be attached to contemporary social mores[74]. Indeed professionals can and should "not merely react to the attempts of others to develop Convention rights, but should attempt to influence such development positively in the interests of the service to which they are custodians"[75]. They can do so in developing their own local policies with human rights values at their core as a matter of best practice rather than risk avoidance, thus making human rights principles the tools with which patients and other service users can negotiate effectively with public authorities for better care and treatment. We see this as the core of a value system that should underlie the development of services under current and future mental health legislation.

5.2   In this chapter we seek to address the question of what – or whose – values should prevail in mental health services, and particularly in those that involve compulsion of patients. In Chapter 6 we highlight some specific ways in which Government and other authorities might foster such a value system.

The role of Values-Based Practice

5.3   The increasing awareness of human rights issues is likely to, and indeed should, increase patients' expectations that their choices and values will be accommodated within mental health services. The principle of patient-centred services has been strongly endorsed in

---

[73]   Lord Woolf, lecture to the British Academy, 15/10/02, quoted in Hansard 28/10/02 col 607

[74]   Persaud A, and Hewitt D (2001) European Convention on Human Rights: effects on psychiatric care *Nursing Standard*, 15, 44, 33-37

[75]   *ibid*

Government policy[76]. Of course, patients who are compelled to engage with services experience a fundamental denial of their choices and values from admission. If such patients are not to be excluded from patient-centred approaches to healthcare provision, specific difficulties must be overcome.

5.4   We are pleased that the National Institute for Mental Health for England (NIMHE) has recognised and sought to address these issues through the promotion of values-based practice, which it has signaled with the appointment this year of a NIMHE National Fellow for Values-Based Practice, Professor KWM Fulford. We think that the approach of Values-Based Practice (VBP) has strong potential to improve and, in some cases, radically transform psychiatric practice. We are aware that the approach is already looked upon with enthusiasm by many stakeholders in mental health, both from service user and provider perspectives, and are pleased that Government is adopting its promotion at policy level[77].

5.5   Values-Based Practice (VBP), the principles of which are summarised in Figure 4 below, is the theory and skills-base of effective healthcare decision-making where legitimately different, and hence potentially contested, values are in play[78]. VBP, in focusing on contested decision-making, is well suited in principle to the particular difficulties raised by compulsion. From our perspective VBP is a helpful approach in three specific respects: it is, (i) patient-centred, (ii) collaborative, and (iii) concerned with assessment. We will comment briefly on each of these features of VBP and then indicate the potential role of this approach in relation to future mental health legislation.

5.6   First, then, the three features of VBP that are of particular relevance to compulsion.

(i) **Values-Based Practice is patient-centred.**

VBP is like Evidence-Based Practice (EBP) to the extent that both are responses to the growing complexity of decision-making in healthcare. VBP and EBP are indeed complementary in this respect (see principle 1, Figure 4 below): VBP is a response to the growing complexity of the values bearing on healthcare decision-making, EBP a response to the growing complexity of the corresponding facts. Bioethics, too, is a response to values-complexity. But where bioethics focuses on good outcomes, or prescribing the "right" values by which decisions should be guided, VBP focuses on good process, on the skills-base of decision-making that seeks to balance legitimately different value perspectives. (These skills are summarized in principles 6-9, Figure 4 below.)

The respect for individual values thus embodied in VBP gives particular cogency to the National Service Framework policy of patient-centred practice. Patient-centred practice, after all, is nothing if not patient-values centred practice[79]. This is important for mental

---

[76] see, in particular, the National Service Framework for Mental Health (Department of Health (1999) *National Service Framework for Mental Health – Modern Standards and Service Models.* London: Department of Health).

[77] see the *NIMHE Values Framework (draft)* www.connects.org.uk/conferences

[78] see Fulford, K.W.M. (forthcoming) 'Ten Principles of Values-Based Medicine (VBM)' in Radden, J. (ed) *Companion to the Philosophy of Psychiatry,* Oxford: Oxford University Press, and Fulford, K.W.M. (forthcoming) *Ten Principles of Values-Based Practice.* Cambridge: Cambridge University Press.

[79] see Allott, P., Loganathan, L and Fulford, K.W.M. (Bill), (002, in press) 'Discovering Hope For Recovery From A British Perspective'. In Lurie, S., Mc Cubbin, M., & Dallaire, B. (Eds) *International innovations in community mental health [special issue].* Canadian Journal of Community Mental Health, 21(2).

health: the relative powerlessness of people with severe mental disorders renders them vulnerable not only to the overtly abusive consequences of fear and stigmatisation (see Chapter 6.34 *et seq* below), but also to well-intentioned, though no less abusive, denials of their values and choices in their "best interests".[80] The skills-based approach of VBP could do much to remedy this. Specifically in relation to compulsion VBP, shifts the emphasis in decision-making from (a negative) denial of patients' values to (a positive) balancing of patients' current values against their own future values and the values of others. We return to this point below, at 5.6(iii). First we consider VBP's particular approach to balanced decision-making.

(ii) Values-Based Practice is Collaborative.

One tried and tested approach to balanced decision-making, particularly in legal proceedings, is advocacy. A disadvantage of advocacy, though, especially if it is the only approach available, is that it tends to become adversarial, a blunt-edged contest for values, determined as much by the skills of the advocate as by the substance of the case. VBP, by contrast, by starting from respect for differences of values, is inherently collaborative. In VBP, different value perspectives, brought together particularly through good communication skills, become a resource for balanced decision-making.

In modern clinical practice an important resource of different value perspectives is provided by the multidisciplinary team or MDT (a form of service delivery endorsed by the National Service Framework) [81]. A danger with such teams is that they can become too 'cosy', allowing genuinely collaborative decision-making to degenerate into a narrowly collusive consensus. Hence we believe that it will always be important to maintain a degree of independent scrutiny. But a well-functioning team, skilled in VBP as well as EBP, and particularly if supported by relevant voluntary organisations and "experts by experience"[82], could, we believe, play an increasingly important role in providing a balanced approach to decisions involving compulsion.

(iii) Values-Based Practice is concerned with assessment.

Ethical aspects of compulsion in psychiatry are widely considered to be limited to matters of 'disposal' (admission and/or treatment under the 1983 Act, for example). But decisions about compulsion turn centrally on assessment, broadly conceived as encompassing not only medico-legal concepts, such as "capacity" and "risk", but also diagnostic concepts (eg "mental disorder" in the 1983 Act). VBP argues (Principle 1, Figure 4 below) that assessment, although usually considered a matter exclusively for value-free scientific evidence[83], also involves (often covertly but always importantly) value judgments.

---

[80] Thus the Egyptian psychiatrist, and current President of the World Psychiatric Association, Professor Ahmed Okasha, has pointed out the extent to which the value of individual autonomy, as promoted by Western bioethics, conflicts with the family and community-centred values of many non-Western cultures (Okasha, A. (2000) *Ethics of Psychiatric Practice: Consent, Compulsion and Confidentiality*. Current Opinion in Psychiatry. Vol 13, 693-698).

[81] see Colombo, A., Bendelow, G., Fulford, K.W.M., and Williams, S. (2003) *Evaluating the influence of implicit models of mental disorder on processes of shared decision-making within community-based multi-disciplinary teams.* Social Science & Medicine, 56: 1557-1570

[82] see for example Jan Wallcraft's paper at www.connects.org.uk/conferences; Jan Wallcraft is National Fellow for Experts by Experience. The role of such experts could be particularly vital in cross-cultural contexts.

[83] The current Mental Health Act Code of Practice, although providing extensive advice on all other aspects of compulsion, including assessment, has nothing at all to say about diagnosis.

This is not the place to argue this point in detail.[84] But if it is right, it has two key consequences for compulsion in psychiatry. First, taken with the model of collaborative decision-making outlined in 5.6(ii) above, it extends the role of the multidisciplinary team from management to diagnosis (we return to this in 5.7 below). Second, it provides a basis for a model of assessment that is more respectful of patients' values. Current models of compulsion are deficit-driven, relying on expert evidence of incapacity or mental disorder to discount the values of the patient concerned. VBP, while recognizing the diagnostic importance of genuinely pathological value judgments[85], relies primarily on the balancing of legitimately different value perspectives. VBP, therefore, while no less decisive when it comes to the need for compulsion, is decisive within a framework of respect for, rather than denial of, patients' values.

5.7   It is important that Values-Based Practice is incorporated fully into the detained patient's experience of services and we believe that proposed new mental health legislation, with modifications, and taken together with the values-focus of the Human Rights Act, could and should achieve this. Again, this is not the place for a detailed discussion of the issues, but we will comment briefly on the relevance of the three features of VBP outlined in 5.6 above from the perspective of the Commission.

(i) Patient-centred practice and mental health legislation.

Although we should not seek to disguise or ignore the brute fact of compulsion at the core of mental health legislation, we believe that such compulsion is most likely to succeed in its primarily therapeutic objectives where it is used with understanding of and respect for the person concerned. Developing the skills-base of Values-Based Practice within multi-disciplinary teams could thus make an important contribution to improving the way in which compulsory powers are employed in practice. Correspondingly, we welcome the NIMHE Values Framework (footnote 77) and related training initiatives in VBP (footnote 88, below) and believe that new mental health legislation and the ensuing Code of Practice should be consistent with and complement these important and positive aspects of the Government's policies on mental health as set out particularly in the NSF.

(ii) Collaborative decision-making and mental health legislation.

Much of the debate about proposed new mental health legislation has focused on the extent to which it will shift the basis of clinical decision-making from patient care to public safety. To the extent that this legislation seeks to make public safety paramount, VBP suggests that mental health stakeholders have been fully justified in uniting against it – for in VBP, making any one value paramount is a recipe for abusive practices. But the danger, now, Values-Based Practice would suggest, is of an adversarial adoption of extreme positions, with stakeholders in mental health seeking to oppose one absolute value (public safety) with another, such as patient care or individual choice.

In the collaborative model suggested by VBP, by contrast, mental health legislation should aim to provide a framework within which these values can be appropriately

---

[84]   see Fulford, K.W.M. (1989) *Moral Theory and Medical Practice*. Cambridge: Cambridge University Press; also Sadler, J.Z. (2002) (ed) *Descriptions and Prescriptions: Values, Mental Disorders, and the DSMs*. Baltimore: The Johns Hopkins University Press; and Sadler J.Z. (forthcoming) *Values and Psychiatric Diagnosis*. Oxford University Press. Again, we welcome the Government's initiative in supporting through the NIMHE the establishment of an international research network to examine the role of values in psychiatric diagnosis and assessment.

[85]   see, eg., Fulford, K.W.M. (1991) *Evaluative Delusions: their Significance for Philosophy and Psychiatry*, British Journal of Psychiatry, Volume 159, p 108-112, Supplement 14, Delusions and Awareness of Reality.

balanced in particular cases. Many of the proposals in the Mental Health Bill of 2002, taken together with the HRA, could provide the basis for such a framework. There remain aspects of the drafting which are inconsistent with balanced decision-making. For example, the lack of discretion provided to clinicians by the draft Bill[86] was an extreme case of how legislative measures might undermine values-based approaches. We are pleased to note that the Government has reconsidered its proposals in this respect[87] and we will look carefully at the revised Bill when it is published. We believe that a collaborative (in the specific sense of the term defined by VBP) rather than an adversarial approach is the way forward. Clinicians and users, after all, no less than the Government, have an interest in improving public safety in relation to mental disorder as well as providing the best possible care tailored to individual patient need.

(iii) **Diagnostic assessment and mental health legislation.**

Mental health professionals cease to collaborate (in the VBP sense of the term) and become collaborators (in the pejorative sense of the term) when they adopt a public safety role other than in relation to mental disorder. Mental health stakeholders were thus right to be concerned that the White Paper preceding the draft Bill of 2002 sought to establish a concept of 'dangerous severe personality disorder' defined solely in terms of a propensity for dangerous behaviour. One approach to defining the proper role of mental health professionals is by reference to specific procedures considered to be "therapies". VBP pushes the definition back to diagnosis. In VBP it is not the *nature* of a procedure that makes it "therapeutic" but its *object*, i.e. preventing, curing or ameliorating a medical disorder. As noted in 5.6(iii) above, mental health legislation has traditionally avoided defining mental disorder other than by providing a framework for expert evidence. VBP endorses this approach but argues that it should be supplemented by secondary legislation and/or an extended code of practice allowing advances in the assessment of mental disorders (including such concepts as capacity and risk) to be incorporated from time to time as they emerge from current and future research and stakeholder experience.

5.8 It is important to recognise that the issues raised by values in mental health are not specific to mental health but generic to all healthcare. Thus, for example, even compulsion is used in the interests of public safety in relation to some infectious diseases. Principle 3 of VBP suggests, furthermore, that as scientific progress opens up an ever wider range of choices in healthcare, issues of values, and of *conflicting* values, will increasingly become matters of urgent practical concern no less in bodily medicine than they are currently in mental health. In developing the theory and skills-base of VBP, therefore, we believe that mental health, which in the twentieth century ran ever in second place to bodily medicine, could be establishing an important model for the future of healthcare generally. This "mental health first" outcome would carry a powerful anti-stigma message which the Government, in supporting these developments, would have a played a key role in delivering. In the following chapter we look at other opportunities and constraints in promoting a values culture within mental health services that operate compulsion.

---

[86] see, for example, Department of Health (2002) Draft *Mental Health Bill* 2002, Cm 5538-I, clause 17.

[87] Adam James *Government powers plan 'shameful'.* Guardian 11 June 2003.

Ten Principles of Values-Based Practice (VBP)

Theory

1   All decisions rest on values as well as on facts, including decisions about diagnosis.

2   Values are noticed only when they are diverse or conflicting and therefore likely to be problematic.

3   In opening up choices, scientific progress is increasingly bringing the full diversity of human values into play in all areas of healthcare.

4   VBP's "first call" for information is the perspective of the patient or patients concerned in any particular decision. This complements the objective and perspective-free approach of Evidence-Based Practice (EBP).

5   In VBP, conflicts of values are resolved primarily by processes designed to support a balance of legitimately different perspectives, and not by reference to rules prescribing the "right" outcome.

Practice

6   Awareness of values can be developed through careful attention to language use in context.

7   Knowledge of different values is available through empirical sources (e.g. "user" narratives, surveys, literary and academic sources) and philosophic sources (e.g. phenomenology, hermeneutics etc).

8   Ethical reasoning is used in VBP primarily to explore differences in values rather than to determine "what is right", as in quasi-legal bioethics.

9   Communication skills (e.g. listening to patients and exploring their values with them, coming to a balance of views in situations of conflict, etc) have a substantive role in decision-making for VBP, rather than a merely executive role as with quasi-legal bioethics.

10 VBP, although involving a partnership with ethicists and lawyers (equivalent to the partnership between scientists and statisticians in EBP), puts decision-making back where it belongs, with users and providers at the clinical coal face.

Fig 4: Ten Principles of Values-Based Practice[88]

---

[88] adapted from Fulford, K.W.M (forthcoming) *Ten Principles of Values-Based Practice (VBP)* in Radden, (ed) *Companion to the Philosophy of Psychiatry.* Oxford: Oxford University Press; for a training programme in VBP, developed jointly between the Sainsbury Centre for Mental Health and Warwick University within the Capabilities Framework, see Fulford, K.W.M., Williamson, T. and Woodbridge, K. (2002) *Values-Added Practice (a Values-Awareness Workshop),* Mental Health Today, October, pps 25-27

6

Achieving a human rights-based service

6.1   Patients whose fundamental rights are curtailed under powers provided by mental health legislation should be able to expect the law to be operated transparently, predictably and under the scrutiny of an independent body. We discuss the question of scrutinising the use of the law at Chapter 20 below. We believe that transparency in the use of powers of compulsion – which requires authorities to operate their power in such a way that is largely uniform and predictable – can best be assured by enacting principles in legislation, and issuing regulation and guidance on specific matters relating to the use of coercion.

6.2   In Chapter 2 of this report we acknowledged that a culture of human rights cannot be imposed upon services from above, but that Government nevertheless has an important role in establishing the boundaries within which services work. By establishing such ground-rules, and by doing so with a particular regard to human rights issues, Government can at least partially fulfill its obligation to ensure that powers used in its name are implemented in accordance with principles of the European Convention. In this chapter, we mainly focus on the means available to establish such ground-rules in current and future legislation.

Developments in primary legislation

6.3   Although we have touched upon concerns over the stalling of the human rights agenda and of Government's role in promoting human rights concerns (see Chapter 2 above), we do acknowledge the achievement of Government in introducing the Human Rights Act 1998, which established in domestic law the very rights and duties that we discuss. In our view, one of the most significant pieces of human-rights based legislation since that time has been the Race Relations (Amendment) Act 2000, particularly because this unequivocally underlines the positive duties on authorities to comply with human rights principles. We discuss this further at Chapter 16.

6.4   We are pleased to acknowledge the likely positive effects for detained patients and their families or carers of certain planned legislation:

* At paragraph 11.58 below we discuss the **Sexual Offences Bill,** which should increase the protection offered by the law against the sexual abuse of all psychiatric patients.

∗ As this report is being written, the Government has announced its intention to provide **Civil Partnership** arrangements so that gay and lesbian couples may have a legal right to recognition[89], which should further consolidate the changes made to rules regarding the identification of Nearest Relatives discussed at Chapter 3.25 *et seq* above.

∗ We also welcome the introduction of the **Mental Incapacity Bill**, although we set out some concerns about particular proposals in the Bill at Chapters 8.12 *et seq* and 11.59 in this report.

∗ Although we are sympathetic towards the concerns expressed by the Mental Health Alliance and the Parliamentary Joint Committee on Human Rights (JCHR) over the draft **Mental Health Bill** of 2002 (see Chapter 4.12 *et seq*), we share the view of the JCHR that aspects of proposed changes to mental health law relating to compulsion should be welcomed as positive attempts to ensure that such compulsion is compatible with a culture of respect for human rights. At the time of going to press we are uncertain as to whether the major flaws in the draft Bill of 2002 will have been addressed by the time that a Bill is introduced to Parliament.

The need for clarity in law

6.5   In January 2001 the European Court of Human Rights stated that:

"it is …essential that the conditions for deprivation of liberty under domestic law should be clearly defined, and that the law itself be foreseeable in its application, so that it meets the standard of lawfulness set by the Convention". (*Kawka v Poland* [2001], para 49).

The UK Court of Appeal, in its *Munjaz* judgment of July 2003, also stressed the importance of transparency and predictability in the operation of domestic law that engages with fundamental Convention issues (see Figure 2, Chapter 3.8 above, and 6.17-23 below). Paradoxically, just as the Courts have insisted on this stability of law, many practitioners charged with powers and duties under the 1983 Act are increasingly bewildered by the pace and unpredictability of legal change.

6.6   In part, this "remarkable surge in mental health caselaw"[90] is due to legal challenges that use the ECHR as a lever to overturn long-held interpretations of law. This is evident in a number of cases discussed in Chapter 3 above involving Tribunal practice and procedure[91]. In other cases, the ECHR's leverage has been most evident simply in getting challenges heard. Many of these cases (such as, for example, *R (on the application of B) v Ashworth* [2003], discussed at Chapter 3.40 *et seq* above) could be cited as good examples of the Human Rights Act working as it was intended, in allowing challenges to be made and establishing the parameters of argument on the interpretation of domestic statute, whether or not the final judgments rely directly on the detail of the ECHR.

6.7   Alongside what might be called the cultural influence of the Human Rights Act on the judiciary, another factor in the apparent increase in judgments which reverse established

---

[89]   Women & Equality Unit (2003) *Civil Partnership: a framework for the legal recognition of same-sex couples.* Department of Trade & Industry June 2003.

[90]   Jones, R (2003) *Mental Health Act Manual*, Eighth edition. London: Sweet & Maxwell, preface

[91]   see, for example, Chapter 3.9 & 3.24 above.

practice may be the Government's commitment to introduce a new Mental Health Act in the near future. With such an announcement, Government inevitably signals that the existing legislation is, in some sense, no longer fit for purpose. This is perhaps bound to lead to more challenges by patients treated under the present law, and may also influence the number of such challenges that are successful.

6.8   An interesting example of these possible effects is discussed at Chapter 9.47 *et seq*, in relation to renewing the detention of patients on leave. The series of recent cases on this issue show not only the judiciary's willingness to reverse its previous determinations on an issue, but also a curious reversal in the respective positions of practitioners and the State over the question of community-based compulsion. In the early years of the Act, the *Hallstrom* judgment (1986)[92] was the judicial answer to practitioners' attempts to interpret the Act's powers as a community treatment order. That answer was a resounding 'no', despite arguments from the Royal College of Psychiatrists and others that such a use of the Act could be in patients' interests. The position established by the courts was that Parliament had appeared to make an intentional link between compulsory treatment and detention in hospital, and it was not for the courts to reinterpret and effectively reverse legislation passed with that intention. The positions of Government and professional bodies over the question of community treatment orders appear to have switched places at some point over the last two decades.[93] Government now stresses community powers as the cornerstone of its proposed legislation, to the disquiet of the professional bodies grouped under the Mental Health Alliance[94]. Amidst this debate over proposals for statutory change, court judgments have gradually eroded the assumed link between detention as an inpatient and compulsory treatment, culminating in the *D.R.* case, which effectively allows patients to be discharged from inpatient care whilst remaining liable to detention and therefore compulsory treatment[95]. The judiciary has moved from a position where it considers inpatient treatment to be the necessary precondition to the renewal of detention under section 20(4)(c), to a position where it considered such a reading to be an illogical and impermissible gloss on that section of the 1983 Act. The lesson that we draw from this, in respect of our present discussion, is that the courts are far from impermeable to the shifts of opinion and influence in politics and society outside of the courtroom. Whilst in Chapter 5.1 above we welcome this in relation to the "living instrument" of the ECHR, it also raises some issues that we highlight below.

6.9   It is difficult for even the most legally-minded practitioner to keep up with frequent changes to the law emanating from the courts. Court judgments, by their very nature, appear to many practitioners as if from on high, with little or none of the forewarning, or preceding debate and even consultation that is often involved in changes to statute law. When caselaw decisions reverse long-held legal positions, even those practitioners who follow the law closely may wonder at the apparent arbitrariness of the legality of their practice.

---

[92]   *R v Hallstrom, ex parte W No 2; R v Gardner ex parte L* [1986]

[93]   Probably around the time of the Mental Health (Patients in the Community) Act 1995.

[94]   Mental Health Alliance (2003) *Reforming the Mental Health Act: the key issues.* Website address: www.mentalhealthalliance.org.uk.

[95]   *R (on the application of D.R.) v Mersey Care NHS Trust* [2002]. See chapter 9.47 *et seq* below.

6.10 We are very concerned that practitioners may be discouraged from taking the legal aspects of their practice seriously by rapidly changing law. Many practitioners already have only a sketchy knowledge of the extent of the powers that they operate and the duties that this places upon them. In a book-length study published this year, Jill Peay outlined research and conclusions based upon professionals' responses to three detailed but imaginary psychiatric case histories[96]. The results show that there is certainly no uniformity of approach, even within particular professional groups, towards the question of whether legal powers of compulsion should be engaged in particular circumstances. Peay has demonstrated that many practitioners, including those who have longstanding experience in operating the powers of the 1983 Act, have a limited understanding of the law as it relates to their practice. This research not only suggests that there is an urgent need for training across all professional groups and individuals who operate the law (it is ironic, for example, that the present law has training requirements for doctors who recommend patients' compulsory admission, but none for the doctors who receive such patients and are responsible for their care and treatment under compulsion), but also shows that the law relating to psychiatric detention and treatment is not uniformly applied, and therefore cannot be foreseeable in its application.

> **Recommendation 4:** The next Mental Health Act should extend the statutory training requirements applicable under the 1983 Act to "approved" doctors and social workers to all professionals who have responsibilities for the operation of its powers.

6.11 Peay concludes that professionals charged with applying the 1983 Act have a "sense of desperation" and a need for "clarity in legislation and defined limits on the responsibilities of practitioners"[97]. Before discussing the tools available to Government to deal with the problems of clarity of law, we should acknowledge its limitations. It is, of course, the judiciary's role to interpret legislation, and the executive cannot provide authoritative guidance on legal positions where these have not been clearly established. It is unfortunate in this respect that the courts frequently narrow the scope of their rulings as far as possible, leaving wider and sometimes fundamental issues unresolved, even when the case is being heard on grounds that there are matters of public interest at stake. Particularly when executive agencies such as the Department of Health are parties to the judicial review of wide-ranging issues of public interest in mental health law, the courts should be encouraged by counsel representing executive interests to engage with and determine as wide an aspect of the cases before them as is consistent with the needs of justice.

Ensuring the principled application of compulsory powers

6.12 In our response to the draft Mental Health Bill of 2002, we suggested that the scope and purpose of mental health legislation should be defined through a clear statement of principles embedded at the start of its provisions. There are clear precedents for such principled statements within legislation (principally the Children Act 1989, section 1). The

---

[96] Peay, J (2003) *Decisions and Dilemmas: working with mental health law*. Oxford, Hart Publishing

[97] *ibid*, p 159

principles should be universally applicable. We were particularly disappointed that the draft bill sought to relegate statements of principle to a Code of Practice and allowed that even such principles need not have universal application, but could be conditional and not applicable in certain circumstances.

6.13   We suggested the following draft principles to Government:

* That informal treatment is always to be preferred over compulsion when circumstances permit.

* That treatment and care should be provided in the least restrictive manner compatible with ensuring the health or safety or the safety of other people.

* That treatment and care should, insofar as is possible, be determined by or reflect the wishes of the patient concerned.

* That treatment and care must be provided in such a way as to respect the qualities, abilities and diverse backgrounds of individuals, and properly takes account of age, gender sexual orientation, social, ethnic cultural and religious backgrounds without making general assumptions on the basis of any of these characteristics.

* That all powers under the Act shall be exercised without any direct or indirect discrimination on the grounds of physical ability, age, gender, sexual orientation, race, colour, language religion or national, ethnic or social origin.

Recommendation 5: The next Mental Health Act should be founded upon principles covering the areas outlined above, and which are explicitly stated on the face of legislation.

Reducing uncertainties in Primary Legislation

6.14   One of the Commission's criticisms of the draft Mental Health Bill of 2002 was that, whilst the draft was complex and lengthy, broad areas of detail relating to the application of the powers were left very ambiguous by primary legislation. Too much detail was left to be determined at a later stage by Regulations or a Code of Practice, and too much responsibility was vaguely invested in the relevant Minister, with little or no indication of how powers were to be exercised in practice.[98]

6.15   The Commission accepts that it is not in the power of Government to foresee and resolve all questions of legal interpretation relating to primary legislation. However, it is possible to ensure that primary legislation is as clear as possible, both in intention and in the details of its execution. Where it is inappropriate to determine matters of detail at the level of primary legislation, statutory regulation and an appropriately robust Code of Practice can provide these, but the broad outlines within which such regulation is made should be established by the Act itself. On a basic level these could be established by the inclusion of principles on the face of primary legislation, but these should also be elaborated in the Act itself in relation to specific powers and duties.

---

[98]   Mental Health Act Commission (2002) *The Mental Health Act Commission's Response to the Draft Mental Health Bill Consultation.* MHAC, September 2002, page 5 *drafting concerns*

Recommendation 6: The Commission urges Government to ensure that the Mental Health Bill introduced to Parliament provides a clear framework for the operation of compulsory powers and does not leave key issues of legal interpretation for determination through Regulations or a Code of Practice.

Regulation of specific areas of compulsion

6.16   The Department of Health has acknowledged that authorities treating patients under compulsion acquire reciprocal duties to ensure that such treatment is provided safely and in accordance with good practice. Whilst we would agree that "higher levels of risk [and] loss of liberty… suggest a greater need for clinical audit and monitoring than usual, with particular attention paid to areas such as: observation; seclusion; restraint and rapid tranquillisation"[99] we suggest that Government should itself seek to ensure that issues such as seclusion and restraint are operated on its behalf in ways that are safe and appropriate. Following the *Munjaz* judgment of 2003, discussed below, the Code of Practice can be used to provide practical guidance that will be generally binding on authorities. We suggest, in addition to such guidance in a Code of Practice, that Government should take the opportunity of new legislation to consider statutory regulation of aspects of particularly invasive or contentious practices. Such regulation could, at the very least, institute record keeping and reporting requirements utilising statutory documentation. It could also ensure training standards in relation to, for example, the physical restraint of patients, and introduce safeguards in relation to certain treatments, such as naso-gastric feeding of anorectic patients, or following rapid tranquilisation of any patient, etc. We also suggest that core requirements regarding seclusion practice (such as particular triggers for multidisciplinary review and particular reporting procedures) could be given unequivocal legal force by use of secondary legislation under a new Act.

The status, use and upkeep of the Code of Practice

6.17   In many chapters of this report we have argued the central importance of Government guidance in relation to the use of powers of compulsion. The Government's role in this is exemplified through the arrangements for preparing and publishing a Code of Practice. As we noted in Chapter 2.9 above, our analysis of the effects of human rights legislation on Government responsibilities was echoed by the Court of Appeal in the *Munjaz* judgment of July 2003[100], which specifically considered the status of the Code of Practice. We have set out the court's determination at Figure 2, Chapter 3.8 above.

6.18   The Court of Appeal has stated that the Code of Practice is one of the positive steps that the State takes to protect the health and rights of persons deprived of liberty. In part, this means that the State is responsible for ensuring that authorities exercising its powers do so in

---

[99]   Department of Health (2002) *Mental Health Policy Implementation Guide: National Minimum Standards for General Adult Services in Psychiatric Intensive Care Units (PICU) and Low Secure Units.* Para 13.3.1.

[100]   *R (on the application of Colonel Munjaz) v Mersey Care NHS Trust & Another, S v Airedale NHS Trust* [2003]

accordance with human rights principles[101]. The Code of Practice is one way in which the State can meet this obligation. The Code can provide transparency and predictability where ECHR compliance requires this but the law is insufficiently defined[102], The Code therefore should be afforded a status consistent with its purpose: "the State should therefore give it some teeth" [103].

6.19 The Court of Appeal gave the current Mental Health Act Code of Practice "teeth" in ruling that, where it deals with issues potentially engaging Convention issues, adherence to its guidance is requirement of compliance with the ECHR. It is therefore possible for a hospital's actions or policies to be in unlawful breach of the Mental Health Act Code of Practice on issues that engage ECHR issues. Therefore the Code of practice should be observed by all authorities unless there is a good reason for particular departures in relation to individual patients. It is not acceptable to depart from the Code as a matter of policy, although policies may identify circumstances when such departures might be considered on a case-by-case basis.

6.20 We hope that Government will now reconsider its approach towards Codes of Practice in mental health legislation, and ensure that they are given a clear status under statute that reflects the position reached through judicial challenge. Both the draft Mental Health Bill of 2002 (clause 1) and the Mental Incapacity Bill (clause 30) provide only that professionals must "have regard to" the respective Codes of Practice. We believe that this reflects a legal position pre-*Munjaz*, and that more emphatic language would now be appropriate. This is not to say that we want the Code necessarily to be statutorily binding on authorities where there are good reasons for departure from its guidance based upon an individual's situation. If authorities are to be forced to follow the Code to the letter irrespective of circumstance then the distinction between the Code and primary legislation would be lost. In our response to the Mental Health Legislation Review Team (1999) we expressed our concern that providing such statutory weight to a Code of Practice would be likely to water-down its provisions until they were a set of minimum standards, rather than a guide to good practice[104].

6.21 It may be that the precedent of section 7 of the Local Authority Social Services Act 1970, which obliges social services authorities to act under the general guidance given by the Secretary of State, could provide a model for legislation that gives a Code 'teeth' in the sense required by the Court of Appeal. We continue to recommend that the next Mental Health Act should at the very least require authorities who operate its powers to record and provide reasons in patients' clinical records for departures from the Code's guidance. We look forward to working alongside the Department of Health in the further development of these issues.

6.22 Both the current and proposed statutory requirements in relation to the preparation or amendment of the Code of Practice establish permissive powers relating to the identification

---

[101]   *ibid*, note 100, paras 59 - 60

[102]   *ibid*, paras 65, 74

[103]   *ibid*, para 56

[104]   Mental Health Act Commission (1999) *The Mental Health Act Commission Submission to the Mental Health Legislation Review Team*, Jan 99, p 10.

of interested parties who must be consulted[105]. We believe that it is vital that consultation reaches across users, carers and all types of healthcare professional concerned with psychiatric compulsion, and trust that such consultation will take place for the Code of any new legislation. The Code also must be regularly reviewed and updated, as it should be a living instrument that is seen to be relevant by all who use it. The current edition of the Code is only the second in the lifetime of the Act and, although not yet five years old, it already requires revision. It is arguably not very important that, in relation to the revision of the Code of Practice, Clause 12 of the draft Mental Health Bill of 2002 is permissive where section 118 of the 1983 Act creates a duty, given that neither legislation sets any specific trigger for revisions. Under the 1983 Act, however, the Secretary of State has statutory arrangements for the Mental Health Act Commission to advise him or her upon the content of the Code and the need for any revisions[106]. Government should ensure that arrangements under the next Act, where the Mental Health Act Commission will be immersed within a wider inspectorate structure, can continue to provide this service. Following the *Munjaz* judgment of 2003, the Code and its provisions are likely to be increasingly central to claims against the Government and its agencies.

6.23   Government therefore has a role through its Code of Practice in providing guidance and standards to ensure that rights are respected by different authorities; to provide transparency and predictability in the operation of the law; and, not least, to help authorities avoid spending time and other resources "re-inventing wheels" in drawing up policies and attending to their own practice.

> **Recommendation 7:** The Commission urges Government to state clearly the legal status of its Code of Practice on the face of primary legislation, and to make statutory provision to ensure that the Code is regularly updated following appropriate consultation.

Code of Ethics for Psychiatry?

6.24   As a part of the development of the National Institute for Mental Health England (NIMHE) values framework, the Royal College of Psychiatrists have been asked to provide a statement of professional values for psychiatry. Some psychiatrists have called for such a statement to be expanded to become a full code of ethics for the psychiatric profession[107]. This would be built upon existing practice guidance, including the General Medical Council's Good Medical Practice (2001); the Royal College of Psychiatrists' Good Psychiatric Practice 2000[108]; and the Mental Health Act Code of Practice.

6.25   We recognise that the call for a specific code of ethics comes in part from psychiatrists' concern over the proposals of the draft Mental Health Bill of 2002. It has been argued that

---

[105] Mental Health Act 1983, s118(3); Draft Mental Health Bill 2002 clauses 8, 13.

[106] SI 1983 no. 892, para 3(2)(d) and SI 1983 no. 894, reg 7(2)(a).

[107] see Sarkar, S.P. and Adshead, G (2003) *Protecting altruism: a call for a code of ethics in British Psychiatry.* British Journal of Psychiatry (2003) 183, 95-97

[108] Royal College of Psychiatrists (2000) *Good Psychiatric Practice 2000* (Council Report CR83). London, RCPsych.

these proposals invite psychiatry to shift its ethical position from traditional altruistic focus on patients' needs to those of society at large, thus treating patients as a means to an end and not an end in themselves[109]. It is suggested that a code of ethics that is specifically owned by psychiatrists could ensure that the needs of individual patients remain the focus of psychiatry.

6.26   The Commission would welcome the development of a code of ethics for psychiatrists, or for any other practitioner whose professional body does not at present provide such a code. Whilst it is certainly the case that, even in the absence of a written code of ethics, doctors working in psychiatry are bound by the law and their training and motivation to act in the interests of patients, we also recognise that the pressures on all branches of medicine, including resources, political pressures, societal expectations etc, can be especially forceful in psychiatric practice. For this reason we look to the continued development of a values-based Code of Practice relevant to *all* mental health professionals operating powers of compulsion, particularly now that such a Code has been given "teeth" by the courts (see 6.17-22 above). This may be even more important under proposed new legislation, where psychiatrists may not be the sole profession given responsibility for the care of patients under compulsion[110]. We strongly urge Government to enact guiding principles on the face of new legislation and to reinforce the Code of Practice, to allow the next generation's mental health law to be based upon firm and irrevocable principles of sound ethical practice.

Recommendation 8: The Commission urges Government to encourage codes of professional ethics relevant to all mental health practitioners

Standards setting

6.27   The Commission recognises the role played by standards in the development and monitoring of mental health services. Such standards range from the general, such as those provided by the National Service Frameworks, to the relatively detailed, such as the National Care Standards Commission's standards for independent hospitals. The Commission was pleased to contribute to the development of the NCSC's standards in relation to the operation of the Act in the independent sector. We also recognise and support Government interventions, such as *A First Class Service*, as the driver of locally-based standards setting under clinical governance arrangements, and the Department-sponsored publications on services for patients from Black and minority ethnic communities discussed at Chapter 16 below. Further standards are set for services by the Social Services Inspectorate[111] and the Commission for Health Improvement. The Commission has been represented in discussions with the Commission for Healthcare Audit and Inspection (CHAI) over future

---

[109] Sarkar, S.P. and Adshead, G, (2003) (see note 107).

[110] Under the draft Mental Health Bill of 2002 (see clause 2(9)), the role equivalent to the 1983 Act's 'Responsible Medical Officer', the 'approved mental health professional', could be performed by professionals other than psychiatrists.

[111] see Social Services Inspectorate (2001) *Detained – inspection of compulsory mental health admissions.* Department of Health, February 2001.

standards and looks forward to the development of standards specific to the operation of mental health law by the CHAI and the Social Care Inspectorate (SCI).

6.28 For a number of reasons, the Mental Health Act Commission does not set standards for services in relation to their operation of the Act. Mental health services are already subject to standards from other bodies, as noted above. We have no wish to add to the burden placed upon service managers and have not been requested to do so by the Department of Health. Services are provided with general standards on the operation of the Act by the guidance of the Code of Practice, and in many cases still strive to achieve these. Although the Commission has not itself added to the rafts of standards applied to mental health services, our Ninth Biennial Report provided 75 recommendations for service improvement, aimed across the range of authorities responsible for operating the 1983 Act, from ward managers to Government[112]. Many of our recommendations suggested to services that they should monitor and seek to improve aspects of care of detained patients that were of particular concern to us, often linked to requirements of the Code of Practice. In some cases we suggested such areas as the focus of local standard setting between service commissioners and providers. We were pleased that, in consultation seminars following publication of the report, hospital managers generally welcomed the report and requested a monitoring tool to measure their services' progress in implementing the recommendations. Roughly a quarter of all mental health services that detain patients have subsequently completed the Commission's monitoring tool and provided us with a copy. These returns have informed a number of our discussions within this report[113]. The monitoring tool is still in use in many services and we are pleased that our collaborative approach has been welcomed in so many services that we visit.

6.29 It therefore remains the case that NHS mental health services are not subjected to any exacting standards regarding their operation of the Mental Health Act. The Commission for Health Improvement's *Final Performance Indicators for Mental Health Trusts 2002/03*[114] do not include any substantive Mental Health Act application standards, although the previous year's standards referred to implementation of MHAC recommendations. Some of this year's CHI standards which relate to health outcomes, such as levels of emergency re-admission, form the start of interesting and useful ways in which the structures of service delivery and outcome might be measured that could be applied to a wide-focus measurement of the effectiveness of episodes of compulsion. Nevertheless, there is no specific high-level indicator for hospitals' administration of the 1983 Act and its Code of Practice in the treatment of patients. Mental health services are therefore star-rated according to a number of measurements which include, for example, financial management and staff sickness rates, but exclude whether or not patients are treated according to practice guidelines issued by the Secretary of State or even within the parameters set by the law.

---

[112] The recommendations from the *Ninth Biennial Report* (2001) are available on the Commission website (www.mhac.trent.nhs.uk). It is hoped that, at the time of publication of this report, the text of that report will be similarly available to download. The Ninth Biennial Report is published by the Stationery Office and available to purchase from the usual outlets as listed on the back cover of this report.

[113] see Figures 12 (Chapter 8.50); 17 (9.30); 19 (9.37); 30 (11.17); and 32 (11.33) below.

[114] Commission For Health Improvement (2003) *Final Performance Indicators for Mental Health Trusts:* www.doh.gov.uk/performanceratings/2003/mh_list.html

6.30 The difficulty facing any future standards-setting regarding the operation of the Mental Health Act in the care of patients is that, where issues of law are concerned, anything less than full compliance is unacceptable and a serious concern. As such, there is no gradation of unlawful practice which might be used to evaluate hospitals by rank or in a 'traffic-light' system. The standards produced by the NCSC (see 6.27 above) are good examples of baseline standards that require the existence of policies, evidence of training and appropriate staffing levels, etc. The question remains over how to measure direct outcomes in the use of compulsion (i.e. that, for any particular patient, all powers were used appropriately, within good practice guidelines and with a satisfactory outcome in the view of both patient and professionals). In 2002 the Commission revised its visiting procedures to provide structured monitoring of specific issues relating to the use of the Act. We discuss these Commission Visiting Questionnaires (CVQs) at Chapter 19.11(c) below, and the initial results from their collation inform much of our discussion in Part Two of this report.

> **Recommendation 9:** The Commission recommends to any successor body further consideration of standards-setting in relation to the exercise of powers and discharge of duties provided by mental health legislation, based upon its experience with establishing quantitative surveys of practice-related issues.

Involving service users and others at policy level

6.31 To avoid policy directives and standards reverting to exclusively top-down measures of control over service provision, it is of course necessary that service users, carers, interest groups and professionals are involved and consulted at all stages of policy-making. We believe the Department of Health, particularly through its policy arm of the National Institute for Mental Health England(NIMHE), to have understood this very well and quite rightly raised expectations, particularly among service users, of opportunities for active involvement in all aspects of its work. We welcome equally the appointment of a NIMHE Fellow for in Experts by Experience (see Chapter 5.6(ii) above). We are fully supportive of the approaches set out in the National Service Framework for Mental Health and subsequent publications[115]. We commend also the National Service Framework for Wales in this respect (see Chapter 18.22 below).

6.32 The user, voluntary and professional groups involved in Mental Health Bill 'stakeholder' meetings with the Department of Health following the closure of the consultation period for the draft Bill of 2002 have reported unanimously their dissatisfaction with the process so far (August 2003). Particular frustrations have been the lack of real information from the Department on the developing plans for the Bill, which has limited the potential for consultees to participate at any meaningful level. We are pleased to note the series of stakeholder consultations starting in autumn 2003 but urge the Department of Health to go further and strive to build bridges between itself as the executive arm of Government and

---

[115]   see, for example, Department of Health (1999) *National Service Framework for Mental Health: Modern Standards and Service Models; (1999) Patient and Public Involvement in the New NHS; (2001) Involving Patients and the Public in Healthcare; a Discussion Document.* All London, Department of Health.

those service user and professional groups who have been critical of its approach to the draft Mental Health Bill of 2002. We are concerned at the outstanding tensions between a number of the most active and forward-thinking voluntary, professional and user-led organisations and the Department of Health, and believe that this can only be detrimental to the progress of the mental health agenda as set out in the NHS Plan and the National Service Framework for Mental Health (see also Chapter 5.7(ii) above). We have similarly encouraged user and professional groups to retain their involvement with Government consultation measures, particularly in relation to the Mental Health Bill, no matter how frustrating they have found this process.

> **Recommendation 10:** We urge Government, and those service-user and professional groups who have been critical of its approach, to participate fully in stakeholder consultation over the redrafting of the Mental Health Bill prior to its presentation to Parliament.

6.33   We discuss service-user involvement at hospital and ward-level in Chapter 9.6 *et seq* below.

Compulsory Mental Health Care and Stigma

6.34   The Commission is a signatory to the Royal College of Psychiatrists' five-year *Changing Minds* campaign, designed to raise awareness of and counter the stigmatising effects of mental disorders, which draws to an end this autumn. We look forward to lending our support to successive initiatives against the stigmatising of the mentally ill. Of all mental health patients, none are so stigmatised as those who receive treatment under compulsory powers, because of widespread ignorance and fear regarding the purpose and usual causes of detention under the Mental Health Act 1983.

6.35   We were pleased that the Department of Health has given its support to the campaign, and we recognise initiatives by the Department of Health and other Government departments, such as the recent consultation by the Social Exclusion Unit on what can be done to reduce social exclusion among adults with mental illness[116]. A number of factors, many of which Government can contribute to positively or negatively, make the anti-stigma initiatives vital in the present climate.

6.36   A number of bodies continue irrationally and perhaps unlawfully to discriminate against people who have been detained under the Mental Health Act 1983. Regrettably, this includes public bodies accountable to Government or established under Government direction. For example, the Department for Education and Skills' *Guides to the Law for School Governors* state "people who can be compulsorily detained under the Mental Health Act 1983… may not serve as governors"[117]. This advice is questionable on a number of grounds, not least in

---

[116] Office of the Deputy Prime Minister / Social Exclusion Unit (2003) *Mental Health and Social Exclusion* Consultation Document, May 2003

[117] There are six guides to the law for school governors. This statement appears, for example, at paragraph 22 of the guide relating to community schools and paragraph 26 of the guide relating to voluntary controlled schools. The guides may be accessed on www.dfes.gov.uk/governor/govguide.htm.

how to determine its meaning, given that detention under the Act is a possibility for anyone provided that certain conditions are met. If this advice accurately reflects a legal requirement we suggest that the law in question should be reviewed, as it is discriminatory. In the Commission's view it is only acceptable to exclude persons who are detained under mental health legislation from public office or other positions where the fact of detention itself prevents them from taking up their role. This is, after all, the position for Members of Parliament and the National Assembly[118], and we can see no justification in any other public office having any more stringent and discriminatory rule.

Recommendation 11: Government should use the next Mental Health Act as an opportunity to outlaw the discriminatory exclusion of persons who have been detained under its powers, including rules in relation to public office.

6.37   The Department of Health's own commissioned study of public attitudes to people with mental illness[119] found that "levels of fear and intolerance of people with mental illness have tended to increase since 1993"[120] and particularly that "attitudes towards people with mental illness …have become less positive between 2000 and 2003"[121]. Fear and intolerance were already noted to be at dangerously high levels prior to 1993[122]. In our view, these findings should serve as a warning to Government that societal attitudes are moving in the wrong direction. We believe that it is within Government's power to alter the course of this movement.

6.38   There is a danger that the emphasis of measures in new legislation that are designed to protect those subject to compulsion from unwarranted interference (such as the increased role of the Tribunal in providing quasi-judicial authority for compulsion) will further alienate from public sympathy those persons who require compulsion. We have no argument against the adoption for the civil commitment process of procedures and standards of proof that are redolent of the criminal justice system, but we are fearful that an unintended consequence of this may be to extend the stigma of criminality to psychiatric patients subject to compulsory powers[123]. This is a particular danger where the purpose of compulsory powers is presented as primarily a matter of social control or managing public risk.

---

[118]   see Mental Health Act 1983, section 141. The parliamentary seat of a Member of the House of Commons, Scottish Parliament or National Assembly of Wales who is detained under the Act on grounds of mental illness will become vacant only after its occupant has been so detained for a period of six months.

[119]   National   Statistics   (2003)   *Attitudes   to   Mental   Illness   2003   Report.*   May   2003, www.doh.gov.uk/public/england.htm; see also Department of Health (2003) Statistical Press Release 2003/0239, 27 June 2003.

[120]   National Statistics (2003) *Attitudes to Mental Illness 2003 Report*, para 2.4, chart 6

[121]   *ibid*, para 2.1, chart 2

[122]   Campbell, T.D. & Heginbotham, C.J. (1991) *Mental illness: Prejudice, Discrimination and the Law* Aldershot: Gower.

[123]   see McGarry & Chodoff *The Ethics of Involuntary Hospitalisation* in Bloch/Chodoff (eds) (1981) *Psychiatric Ethics.* Oxford University Press, p 205

6.39 We are pleased to see that NIMHE's presentation of the policy framework for mental health highlights that the predominant core value of any future legislation must remain centred on health[124]. We also support the Government's adoption of frameworks of Values-Based Practice (see Chapter 5 above). However, insofar as the Government has emphasised issues of public safety over healthcare issues in its presentation of plans for future mental health legislation, we believe it to have done justice neither to the real purpose of such legislation nor to the patients whose care will be regulated under its powers.

> **Recommendation 12:** We urge Government and health service providers at all levels to avoid stereotypical and inaccurate presentations of mental health service users, especially in relation to public risk.

---

[124] Department of Health (2003) *Cases for Change: Policy Context.* NIMHE, p 4

Part 2

Issues arising from the application of the Mental Health Act 1983

7

The Scope of the 1983 Act

7.1 There are a number of actual or perceived limitations on the scope of the Mental Health Act 1983 in relation to the detention of certain types of patients.

Patients with Head Injuries

7.2 To be detained *for treatment* under the 1983 Act (i.e. under section 3 or a hospital order such as section 37), a patient must be certified as suffering from either mental illness, psychopathic disorder, mental impairment or severe mental impairment. It is generally accepted that brain injuries acquired in adulthood fall into none of these categories.

7.3 An injury to the brain may give rise to mental illness or psychopathic disorder, but it is neither of these things in its own right. Adult brain injuries are generally excluded from the categories of mental impairment because an adult brain is fully developed, and a mentally impaired patient must be suffering from "a state of *arrested or incomplete development* of mind" according to the Act's perhaps rather arbitrary definition.

7.4 The 1983 Act does allow that a patient may be "mentally disordered" in a non-specific sense that is applicable to brain injury patients, although the only powers of detention applicable to patients falling into this general category are short-term holding or assessment powers[125]. These powers may be useful for crisis management, but provide no secure footing for the long-term care that brain injury patients may need. The Commission is often approached for advice on these matters, although it can do little more than set out the law as it is understood now. The apparent limitations of the 1983 Act in relation to brain injuries provide one clear example of why it may be helpful to adopt a generic definition of mental disorder as a criterion for compulsion in the next Act, provided that suitably robust thresholds for the use of compulsion can be agreed upon (see Chapter 8.15 *et seq* below).

Drugs and Alcohol

7.5 In its consultation document on the draft Mental Health Bill of 2002, the Department of Health suggested that clinicians may be deterred from using the 1983 Act to detain mentally disordered people who are at immediate risk of suicide but whose main diagnosis is nevertheless alcohol dependence[126]. This suggestion seems to us unlikely, even though there is

---

[125] i.e. sections 2, 4, 5, 135 and 136 of the Act

[126] Department of Health (2002) *Mental Health Bill Consultation Document* Cm 5538-III para 3.23

little doubt that persons with substance abuse problems are often denied access to appropriate mental health services. We do not believe that such barriers to care are created by the law.

7.6   Section 1(3) of the 1983 Act states that nothing in the Act shall be construed to imply that a person suffers from mental disorder by reason only of dependence on alcohol or drugs. We have seen little evidence that this exclusion has been misinterpreted so as to prevent patients with dual diagnoses (i.e. both mental disorder and substance abuse problems) from the reach of the Act. We believe it to be more likely that such patients are often excluded from treatment because of the lack of effective services.

7.7   The Department of Health's *Dual Diagnosis Good Practice Guide*, published three months before the draft Mental Health Bill of 2002 Bill, acknowledged that patients (or potential patients) with dual diagnosis have "almost certainly been excluded from all the available services" because of a lack of integration between mental health and substance misuse services, clear care co-ordination pathways and a clear operational definition of dual diagnosis[127].

7.8   We congratulate the Department of Health on its *Dual Diagnosis Good Practice Guide* and will follow with interest its effect on services for detained patients. We discuss issues relating to drugs and alcohol with detained patients at Chapter 11.51 below.

Exclusion clauses in the next Mental Health Act

7.9   The 1983 Act not only excludes from the definition of mental disorder (and therefore from the scope of its powers of compulsion) drug or alcohol dependence, but also "promiscuity or other immoral conduct" and "sexual deviancy". We have urged Government to retain the principle of the 1983 Act's exclusions in the next Mental Health Bill whilst updating the language to reflect modern attitudes towards and understanding of sexuality. Continuing to mark such explicit exclusions would help to ensure that the Government's intention that the next Mental Health Act should not be used as a means to promote social control[128] is observed in practice whilst the law remains on the statute books.

> **Recommendation 13:** We continue to suggest that the following exclusions should be stated in the next Mental Health Act:
>
> (i)   No person may be dealt with under this Act as suffering from mental disorder solely on grounds of dependence upon, or use of, alcohol or drugs;
>
> (ii) no person may be dealt with under this Act as suffering from mental disorder solely on grounds of sexual behaviour or orientation; and
>
> (iii) no person may be dealt with under this Act as suffering from mental disorder solely on grounds of commission, or likely commission, of illegal or disorderly acts

---

[127] Department of Health (2002) *Mental Health Policy Implementation Guide: Dual Diagnosis Good Practice Guide.* April 2002, section 1.1

[128] Department of Health (2002) *Mental Health Bill Consultation Document Cm* 5538-III para 3.22

Psychopathic Disorder

7.10   It is now over a quarter of a century since the Butler Committee recommended that the 1959 Mental Health Act's legal category of "psychopathic disorder" was no longer appropriate and that legislation should refer instead to "personality disorder". The opportunity to adopt this recommendation with the passing of the 1983 Act was missed, and the term remains at section 1(2). The next Mental Health Act seems unlikely to refer specifically to either psychopathic or personality disorders, given the proposed adoption of a single, generic category of Mental Disorder. This, at least, should allow the legal concept of a "psychopath" to fall into belated disuse and so become considered as much of an archaism as the terms "moral imbecile" and "moral defective" that it replaced. Disappointingly, however, any benefit that might be gained with the loss of this ill-defined and therefore pejorative terminology is under threat by the creeping adoption of the phrase "Dangerous Severe Personality Disorder" or "DSPD" in its stead.

7.11   Psychopathy is a notoriously slippery term. The epidemiology of psychopathy is often equated incorrectly with that of anti-social personality disorder, to which it is linked. DSM IV identifies eleven separate personality disorders, though many patients are defined as having more than one. For practical purposes the eleven classifications are now grouped into three broad clusters which are used to aid diagnosis. Nonetheless the notion of eleven overlapping disorders is in itself confusing and causes significant problems epidemiologically, not least because of the imprecision of case definitions.

7.12   Psychopathy, on the other hand, is defined in a rather circular way against violent and anti-social behaviours. The epidemiology of violence in relation to psychopathy is flawed because the condition is defined in part by a history of violence and a propensity to violence. Within personality disorders, anti-social personality disorder (ASPD) is often equated with psychopathy, yet these two conditions are not equivalent. ASPD may have some elements of tendency to violence but is not defined wholly in that way. The problems of re-defining patients as having psychopathic disorder (whatever that might be, given the problems of case definition, diagnostic categorisation and epidemiology) only serves to underline the difficulties inherent in using such classification and the potential for their misuse.

7.13   Government first introduced the term Dangerous Severe Personality Disorder (DSPD) in 1999 as "a working definition"[129] to describe its proposals for policy development[130]. "DSPD" is therefore a term of politics rather than medicine, having no aetiological grounding and therefore no precise clinical meaning. It is therefore just as inappropriate a description of a patient's medical condition as "psychopathy" and its predecessors are now widely accepted to be. Whilst we acknowledge that the term "DSPD" was sensibly absent from the draft Mental Health Bill of 2002, and is largely absent from the NIMHE policy guidance on personality disorder services (see 7.17 *et seq* below), we are extremely concerned that it has been adopted for the official title of personality disorder units in the high security services, and has now been reinforced as such by statutory regulation[131].

---

[129]   Home Office (2001) *DSPD Programme Progress Report.* November 2001, page 3.

[130]   Department of Health (1999) *Managing Dangerous People with Severe Personality Disorder: Proposals for Policy Development.* July 1999.

[131]   The Safety and Security in Ashworth Broadmoor and Rampton Hospitals Amendment Directions 2003 refer to the hospitals' "DSPD facility" (Regulation 3).

Nevertheless, it is not too late to abandon this unnecessarily stigmatising and unhelpful terminology for forensic and/or high security personality disorder centres.

> **Recommendation 14:** Government, and all other authorities involved in the care of personality disordered patients, should cease any direct or indirect promotion of the terms Dangerous and Severe Personality Disorders or DSPD. Personality Disorder services could be distinguished according to security level or forensic input, as with other mental health services.

"Treatability" and exclusion from care

7.14 Research carried out in 1993 established that most forensic psychiatrists supported the inclusion of personality disordered patients within the scope of mental health legislation, and that there was already considerable support amongst forensic psychiatrists for the development of specialised personality disorder facilities in prisons and high security psychiatric hospitals[132]. A decade later, whilst Government has sanctioned the development of such an infrastructure for the care and treatment of severely personality disordered patients (see Chapter 12.63 *et seq*), its proposals for legal powers of detention for such patients is opposed by, amongst others, the Royal College of Psychiatrists and the British Medical Association.

7.15 The issue of contention is, of course, the Government's proposal for the "abolition of the so-called 'treatability test' in relation to psychopathic disorder"[133]. At the time of writing it is unclear what provision regarding this may be made in any Mental Health Bill brought to Parliament: our recommendation is discussed at 7.23 below.

7.16 The "treatability test" is actually the 1983 Act's requirement that patients who are classified as suffering from either psychopathic disorder or mental impairment should only be detained in hospital for treatment if that treatment is "likely to alleviate or prevent a deterioration in their condition". It is true that some clinicians are pessimistic with regard to the effectiveness of available treatments for some personality disorders. However, the *Reid* case[134] held that "medical treatment" in respect of the treatability test includes the management of the patient in a structured setting so as to provide symptomatic treatment, even if the underlying disorder remains unaffected. *R (on the application of Wheldon) v Rampton Hospital Authority* [2001] further established that the actual benefit to the patient

---

[132] Cope, R (1993) *A survey of forensic psychiatrists' views on psychopathic disorder* in <u>The Journal of Forensic Psychiatry</u> Vol 4 No2 215-235. Based on questionnaires returned by 90% all forensic psychiatrists working in England, Scotland and Wales (N = 86), 81% overall supported the continued extension of compulsory mental health powers to personality disordered patients (defined generally as persons whose mental disorders are only manifested by abnormally aggressive or seriously irresponsible behaviour), whether through specific inclusion in the Act (53%) or the adoption of terminology that encompasses personality disorder as in section 17(a)(i), Mental Health (Scotland) Act 1984 (28%). 79% supported more facilities in prison, 59% in HSHs and 41% in RSUs.

[133] Department of Health (2003) *Personality Disorder – No Longer a Diagnosis of Exclusion; Policy implementation guidance for the development of services for people with personality disorder.* London: NIMHE April 2003, Para 61

[134] *Reid v Secretary of State for Scotland* [1999]; *Reid v UK* [2003]

of treatment may be "very limited", for the treatability test to be satisfied, and it can be enough for beneficial results to be considered probable at some time in the future (although, as we note at 7.25 below, there is an argument that these judgments may only be confidently applied to patients subject to restricted court orders).

7.17   The *Reid* case also confirmed that treatability was a matter that Mental Health Review Tribunals must consider when hearing the appeal of a psychopathic disordered or mentally impaired patient. In *R (on the application of P) v MHRT for the East Midlands and North East Regions* [2002], a patient challenged the Tribunal's decision not to discharge him from his detention as a patient suffering from psychopathic disorder, arguing that he had not acted recently in a dangerous or irresponsible manner and therefore no longer fell within the Act's definition of the legal classification. The court held that it was sufficient that the MHRT considered susceptibility to such conduct, and not whether it had actually occurred or was occurring. Thus a patient may be detained as suffering from psychopathic disorder on evidence of past behaviour alone, and that the risk of such behaviour reoccurring if the detention ended is enough to justify its continuance.

7.18   The Commission would have liked to see advice based upon case law relating to the "treatability test" provided by NIMHE's 2003 policy implementation guidance *Personality Disorder – No Longer a Diagnosis of Exclusion*, particularly given this document's assertion that "the current 1983 Act is often interpreted as excluding those with personality disorder from compulsory detention because of the requirement that the mental disorder be 'treatable'"[135]. We doubt that this assertion is in fact the case among most mental health professionals who might be in a position to use the Act's powers in detaining personality disordered patients, although this is not to deny that there are barriers in the provision of suitable treatment for such patients. As we have noted in relation to the treatment of patients with dual diagnoses of mental disorders and substance misuse problems (7.6 above), the barrier to appropriate care is not so much any technicality of law but rather insufficient facilities and mental health professionals with suitable training, or insufficient access to such facilities and professionals from mainstream mental health services.

7.19   The NIMHE guidance, whilst providing much useful material on personality disorder service models, conflates the issues of legal requirements for detention and access to appropriate services in a manner that seems unlikely to win over the professionals that it seeks to advise. It is not helpful to suggest that clinicians' views about the treatability of personality disorder "will change with the new mental health legislation… which removes the treatability clause and provides a generic description of mental disorder"[136]. Clinicians' views about the potential benefit to any patient of detention in hospital are not be determined by technicalities of law, but by clinical experience, theoretical approach and an understanding of the realities of service provision.

7.20   Clinicians will feel ethically bound to only recommend treatment that will be of some therapeutic benefit to any potential patient. In assessing the most suitable placement for a

---

[135] Department of Health (2003) *Personality Disorder - No Longer a Diagnosis of Exclusion; Policy implementation guidance for the development of services for people with personality disorder.* London: NIMHE April 2003, para 27.

[136] *ibid.*, para 27

mentally disordered offender with severe anti-social personality disorder, the effective choice may be whether the person is better suited to hospital or prison, and prison may be the most suitable option from available services. At present, by the Department of Health's own calculations, for every patient in hospital who could be classed as "DPSD", there are at least four "DPSD" prisoners[137]. It is likely that the Government's planned restructuring and development of services for severe personality disorders will therefore have far more effect on clinical decisions than any change in the law.

Replacing the "treatability" clause

7.21   At Chapter 4 we discuss human rights issues that may arise in future legislation, and note US Court determinations that some form of treatment is a requirement to justify psychiatric detention with due process of law (see Chapter 4.17 on *Wyatt v Stickney*). This, we suspect, echoes the practical approach taken by clinicians now, not least because they quite understandably resist being given responsibility for 'patients' over whose conditions they have no control and can have no effect. However, it has been forcefully argued that, on the basis of cases already decided in relation to the European Convention of Human Rights, the ECHR makes no practical requirement for a patient to be treatable to make detention lawful[138]. On a similar basis, it may be that argued that the requirements of 'treatability' under the 1983 Act have been diluted by case law (see 7.17 above) to the point where they have no more of an influence on legal thresholds for compulsion than would have been provided by the vague criteria suggested in the draft Mental Health Bill of 2002[139].

7.22   The Commission was particularly concerned by the 2002 draft Mental Health Bill's suggested criterion that "treatment must be available in the patient's case" for the threshold of compulsion to be met (Clause 6(5)). If this was intended to address questions of treatability or reciprocity, we considered it ill-defined for such a purpose, and could even be used to exclude patients inappropriately from services by limiting authorities' responsibilities towards patients requiring specialist services that are difficult to access[140].

7.23   In our response to the 2002 Draft Mental Health Bill, we suggested that the Government's own concept of *therapeutic benefit* could be considered as an acceptable alternative to the 1983 Act's "treatability" requirements that would still provide a certain measure to determine the necessity of compulsion. Therapeutic benefit was defined in the White Paper *Reforming the Mental Health Act* as encompassing "improvement in the symptoms of mental disorder or slowing down deterioration and the management of behaviour arising from the mental disorder"[141].

---

[137]   *ibid.,* paragraph 3.

[138]   Hewitt, D (2002) *Treatability Tests,* Solicitors Journal, 4 October 2002, pp 886-887

[139]   for example, Hewitt (2002) *Treatability Tests, ibid,* does take the position that the draft Mental Health Bill of 2002 (Clause 6) addresses treatability by the 'relevant conditions' that medical treatment is required, available and cannot be given without compulsion.

[140]   Mental Health Act Commission (2002) *The Mental Health Act Commission Response to the draft Mental Health Bill Consultation.* MHAC, September 2002, para 4.14

[141]   Department of Health (2000) *Reforming the Mental Health Act. Part I: The new legal framework.* Cmnd 5016-I. Para 3.21.

Recommendation 15: The Commission commends to Government the concept of "therapeutic benefit" as one particular criterion for the compulsion of psychiatric patients.

Preventive detention, prediction and proof; "seven-tenths of the human race..."

7.24   On 3 October 1838 the Lunacy Commission, acting in a role that is roughly equivalent to today's Mental Health Review Tribunal, resorted to a vote to decide whether to discharge a patient after a three-day hearing. It was the first time that they had decided a case by voting in their ten-year existence. Lord Ashley (later the Earl of Shaftesbury) wrote in his diary that the patient in question:

> "...had been seized only a few days when we proceeded to inquire into his alleged insanity and the grounds of his detention; a more heartless ruffian, one more low in mind and coarse in language, though a man of talent and education, never entered the walls of a prison or a madhouse. The opposite party, however, could not prove against him one single act of violence; his words, his manner, his feelings, were awfully wicked; but he had never as yet (although their charge extended over several years) broken out into action. In fact, a decision on our part, that he was rightfully detained, would have authorised the incarceration in Bedlam of seven-tenths of the human race who have ever been excited to violence of speech and gesture."[142]

The Lunacy Commissioners voted to discharge the patient on a division of six to four. Ashley's diary entry also ruefully noted that "we can lay down no fixed rules for decision; we must take our course, according to doctors' prescriptions, *pro re nata*"[143].

7.25   The Lunacy Commission's debate of 165 years ago has been revived by proposals for new legislation during our reporting period[144]. The Joint Committee on Human Rights (JCHR) has questioned whether any law that makes provision for the non-therapeutic detention of persons without conviction of an offence, on the grounds of "speculation about possible future behaviour and resulting risk to identified persons", will be compatible with the European Convention[145]. The JCHR noted that explicit powers of preventive detention established by the Mental Health (Public Safety and Appeals) (Scotland) Act 1999 had been deemed compatible with ECHR Article 5 by the Judicial Committee of the Privy Council[146], but pointed to the fact that these powers related only to restricted patients who have been convicted of serious offences and set no clear precedent for patients who have had no contact with the criminal justice system.

---

[142]   quoted in Hodder E (1890) *The Life and Work of the Seventh Earl of Shaftesbury KG.* Cassell & Co, 1890. p124

[143]   Hodder (1890), as above. *Pro re nata* - 'as the occasion arises'.

[144]   see, for example, Peay, J (2003) *Decisions and Dilemmas; working with mental health law.* Oxford, Hart Publishing, pp154; Sugerman, P A (2002) *Persons of unsound mind, dangerousness and the Human Rights Act 1998* in The Journal of Forensic Psychiatry, Vol 13 No.3, December 2002, 569-577

[145]   House of Lords, House of Commons Joint Committee on Human Rights (2002) *Draft Mental Health Bill: twenty-fifth report of session 2001-02.* HL Paper 181, HC 1294. London, The Stationery Office, November 2002. para 46.

[146]   Anderson, *Reid and Doherty v the Scottish Ministers and the Advocate General for Scotland* [2001]. This may yet be appealed to the European Court of Human Rights.

7.26 The JCHR has suggested to Government that, when introducing a Bill to Parliament in relation to preventive detention, it should make publicly available an account of risk factors to be used in assessing dangerousness and their reliability[147]. In the US, 'dangerousness' must be "based upon a finding of a recent overt act, attempt or threat to do substantial harm to oneself or another" (*Lessard v Schmidt* 1972). Peay (2003) suggests this as a potential precursor for a similar finding under UK law[148]. Given the very real difficulties of predicting future violent behaviour, it is difficult to see how the Lunacy Commission's dilemma might be resolved by any proposal made so far.

7.27 It has been suggested that the forthcoming Mental Health Bill will extend current provisions for the courts in making hospital orders so that these may be applied to persons not charged with imprisonable offences[149]. This may be an unnecessary blurring of civil and criminal-justice powers. We are sympathetic to the concern that it would be a disproportionate use of powers for courts to order the detention in hospital of persons charged with petty offences.

The limited usefulness of legal classification in relation to personality disorders and mental illness

7.28 It is the case that significant numbers of people with a primary diagnosis of personality disorder are detained under the Mental Health Act 1983. Figure 5 below provides a snapshot of the number of patients detained in England on the 31 March 2002 by Mental Health Act category (equivalent figures are not available for Wales). The 654 psychopathic disorders amount to 5% of all classified disorders in the table[150]. The significant proportion of women patients (197) indicates that there is likely to be a range of personality disorders subsumed in this legal category[151]. Not all patients detained as suffering from "psychopathic disorder" will be suffering from severe antisocial personality disorder (the closest description of "DSPD" that is clinically meaningful). Detained patients of either sex may be suffering from any of the other nine recognised clinical categories, including borderline personality disorders and other disorders. Many of these patients may be "dangerous" only to themselves through self-harm and suicide, even among those placed within high secure services. We discuss the placement of personality disordered patients within the health service at Chapter 12.63 *et seq*.

7.29 Currently available statistics do not show the number of patients detained with a classification of more than one mental disorder category, as only a patient's "primary" diagnosis is recorded for statistical collation. It seems likely that a number of patients classified as suffering from mental illness in the above table will also have a subsidiary classification of psychopathic disorder. This is suggested from anecdotal observation on Commission visits

---

[147] *ibid* note 145 above, para 47.

[148] Peay, J (2003) p163n; see also Chapter 4.14 above for the U.S. as a precursor for future directions in UK law.

[149] Adam James *Government powers plan 'shameful'* Guardian, 11 June 2003.

[150] A category of disorder does not need to be assigned to patients detained under sections 2, 4, 5(2), 5(4), 135 or 135: such patients will show in the "not specified" category of Figure 5 above.

[151] see, for example, Coid, Kahtan, Gault and Jarman (2000) *Women admitted to secure forensic services: II identification of categories using cluster analysis*. Journal of Forensic Psychiatry Vol 11 No 2 Sept 2000 296 – 315.

Classification	Male	Female	Total
Mental Illness	7,088	3,791	10,879
Psychopathic Disorder	457	197	654
Mental Impairment	730	181	911
Severe Mental Impairment	132	38	170
Not specified (see footnote 150)	422	423	845
Total	8,829	4,630	13,459

Fig 5: Detentions under the MHA 1983, 31/03/02, by legal category of mental disorder

Data Source: DOH (2002) Statistical Bulletin In-patients formally detained in hospitals under the MHA 1983 and other legislation, England: 1991-92 to 2001-02 (Bulletin 2002/26)

as well as the Government's contention that psychiatrists are reluctant to admit to hospital personality disordered patients who cannot also be classified as mentally ill[152].

7.30   It seems likely that actual co-morbidity between mental illnesses and personality disorders is extremely common. One 1998 study of 713 personality disordered offenders in High Security Hospitals found that 59% had one or more additional diagnoses[153]. Such clinical levels of co-morbidity are not reflected in the formal classification of disorders under the Act. A study published this year[154] found that, in a random sample of patients from Ashworth Hospital, the prevalence of personality disorders among patients with a primary Mental Health Act classification of Mental Illness was the same as for those patients classified primarily under Psychopathic Disorder. For example, over three-quarters of patients in both the Mental Illness and Psychopathic Disorder groups were found to meet the diagnostic criteria for antisocial personality disorder. Two thirds of the Psychopathic Disorder group met the criteria for depression, over half met the diagnostic criteria for anxiety, and 11% met the diagnostic criteria for psychosis. We refer to this study again in Chapter 12.67 below in relation to its implications for service development.

7.31   If there is widespread co-morbidity between personality disorders and mental illness irrespective of Mental Health Act classification, then "the dichotomy imposed by legal classification is misleading and obscures the multiple problems shared by patients in the two categories"[155]. This would suggest that the Government is correct in seeking to abandon the

---

[152]   Department of Health / Home Office (1999) *Managing Dangerous People with Severe Personality Disorder; Proposals For Policy Development.* July 1999, page 10, para 13.

[153]   Taylor, Leese, Williams, Butwell, Daly and Larkin (1998) *Mental disorder and violence: a special (high security) hospital study.* British Journal of Psychiatry 172, 218-224 , table 1b.

[154]   Blackburn, Logan, Donnelly and Renwick (2003) *Personality disorders, psychopathy and other mental disorder: co-morbidity among patients at English ands Scottish high security hospitals.* Journal of Forensic Psychiatry and Psychology Vol 14 No 1 April 2003 111-137.

[155]   *ibid.* p114

legal classifications in the next Mental Health Act. In the meantime, following *B v Ashworth Hospital Authority* [2003], which we discuss at Chapter 3.40 *et seq*, "the question of reclassifying patients to include other disorders will assume a far greater importance than hitherto it has had"[156].

7.32   *B v Ashworth* has therefore given increased legal importance to the 1983 Act's differentiation of Mental Disorder into discrete categories just as proposals are in hand for the Act's successor to dissolve these into a generic definition of "Mental Disorder". This clearly raises important issues relating to the circumscription of legal powers over patients which will need careful consideration. It may be argued that the artificial categories erected by the 1983 Act provide neither clear guidelines for professionals nor protection for patients, and the Mental Health (Scotland) Act 1984 clearly operates without such categories. On the other hand, the abolition of distinct legal categories of mental disorder by the 2002 draft Mental Health Bill would seem to return patients to a position where they might be compelled to accept treatment for any mental disorder, and not just that which has been accepted as justification for compulsion. Whilst the Tribunal may be able to regulate practice in respect of long-term treatments under the proposals for the next Act, we envisage future legal difficulties for new legislation unless this matter is addressed.

---

[156]   Simon Brown LJ, *R (on the application of B) v Ashworth Hospital Authority* [2003], para 81

The Threshold for the Use of the 1983 Act

Informal Treatment and the Incapable Patient

8.1 The recognition that informal, consensual psychiatric treatment can be achieved and is to be preferred over compulsion wherever possible is one of the clear advances in mental health legislation in the twentieth century, and a legacy that society should seek to preserve.

8.2 This legacy is a system that contains conflicting tensions around the threshold at which formal powers should be imposed upon patients. The imposition of formal powers over patients is a serious interference with human rights and must be a last resort, and yet patients who fall below this threshold are denied access to the safeguards embedded within formal powers and duties and may even, as a consequence, receive inadequate care.

8.3 From its establishment the Commission has raised the plight of a particular group of such patients: those who are subject to "de facto" compulsion[157]. We have been concerned that some patients who are not subject to formal powers of compulsion (and who are excluded from our remit as a consequence) may still be denied autonomy within psychiatric services, either because of the incapacitating effects of their illness, or because of hidden compulsion in such services, or through a combination of both.

8.4 It is well established that, in practice, informal patients who volunteer to enter hospital may well feel that they have little option but to do so, as otherwise powers of compulsory admission will be used. Patients commonly complain that they feel forced into admission or treatment even when there are no formal powers implemented in relation to their care[158]. It seems unlikely that there could ever be a legislative remedy to the dilemma of 'hidden compulsion', especially in relation to mentally competent patients, which did not undo the gains in UK law of the last half-century. However, the safeguard of monitoring oversight could be made available to such informal patients, focusing in particular on whether restrictions on such patients' liberties were being applied and ensuring that care is provided to an appropriate standard (see Chapter 20.11 below).

---

[157] see Mental Health Act Commission (1985) *First Biennial Report 1983-5*, page 11; MHAC (1989) *Third Biennial Report 1987-89* p35; MHAC (1991) *Fifth Biennial Report* 1997-9 p47,56; MHAC (1999) *Eighth Biennial Report* 1997-9 p254; MHAC (2001) *Ninth Biennial Report* 1999-01 p 80. London: Stationery Office

[158] Legemaate, J (1992) *Compulsion and patients' rights in psychiatry: an international perspective in Law and Mental Health; Historical, legal, ethical diagnostic and therapeutic aspects.* Proceedings of the 17th International Academy of Law and Mental Health, 1991. Leuven, Belgium.

8.5   We recognise and support the Government's intention to provide safeguards for incapacitated but compliant patients in the next Mental Health Act and a Mental Incapacity Act[159], but we are also mindful that five years have passed since the House of Lords' ruling in *Bournewood*, which established the current legal position whilst noting that it left "an indefensible gap in mental health law"[160]. In our Ninth Biennial Report (2001) we urged the Government to consider ways in which patients may be protected whilst legislation is awaited[161], and we regret that no action has been taken on this recommendation. In the meantime, the Courts have further expanded the available powers of compulsion over incapacitated persons to encompass the social and personal sphere as well as medical treatment, without any concomitant expansion of safeguards[162]. We are pleased that the Mental Incapacity Bill will do something to address this imbalance (although see Chapter 8.12 - 14 below).

8.6   At the time of writing, a decision was awaited from the European Court of Human Rights in the *Bournewood* case, and it is therefore possible that the legal position debated below will have changed by the time this report is published.

8.7   During our reporting period we have encountered great concern and considerable debate over the application of present law in this area. There have been many disputes between medical and social work professionals over whether the Act may be applied to particular patients or in particular circumstances. The *Bournewood* ruling stated that mentally incapacitated patients who were compliant with admission to hospital could be admitted under the common law. Government advice on practice following the ruling suggested that, where a patient has been admitted informally to hospital under such circumstances, but then fails to accept necessary treatment or refuses to co-operate with those caring for him or her, consideration should be given to either discharge from hospital or assessment for detention under the Act[163]. In this way, although the law only requires consideration to be given to compliance to hospital *admission*, professionals are encouraged to take a broader view in assessing the wishes of patients and their attitude towards their total experience of hospitalisation, including forms of treatment proposed. We have sought and received confirmation from the Department of Health that it stands by its 1998 guidance that "non-compliance may be evidenced by a patient who resists necessary treatment or persistently and purposefully tries to leave hospital".

8.8   In many cases disputes arise over the question of a patient's "compliance" with hospital admission:

＊ It is sometimes the case that medical professionals argue for use of the Act solely because they are uncomfortable in giving certain treatments for mental disorder (particularly

---

[159]   *Draft Mental Incapacity Bill* Cm 5859-1, June 2003. The Commission also welcomed the attempt by Helen Clark MP on the 13 February 2003 to introduce a *Patients Without Legal Capacity (Safeguards) Bill* to Parliament under the ten-minute rule. The attempt was unsuccessful.

[160]   Lord Steyn in *R v Bournewood Community & Mental Health NHS Trust ex parte L* [1998]

[161]   Mental Health Act Commission (2001) *Ninth Biennial Report* 1999-2001. London: Stationery Office, chapter 6.68-9, recommendation 72.

[162]   *Re F (Adult: Court's Jurisdiction)* [2000] 3 WLR 1740. See Hewitt, D (2000) *Widening the 'Bournewood Gap'?* Journal of Mental Health Law, November 2000, pp 196-204.

[163]   Health Service Circular 1998/122

ECT) under the common law. In the Commission's view, this is not an adequate reason for invoking formal detention under the Act. We can see no reason in law why a patient who is incapable of consent but is compliant to hospital admission should not receive ECT or medication for mental disorder under common-law powers. If doctors wish to provide such patients, or themselves, with some level of safeguards against unwarranted treatment, they could seek a clinical second opinion from a colleague.

* In other cases, professionals may disagree as to whether a patient's attitude towards treatment can be considered relevant to the question of his or her compliance with hospital admission. Some professionals adopt a disjunctive approach to consent to admission and consent to treatment following admission, on the basis that the law only requires consideration of the former. Certain lines of argument in the Seventh and Eighth editions of the *Mental Health Act Manual* have been cited to support this approach, particularly the view that patients who have not objected to their admission to hospital can and should remain as informal patients even if their treatment for mental disorder is subsequently administered by force under the common law[164]. Whilst there are undoubtedly situations where this approach is correct in law and defensible in practice (dependent on the situations and, perhaps, on the nature and duration of force used), we do not encourage professionals to make inflexible distinctions between admission and treatment. In our view patients may evidence non-compliance with hospital admission through resistance to receiving necessary treatment in hospital. It is not realistic to expect incapacitated patients to distinguish in thought or action between their admission to hospital and the treatment that such admission serves to provide. The question of whether a patient is compliant is therefore a clinical judgment that should take account of a patient's stated views and behaviour to both remaining in hospital and to accepting the treatment that is offered there.

8.9 The Commission has been approached for guidance in defining "non-compliance", particularly by professionals whose patients display little or no *active* resistance to detention or treatment. In effect, this is a question of whether non-compliance has to be evidenced by a positive act of resistance. This question may arise with non-catatonic patients who are nevertheless uncommunicative, mute and withdrawn. Such patients may be refusing food and water, often will be elderly and, if so, may well be being considered for treatment with ECT. The type of treatment for mental disorder proposed should have no bearing on the question of whether such a patient may be treated informally or under detention (see 8.7 above). However, we do consider it possible for professionals to decide appropriately that a patient is non-compliant, even in the absence of a demonstrable refusal. We think that this is properly a matter for the professionals concerned to evaluate, and that guidance which limits professional discretion may be counter-productive, although non-prescriptive guidance may be useful to services. Existing Department of Health guidance does state helpfully that "compliance should not be assumed if the patient's intentions are not clear", from which it seems to us reasonable that subtler forms of resistance should be recognised alongside the more overt forms. In our view it is proper, where doubt over these issues exists in relation to any particular patient, to arrange a Mental Health Act assessment to test the issues in practice.

---

[164] see, for example, Jones (2003) *Mental Health Act Manual* para 1-688. The Manual does, however, temper this advice with support the Department of Health advice of HSC 1998/122 (see para 8.7 above).

Recommendation 16: We invite the Department of Health to consider suitable guidance on the issues surrounding the determination of non-compliance in patients for current services and for the next Code of Practice.

8.10   In 1986 the Commission first requested the Secretary of State to exercise the power under section 121(4) and direct that the Commission should keep under review aspects of the care and treatment of informal psychiatric patients, including patients subject to Child Care Orders[165]. Our request was that the specific foci of such an extended remit would be limited to monitoring any restraint placed upon patients' movement, including leaving hospital; intentional deprivation of the company of other patients or of amenities enjoyed by others; and the imposition of certain forms of medical treatment. This and subsequent Commission suggestions that its remit be extended to informal patients under certain circumstances have been rejected.

8.11   Under the Draft Mental Health Bill of 2002, the care plans of informal psychiatric patients without mental capacity would be subject to the overview of the Tribunal through the agency of a Tribunal-appointed doctor, equivalent in many ways to current statutory Second Opinion provisions for detained patients. We trust that such arrangements will be complemented by general monitoring oversight of the successor body to the Commission, as suggested at Chapters 8.10 and 20.11 of this report.

Recommendation 17: The next Mental Health Act should provide specific monitoring powers to the MHAC successor body in relation to patients subject to *de facto* psychiatric compulsion.

The relation of proposed mental incapacity and mental health legislation

8.12   The proposed interrelation between the proposed Mental Incapacity and Mental Health Acts is not entirely clear. We recognise that the Mental Incapacity Bill's primary purpose is to clarify and reform common law provisions relating to decision-making on behalf of mentally incapacitated persons, and that it will therefore replace Part VII of the current Mental Health Act (relating to the management of patients' property and affairs) whilst not seeking to concern itself with detention or compulsory treatment[166]. We are concerned that the drafting of the two Bills is not sufficiently precise to ensure that this is how they are put into practice.

8.13   Although there are plausible arguments for restricting the scope of powers of attorney under mental incapacity legislation to patients who are compliant with psychiatric treatment, especially given that non-compliant patients' care would fall within Part V of the

---

[165] Under the then extant Child Care Act 1980. The Commission is currently seeking similar extension of its remit to psychiatric patients subject to residence orders of the Children Act 1999

[166] Department of Constitutional Affairs (2003) Mental Incapacity Bill, explanatory notes 5 & 9. Cm 5859-II

draft Mental Health Bill and so be regulated (and authorised) by the Mental Health Tribunal, this is clearly not the effect of the Mental Incapacity Bill as set out at clause 10[167]. As drafted, mental incapacity legislation could allow a person with powers of attorney over an incapacitated person to provide the authority for that person to be admitted to psychiatric care despite their resistance. It is possible that such powers would work in tandem with the safeguards proposed under Part V of the draft Mental Health Bill of 2002, whereby the Tribunal must approve care-plans for such patients for them to be lawful. However, without further clarification it would seem that potentially the two powers conflict.

8.14   The powers proposed under the draft Mental Health Bill of 2002 and the Mental Incapacity Bill may conflict in another way. Clause 27 of the Mental Incapacity Bill prevents that legislation from providing authority to give a person treatment for mental disorder if that treatment is regulated by Part IV of the Mental Health Act. This would appear to be designed with a dual purpose: to ensure that patients in relation to whom another person has lasting powers of attorney will still be subject to the safeguards of the Mental Health Act in relation to ECT, neurosurgery or medication for mental disorder; and to ensure that the powers of the Mental Health Act are not negated by advance directives made under the Mental Incapacity Act. However, Part IV of the draft Mental Health Bill of 2002 includes, at clause 117, a definition of medical treatment that is as broad as that currently applied to Part IV of the Mental Health Act 1983 under the powers of section 63. Just as section 63 of the 1983 Act extends to nursing care, rehabilitation etc, so clause 117 of the draft Bill would seem to apply to a patient's entire care-plan. If this analysis is correct, it is difficult to envisage any aspect of the psychiatric care of mentally incapacitated patients that would be left within the scope of the Mental Incapacity Act. We believe that further consideration needs to be given to both draft Bills to ensure that these matters are resolved.

Recommendation 18: Potential conflicts between the Mental Incapacity Bill and proposals for a new Mental Health Act should be reviewed and addressed by Government.

The threshold for compulsion under proposals in the draft Mental Health Bill of 2002

8.15   The Commission argued in its response to the consultation over the draft Mental Health Bill of 2002 that the conditions for compulsion set out at clause 6 of that Bill are insufficiently defined to provide a threshold for compulsion under the new Act. Although we appreciate that the criteria for compulsion are being reconsidered for the redrafted Bill, in the following paragraphs we set out our concerns over the criteria proposed so far.

8.16   Draft Mental Health Bill 2002:
The first condition of compulsion is that the patient is suffering from mental disorder
We do not object to having a generic category of mental disorder as the foundation of a new

---

[167]   Clause 10 of the Mental Incapacity Bill authorises a person with lasting powers of attorney to use or threaten to use force to secure the commission of an act resisted by an incapacitated person, or to restrict the liberty of movement of an incapacitated person, provided that it is necessary to do so to avert a substantial risk of significant harm to the person concerned. The powers extend to making decisions about medical treatment, subject to any advance directive.

Mental Health Act (see Chapter 7.4 above). Prior to *B v Ashworth* [2003], discussed at Chapter 3.40 above, we were not convinced that the further division of mental disorders into subgroups had any positive purpose in the operation of the law. It may be that new legislation can afford patients equivalent protections to those established in *B v Ashworth* without reintroducing categorisation of mental disorders, through suitably robust criteria for the imposition of compulsion.

8.17   Draft Mental Health Bill 2002:

The second condition for compulsion is that the mental disorder is of such a nature or degree as to warrant the provision of medical treatment

This is inadequate as the Bill's own definition of medical treatment (clause 2(5)) is so broad that all mental disorders, by definition, could be said to "warrant" medical treatment of some kind (albeit usually only on a consensual basis, and often without any degree of necessity). This condition therefore has little or no defining purpose that is not served by the first condition and is meaningless as a measure against which any threshold for compulsion might be defined. The measure of such a threshold must be that the nature or degree of the mental disorder is such to warrant medical treatment **under compulsion**. This threshold can only be addressed through criteria such as those set out in the third condition suggested by the draft Bill (clause 6(4)), as discussed at 8.19 below. We therefore recommended that the second condition (Clause 6(3)) should be removed and the concept of "nature and degree" should be introduced into the third condition.

8.18   Draft Mental Health Bill 2002:

The third condition for compulsion is that it is necessary

(a) in the case of a patient who is at substantial risk of causing harm to others, that medical treatment be provided, and

(b) in any other case, that treatment is necessary for the health and safety of the patient and could not be provided without the use of compulsion.

The intention of the division of this condition into two parallel sub-clauses appeared to be the avoidance of difficulties in relation to "treatability" and the "necessity" for compulsion of those patients who pose a substantial risk of harm to others (referred to below as 'high-risk patients'). Whilst the Commission understands the Government's concern that such criteria may be used to exclude or excuse some high-risk people from mental health services under compulsion, we believe such concern to be misplaced. We also doubt that the drafting of clause 6(4)(a) achieves the Government's intention.

8.19   The Commission has consistently argued that the issue of health disposals for those persons who present a high-risk of harm to others is only relevant insofar as such a disposal would provide a better chance of reducing that risk by alleviating or preventing deterioration in mental disorder[168]. The management of deviant behaviour alone does not – and should not – fall within any definition of medical treatment. We do not therefore agree that the "treatability test", as it has been developed in case-law[169] can or should be put aside by new legislation. Where such a treatability test cannot be met, disposals of high-risk offenders should be a matter for criminal and not mental health law (see Chapter 7.14 *et seq* above).

---

[168] see, for example, MHAC (2000) *Managing Dangerous People with Severe Personality Disorders; Response of the Mental Health Act Commission to proposals for policy development.* www.mhac.trent.nhs.uk/dspdnew.pdf para iii.

[169] *R v Canons Park Mental Health Review Tribunal ex p. A* [1994]; *R v Secretary of State for Scotland*, 1998.; *R (on the application of Wheldon) v. Rampton Hospital Authority* [2001]

8.20   The conditions set by both (a) and (b) above would allow for a patient to be compelled to accept medical treatment for mental disorder on the grounds that this was necessary for the protection of other persons. Because of this essential similarity, the only substantive difference between clauses (a) and (b) is that the latter requires that treatment can only be provided if compulsory powers are invoked, whereas the former is silent upon this matter.

8.21   We believe that it is unnecessary to introduce a specific condition for high-risk patients that excludes consideration of whether the use of compulsion is necessary to achieve the aim of protecting other persons from the action of the patient. Case-law has set a clear precedent that compulsion can be justified if it is a proportionate response having regard to the risks that would be involved in discharge[170]. We can therefore see no reason why the conditions set out at (b) would prevent the appropriate treatment of high-risk patients. This would particularly be the case where a patient's co-operation with consensual treatment would be unstable and there would be too great a risk involved in holding compulsory powers in abeyance.

8.22   The Commission has suggested that clause (a) above (Clause 6(4)(a) of the draft Bill), is therefore contrary to the principles on which the Bill is said to be based, and should be deleted. Instead, the law should require as a condition of compulsion that:
(a) it is necessary for the health or safety of the patient or the protection of other persons that medical treatment be provided to him; and
(b) the nature or degree of the mental disorder is such that treatment cannot be provided to him unless he is subject to the provisions of this Act.

8.23   Draft Mental Health Bill 2002:
The fourth condition for compulsion is that appropriate medical treatment is available in the patient's case.
We are uncertain of the purpose of this condition. If this was intended to address questions of treatability or reciprocity, it appears ill-defined, and could even be used to exclude patients inappropriately from services by limiting authorities' responsibility for the care and treatment of patients who require difficult to access specialist services.

8.24   We have recommended that a more appropriate condition should be based upon the concept of "therapeutic benefit" that was introduced in the Government's White Paper[171]. In the Commission's view, "therapeutic benefit", which would be defined to encompass "improvement in the symptoms of mental disorder or slowing down deterioration and the management of behaviours arising from the mental disorder"[172], provides a more certain measure against which to determine the necessity of compulsion. We accept, however, that a Tribunal considering the authorisation of or appeal against compulsory treatment should question whether appropriate services are being provided to the patient concerned. As such,

---

[170]   e.g. *R (on the application of H.) v Mental Health Review Tribunal, North and North East London Region* [2001]

[171]   Department of Health (2000) *Reforming the Mental Health Act. Part I: The new legal framework.* Cmnd 5016-I.

[172]   Department of Health (2000) *Reforming the Mental Health Act. Part I: The new legal framework.* Cmnd 5016-I, para 3.21. In 1986, there were 4,602 detained patients resident as of the 31 December, compared with 88,820 informal patients. By 1999 the former figure had risen to 13,000 and, although no comparable figure of informal patients is given, the rise in formal admissions is noted to be steeper than that for informal patients in the intervening period [data sources as below, note 173]

it may be appropriate to incorporate the "condition" that "appropriate medical treatment is available in the patient's case" into Tribunal rules or guidance.

Admission trends under the Mental Health Act 1983

8.25 In our Ninth Biennial Report we noted the general increase in uses of the Act over the last decade. Figure 6 below shows the trend for the lifetime of the 1983 Act so far. Although there is a leveling off in most recent years, this shows that the use of civil compulsion has roughly doubled during the lifetime of the Act. There has been no overall rise in the use of the 1983 Act for patients involved in criminal proceedings or under sentence during the lifetime of the Act: we look in more detail at these trends at Chapter 13 below.

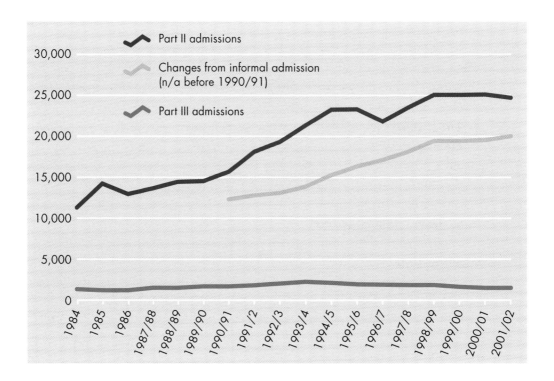

Fig 6: Mental Health Act 1983 admission trends, England 1983-2002 [173]

8.26 The last available figure for the number of detained patients resident at any one time (31 March 2002) showed 13,459 patients subject to the Act. The proportion of inpatients who are detained appears to remain relatively large, and is probably higher than in the early years of the Act[174]. In some medium and high secure units, of course, all or almost all patients are detained, but the rise is also notable in acute and admission wards.

8.27 The general increase in the use of the Act and the proportion of detained patients on some wards may be due to a number of factors:

---

[173] sources: DHSS (1987) *Mental Health Statistics for England 1986* Booklet 11, Legal Status Table D1; Department of Health (1995) *Statistical Bulletin 1995/4*; DH (1996) *Statistical Bulletin 1996/10*; DH (1999) *Statistical Bulletin 1999/25*; DH (2002) *Statistical Bulletin 2002/26*. Data accuracy is compromised by its several sources, mixture of calendar years and financial years and possible discrepancies in categorisation over time.

[174] see Mental Health Act Commission (2001) *Ninth Biennial Report 1999-01*, London: Stationery Office. Chapter 3.1 - 3.2

* In part, this may simply be a reflection of the rise in the use of the Act against decreasing numbers of inpatient beds. A number of patients who might have been informal inpatients in the early years of the Act are now more likely to receive community-based treatment.

* Bed pressures may also lead to only the most severely ill, who are the most likely to be detained, being admitted. Bed pressures may also lead to shorter but more frequent detentions for some patients.

* The promotion of risk-management by mental health policy makers, the criticisms of post-incident inquiries or even generally less permissive societal attitudes may account for some of the rise. These factors may encourage medical and social care professionals to use the Act more readily, either through lowering the perceived thresholds for such use or through fostering defensive professional practice.

* Although there is little research in this area, many practitioners believe that there has been a dramatic increase in illicit drug use by seriously mentally ill people in the last ten to fifteen years. Increases in drug and alcohol abuse co-morbidity might explain apparent rises in severity of mental disordered persons, given that drug/alcohol abuse may make mentally ill persons more disinhibited or may aggravate their symptoms, thus making their detention more likely.

* The environmental conditions on inpatient wards may be responsible for an increase in the detention of patients who would otherwise discharge themselves against medical advice.

8.28   We analyse and discuss the overrepresentation of Black and minority ethnic patients in the above figures in Chapter 16 below.

Section 2 And Section 3

8.29   The majority of civil detentions under the 1983 Act are initiated using either of the admission sections 2 or 3. Section 2 allows detention for assessment and/or treatment for a maximum of 28 days, whilst the renewable powers of section 3 effectively allow for indefinite detention for treatment. The two powers have separate criteria (and therefore safeguards) for use. It is a matter of professional judgment as to that which is appropriate in any particular case. Chapter 5 of the Code of Practice provides guidance on the choice between powers.

8.30   Figure 7 below shows the percentage use of sections 2 and 3 for 2001/02. It is to be expected that, as this data suggests, proportionally more patients should be detained under section 2 than section 3 upon admission to hospital, and that the reverse would be true for informal inpatients made subject to the Act. The key issue determining whether section 2 or 3 is appropriate in many cases is the diagnostic and prognostic confidence of the clinical team in respect of a particular patient.

8.31   The relative use of sections 2 and 3 has not been constant throughout the life of the 1983 Act. Figure 8 below shows that as well as a general increase in the number of uses of the Act, the proportion of uses of section 3 to section 2 has risen dramatically from the time before the first publication of the Code of Practice (1990). It seems likely that this reflects practitioners' use of the Code's guidance in relation to the purposes of sections 2 and 3.

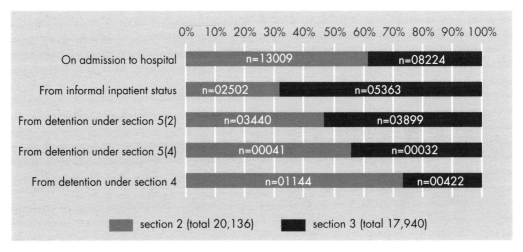

Fig 7: Uses of sections 2 and 3, NHS facilities, England 2001-2002

Data source: DOH (2002) Statistical Bulletin 2002/26 table 8

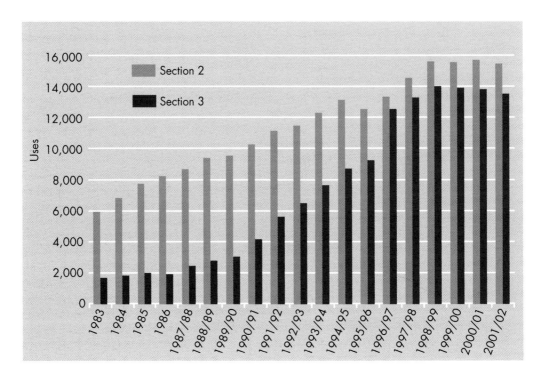

Fig 8: Uses of sections 2 and 3 to admit patients, NHS facilities, England 1983 – 2002[175]

8.32 In past Biennial Reports the Commission has criticised authorities for using section 2 powers for patients known to their clinical teams[176]. We continue to advise authorities to monitor the ratio of uses of the Act and, where section 2 usage is high proportionate to the use of section 3, to look carefully at the reasons for the use of particular sections, considering the following issues:

(i) Although powers of compulsory treatment apply equally to section 2 and section 3 patients, we consider it bad practice to use section 2 as a short-term treatment power

---

[175] Data sources: as for Figure 6 above (note 173).

[176] e.g. Mental Health Act Commission (1993) *Fifth Biennial Report 1991-3* p103-4; MHAC (1995) *Sixth Biennial Report 1993-5*, Chapter 3.1; MHAC (1997) *Seventh Biennial Report 1995-7* Chapter 3.1.1. London: Stationery Office

alternative to section 3. This does not mean that we consider compulsory treatment under section 2 to be bad practice, and indeed the Commission frequently corrects the misconception amongst some professionals that compulsory treatment (particularly ECT treatment) cannot be given to a patient detained under section 2. However, we do consider that section 2 should be seen primarily as an assessment power that allows treatment, rather than as a treatment power in itself. The safeguards offered by the Act's admission criteria in respect of sections 2 and 3 are different for this reason.

(ii) We therefore advise against viewing section 2 as in some way a "less restrictive" version of section 3. Both powers must be rescinded when no longer clinically appropriate, and most section 3 detentions are less than one month in duration. The equation of less formality and less restriction is generally erroneous (see 8.42 below) and ignores the important safeguards provided by the criteria for detention.

(iii) The safeguards and entitlements of detention under section 3 can create perverse incentives against its use. In particular, patients detained under section 3 have a statutory right to aftercare under section 117 that is denied to patients detained under section 2, and Nearest Relatives have a right to object to admission under section 3. It is important that professionals are careful not to determine which power is appropriate according to interests other than those of the patient.

(iv) We accept that patients who are known to services may yet require detention for assessment if, for example, the degree of their disorder is not clear at the time of admission[177]. However, if individual patients are repeatedly detained under section 2 powers over any period of time, this would suggest that the power is being ill-used and the patient's health needs ill-served. Similarly, when a patient who has had previous contact with services is detained under section 2, it is useful to check whether that patient was receiving adequate support prior to detention.

8.33 The latest edition of the *Mental Health Act Manual* suggests that Parliament intended section 2 of the 1983 Act to be the single point of admission to civil detention, excepting emergencies[178]. In part this argument suggests that the Code of Practice is wrong to advise against using section 2 simply because detention is not expected to last more than 28 days, and that the Commission is therefore incorrect to object to the use of section 2 as a short-term alternative treatment power to section 3. We are not aware of any direct evidence supporting this claim regarding Parliament's intention, and therefore advise practitioners to follow the Code of Practice as the extant Government guidance on the issue. Whilst the Commission does not accept the Mental Health Act Manual's arguments at para 1-036, we commend to practitioners its discussion of what may constitute knowledge of a patient sufficient to admit under section 3 as a useful basis upon which to consider their own practice.

8.34 We are pleased that the proposals for the next Mental Health Act suggest a single point of entry into civil compulsion for all patients, equivalent in many ways to the current section 2 powers. We suggested such a model (based upon other UK mental health legislation) in 1993, and have argued for such a change in our submissions on the reform of the 1983

---

[177] see Mental Health Act Commission (1998) *The Threshold for Admission and the Relapsing Patient.* Available from www.mhac.trent.nhs.uk.

[178] Jones, R (2003) *Mental Health Act Manual*, eighth edition London: Sweet & Maxwell para 1-036

Act[179]. Whilst we accept that there are difficulties of interpretation and implementation with the current law, we do not advise practitioners to attempt to resolve these by transposing proposed legislative structures onto existing law. It would be helpful for the Department of Health to confirm or update its guidance in the Code of Practice to provide certainty to practitioners.

> **Recommendation 19:** The Department of Health is asked to confirm or update its guidance at chapter 5 of the Mental Health Act Code of Practice in the light of the above.

Assessment powers not renewable

8.35   Section 2(4) provides an intentional limitation on the duration of detentions for assessment by effectively preventing the 'renewal' of section 2 powers. As such, detention under the Act can only be continued at the end of a section 2 through the use of section 3 powers.

8.36   Some practitioners have raised questions about this, particularly in relation to patients whose diagnoses remain unclear at the end of the 28 days of a section 2. Some patients' presentations can involve indistinct mixtures of diagnostic categories, which may be complicated by substance misuse. Practitioners have found themselves with no option but to argue for continued detention under section 3 as the only way to keep such patients in receipt of care and treatment, even though the patient's assessment continues without material change under the new power. In such circumstances, medical recommendations appear to have been completed upon a balance of probabilities, with doctors stating in good faith that they are of the opinion that a certain diagnostic category applies, even if they do not hold this opinion with absolute certainty. The diagnostic categories may be subsequently re-classified during the course of the detention.

8.37   The law looks set to confront such practices in two ways:

(i) *B v Ashworth Hospital Authority* (2003) (see Chapter 3.40 *et seq* above) has made the question of a patient's diagnostic category much more important, by limiting compulsory treatment (including nursing care, bed allocation, etc) to that which is appropriate in the treatment of the diagnostic category under which the patient is detained. We hope that case law subsequent to this ruling will not set artificial boundaries as to what is appropriate treatment for specific diagnostic categories, but it seems likely that challenges seeking such restriction will follow.

(ii) Although diagnostic categories are likely to be irrelevant to the conditions of compulsion under the next Mental Health Act, which may rely only on the generic term "mental disorder", it seems possible that some degree of uncertainty as to a patient's true condition at 28 days could provide an insurmountable obstacle to a Tribunal's approval

---

[179] Mental Health Act Commission (1993) *Memorandum to the Secretary of State for Health on the Mental Health Act 1983*, reprinted at appendix 16 of MHAC (1993) *Fifth Biennial Report 1991-3*. London: Stationery Office; MHAC (1999) *Submission to the Mental Health Legislation Review Team*; MHAC (1999) *The Mental Health Act Commission Response to the Green Paper Proposals on the Reform of the Mental Health Act 1983*; (2002) *The Mental Health Act Commission Response to the Draft Mental Health Bill Consultation.*

of further detention. This could be an example of where the burden of proof on the detaining authority to justify its action is onerous. In our view there needs to be a careful balancing of civil liberties concerns against the possibility that legal technicalities may cast patients out of services' reach. Government should attend to this balance when considering Tribunal regulations under future legislation.

Re-applying for detention after MHRT discharge

8.38   In the *Brandenburg* case (2001)[180], the Court of Appeal held that a patient can be re-detained soon after his discharge by MHRT, but that the ASW should take account of the decision of the MHRT when deciding whether to make an application. The Tribunal decision would usually be conclusive where re-detention was proposed in a matter of days following discharge. Unless such an application for re-detention can be justified by either a change of circumstance from that pertaining at the time of the Tribunal decision, or information unknown to the Tribunal, the courts would be likely to find it unlawful on grounds of irrationality on an application for judicial review.

8.39   Both the *Brandenburg* case and the subsequent case of *R (on the application of H) v Oxfordshire Mental Healthcare NHS Trust* [2002] involved Tribunal decisions to defer discharge pending the making of certain arrangements. In the first case, the rationale for re-detention was deterioration in the patient's mental state. In the second, the rationale was at least in part due to a failure to identify suitable arrangements to meet the Tribunal's conditions, although here too there was deterioration in the patients' mental state and behaviour, alongside difficulties in obtaining the patient's co-operation in discharge arrangements.

8.40   *Brandenburg* does not provide a precedent for authorities to overrule Tribunal decisions to discharge patients, even where they view such decisions as perverse. The Court of Appeal ruled in another case[181] that the proper procedure for authorities in such circumstances is to apply to the Administrative Court for judicial review and a stay of the Tribunal decision[182].

Emergency admissions (section 4)

8.41   Section 4 of the 1983 Act allows for emergency admission of a patient to hospital based upon a single medical recommendation in situations where there is no time to get the second medical recommendation required by sections 2 or 3. Since 1983 we have sought to ensure that procedures under section 4 are used only when there is a genuine emergency and not for administrative convenience. We have raised this matter on visits and in past Biennial Reports[183].

---

[180] *R v East London and City Mental Health NHS Trust ex p Brandenburg* [2001].

[181] *R (on the application of H) v Ashworth Hospital Authority; R (on the application of Ashworth Hospital Authority) v Mental Health Review Tribunal for West Midlands and North West Region* [2002] EWCA Civ 923

[182] see Jones (2003) *Mental Health Act Manual*, eighth edition. London: Sweet & Maxwell , 1-049, page 32 for details.

[183] see, for example, Mental Health Act Commission (1995) *Sixth Biennial Report 1993-5*, London: Stationery Office. Chapters 3.1 & p149, Chapter 11;

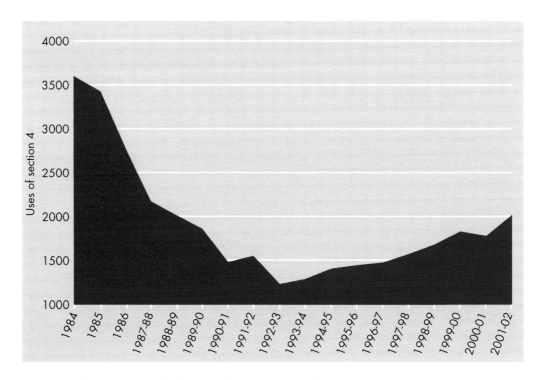

Fig 9: Use of section 4, NHS facilities, England, 1984-2003[184]

8.42 At one time, prior to the 1983 Act, emergency admission became the most common mode of entry into psychiatric compulsion. A Government enquiry in 1966 found a widely held belief that the relative lack of formality was more "humane" than admission powers subject to greater safeguards. As shown at Figure 9 above, the first ten years of the 1983 Act saw a rapid decline in the number of emergency admissions "largely due to pressure from the Mental Health Act Commission" [185]. It is clear, however, that the number of uses of emergency admission is again on the rise.

8.43 In our experience, practitioners today are not likely to prefer section 4 under the erroneous belief that it is the least restrictive option for patients, as there is a wider recognition of the importance of the formal safeguards for patients of the admission procedures under sections 2 and 3. There are many possible reasons for the increase in the use of section 4. It may be that there are simply more genuine psychiatric emergencies, where patients are being brought into hospital at a time of acute crisis at the last possible moment. If this is the case, it may point to failures in community support, outreach and early identification of need, or may simply be a reflection of understandable attempts by professionals to sustain patients in community settings for a little longer than resources or the patients' condition finally permits. It may also indicate that potential service users are reluctant to seek help due to fear of coercion or dislike of services. However, our experience suggests that the use of section 4 is as likely to be determined by difficulties in accessing a second doctor, leading to situations where section 4 admission is the best available option in the interests of the patient (see also 8.69 below).

---

[184] Data sources: as for Figure 6 above (note 173).

[185] Jones R (2003) *Mental Health Act Manual*, eighth edition. London: Sweet & Maxwell para 1-063

Section 5 holding powers

8.44   From 1997 we have expressed concern in our Biennial Reports at the high number of patients who agree to enter hospital on an informal basis but become subject to formal detention during their stay. From around this time the rate of increase in such use of the Act has appeared to slow from its dramatic rise in previous years. Figure 10 shows this in relation to the use of the holding powers of section 5. Figure 6 (8.25) above demonstrates a similar pattern for all changes from informal status, including those patients who move directly from informal status to detention under section 2 or 3. However, whilst the rise in uses may have slowed, the numbers of patients involved remains high.

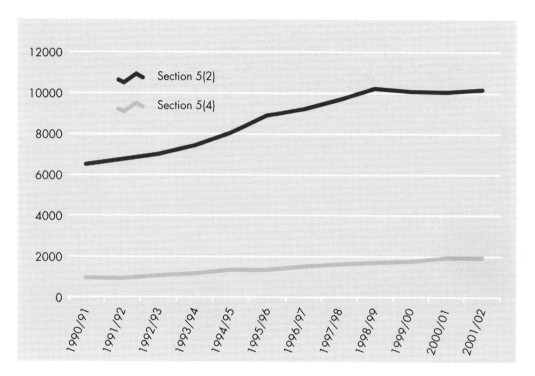

Fig 10: Uses of section 5(2) & 5(4), England, 1990-2002

data sources: as for Figure 6 above (see footnote 173)

8.45   In our last Biennial Report we suggested that the high levels of use in holding powers *may* be a result of clinicians' efforts to allow informal admission wherever possible, in accordance with the principles of the Code of Practice requiring treatment in the least restrictive manner possible, even where they suspect that this may result, eventually, in the use of compulsory powers. We noted the more generally accepted explanation, which is that many psychiatric wards have become places where even those who initially enter voluntarily have to be coerced to stay[186].

8.46   Work undertaken by the Royal College of Psychiatrists' Research Unit at the instigation of the Department of Health has suggested that there may be a lower working threshold for admission to compulsion in relation to those patients who are made subject to formal powers when already informally resident in hospital[187]. This is because:

---

[186] see Mental Health Act Commission (2001) *Ninth Biennial Report 1999-01*. London: Stationery Office Chapter 2.37 - 2.40.

[187] Bindman J, Thornicroft G & Tighe J (2000) *A study of the use of the MHA 1983 in eight sites (a report on Module B to the Department of Health)*. London, Royal College of Psychiatrists Research Unit

∗ In the case of section 5 holding powers, temporary detention may be achieved with only one medical recommendation, rather than the two required for sections 2 or 3; and

∗ Where patients move directly from informal inpatient status to detention under sections 2 or 3, staff already feel a sense of responsibility for them and for their case management[188]. This may make such staff more willing to consider the use of formal compulsion than if such compulsion would result in the patient's physical admission to hospital from the community.

8.47 Just over a third of patients made subject to doctors' holding powers under section 5(2) are returned to informal status within the 72-hour period that the power lasts (see Figure 11 below). Patients who are assessed as requiring formal detention in hospital whilst held under section 5(2) are slightly more likely to be detained under section 3 than section 2. This preference for using section 3 is a reversal of trends apparent before the mid-1990s. It may indicate that patients being held under this power are now better known to services (which suggests that they may have been inpatients for some time or admitted on previous occasions), although it could simply reflect changing patterns in the use of sections 2 and 3 (see 8.31 and Figure 8 above).

8.48 It is important that assessments are undertaken a soon as possible following the instigation of a holding power, to avoid patients being held under this power any longer than is necessary regardless of whether they are to return to informal status or detained further under the Act. It is also important that the expiry date and time of holding powers is accurately recorded in patients notes: in half of 134 episodes of section 5(2) usage examined on Commission visits over 2001/02, no such record could be found[189].

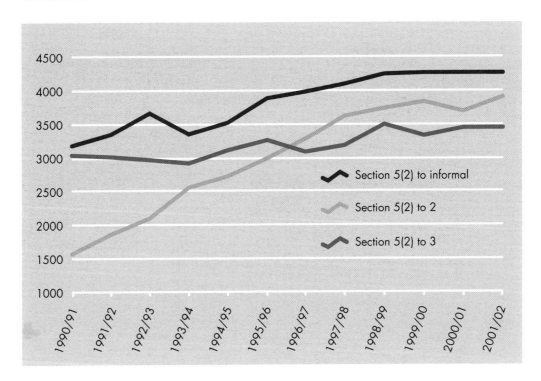

Fig 11: Outcomes of the use of section 5(2), England, 1990 – 2002[190]

---

[188] see Peay, J (2003) Decisions and Dilemmas Oxford, Hart Publishing p128

[189] CVQ data from 2002/03: 68 of 134 available records showed no diary entry or entry in patients' notes detailing date and time of expiry of sections 5(2). See chapter 19.11(c) for discussion of the CVQ exercise.

[190] Data: source: as for fig 10 above.

8.49 Patients and practitioners often express concern that holding powers are kept in reserve over informal patients, for instance as an implied or explicit threat should they attempt to discharge themselves or even just leave the ward. In some circumstances, particularly when a patient who has reluctantly consented to enter hospital would otherwise have met criteria for detention, the implicit threat of detention cannot be avoided. However, practitioners should guard against making explicit threats of using compulsory powers as a default option, which amounts to 'de facto' detention without safeguards. If a patient's consent to admission fluctuates or is given only under explicit threats of compulsion, assessment for formal detention should be considered.

8.50 In our Ninth Biennial Report we recommended that all hospitals should undertake routine collation of detailed statistics on the use of section 5(2), including the time taken to complete assessments whilst the patient is being held. Figure 12 below shows self-assessments of roughly a quarter of all hospitals in England and Wales on this issue. Although this group is self-selecting, as returns were completed on a voluntary basis, it shows encouraging uptake of our recommendation (indicated by both amber and green returns).

Recommendation 20: Future mental health legislation should require recording and monitoring of uses of holding powers initiated by medical staff, using statutory forms to ensure uniformity of data collection and practice.

Use of section 5(2)								
	N/A		Red		Amber		Green	
	n.	%	n	%	n	%	n	%
Are written policies available, understood and followed in practice ?	7	9.7	4	5.6	9	12.5	52	72.2
Is the staff complement adequate in number and training to implement policy ?	7	9.7	0	0	21	29.2	44	61.1
Are there at least annual in-house reviews with Board reporting ?	10	13.9	5	6.9	18	25	39	54.2
Is there on-going audit leading to remedial action on issues raised ?	8	11.1	4	5.6	22	30.6	38	52.8

Fig 12: Self-assessments of 72 hospitals/Trusts in relation to progress in implementing Commission Ninth Biennial Report Recommendation 14

Sections 135 and 136

8.51 Figure 13 below shows the numbers of places of safety detentions in English hospitals in 2001-02. These statistics do not include such detentions in police stations and are therefore substantially incomplete. We consider it to be a serious lack in mental health statistics that there are no total figures available for the uses of these powers. The available statistics show that there are considerable more men than women made subject to the holding powers of sections 135 and 136, and suggest that nine out of ten uses of the power are initiated from a public place (i.e. using section 136 powers), rather than by warrant under section 135 to enter private premises.

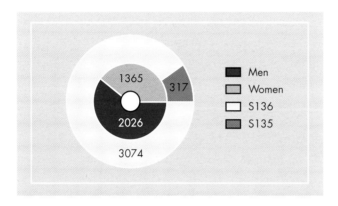

Fig 13: Place of safety detentions in hospitals, England 2001-2[191].

Recommendation 21: Future mental health legislation should require recording and monitoring of uses of holding powers initiated by social services with police involvement, using statutory forms to ensure uniformity of data collection and practice.

Requirements for warrant applications under Section 135

8.52   It would seem that there is increasing confusion over the requirements of Police and Criminal Evidence Act 1984 in relation to warrants under section 135 of the Mental Health Act 1983. It has been widely assumed that the requirements of PACE are applicable to section 135 warrants, given that that section 15(1) of PACE extends those requirements to warrants issued to a constable under *any* legislation. However, PACE goes on to assume that such warrants are *applied for* by constables, whereas Mental Health Act Section 135 warrants, although providing authority for constables to enter premises, are nevertheless applied for by social workers. The current edition of the *Mental Health Act Manual* raises this problem and submits, with the support of the Home Office, that the better interpretation of PACE is that it nevertheless extends to section 135 warrants[192]. As such the raft of requirements applicable under PACE (such as that a warrant application is made *ex parte* and in writing, that it can authorise entry once only, shall expire after one month, etc) would be relevant when applying for and executing warrants under section 135. The Commission has always supported this view.

8.53   This view appears to have been challenged in the approach taken by the Court of Appeal in *Ward v Commissioner for the Metropolitan Police and Epsom & St Helier NHS Trust* [2003].

---

[191] Source: Department of Health (2003) *Inpatients Formally Detained in Hospitals under the MHA 1983 and Other Legislation; NHS Trusts, Primary Care Trusts, High Security Psychiatric Hospitals and Private Facilities: 2001-02.* London: DH.

[192] Jones, R (2003) *Mental Health Act Manual,* eighth edition. London: Sweet & Maxwell 1-1183.

The court found that a warrant form provided under section 135 had "a number of features which were clearly referable to other statutory regimes, in particular the regime relating to search warrants under sections 15 and 16 of the Police and Criminal Evidence Act 1984" and was thus "not entirely appropriate to the relevant statutory provisions" (paragraph 11). The court therefore proceeded on the assumption that sections 15 and 16 of PACE had no relevance to section 135 of the Mental Health Act 1983.

8.54   This ruling, which may yet be appealed, may not change practice dramatically. The court allowed that a magistrate was entitled to make such conditions as to the execution of the warrant as he or she saw fit: "any condition which can sensibly relate to the execution of a warrant in a way which protects the interests of the person liable to be removed whilst furthering the object of the grant of the warrant, may be imposed, if a magistrate considers it appropriate in a particular case to do so" (paragraph 15). By extension, it seems possible that magistrates may be able to impose requirements relating to applications for warrants that mirror PACE requirements. But notwithstanding the practical effects of the judgment, it would appear to challenge widely held assumptions about the requirements of law for the operation of section 135.

8.55   Over this reporting period, and prior to the *Ward* ruling discussed above, there has been confusion over the actual requirements of PACE as they were assumed to relate to section 135 warrants. A misunderstanding over actual requirements of PACE section 15(3) and the Human Rights Act 1998 reportedly alarmed some magistrates into insisting that persons made subject to warrants under Section 135(1) or (2) must be given notice of the application. This Commission received a number of requests for advice on this issue from alarmed social workers, who thought that such notification would undermine the purpose of such a warrant by driving its subject away. The Commission Policy Unit was was able to provide a view that this appeared to be a misunderstanding of PACE requirements, given that section 15(3) of PACE does not require notice to be given to the subject of any application for a warrant. In the Commission's understanding, section 15(3) of PACE simply states that the application should be made *ex parte* and be supported by an "information in writing" (i.e. a statement of the power under which the application is made and the grounds for the application, identifying as far as possible the premises to be searched and the object of the search). Although, following *Ward*, magistrates may impose such conditions as they see fit to the execution of warrants, the Commission doubts that providing as a condition of issue of the warrant that advance notice of it be given to its subject would be seen in many circumstances as 'sensibly relating to its execution' or 'furthering the object of its granting'.

8.56   Especially as the draft Mental Health Bill of 2002 suggests that the next Act will retain a power similar in drafting and effect to that of the current section 135 (see 8.58 below), it would be helpful for Government to provide an authoritative view on the requirements under section 135, PACE and the Human Rights Act on applicants for warrants to take or retake patients.

In 43 local authorities, police required ASWs to complete a risk assessment prior to attending. Twenty-nine police forces did not accept social services' risk assessments but required ASWs to complete a police risk assessment. Many of these would not accept verbal assessments and required the assessment to be faxed or delivered to the police station. Given that police usually assess different aspects of risk it would make sense for ASWs to be offered training on what police need when assessing risk.

Good practice example

In Newham the ASWs use a risk assessment form that has been jointly devised with police.

Attending Assessments

In 32 local authorities, police had not attended when asked to by an ASW. The reasons given were mixed. Staff shortages, availability, priority, timing of assessments and geographical distance appear to be the main problems. Most of the 32 local authorities recognised that police would not come out at hand-over time. However, from Commission visits to local authorities it appears that ASWs do not always take this into consideration when planning assessments.

The Commission has heard anecdotal accounts of at least one police force having notified social services that they would not be available for section 135 call-outs due to the pressure of anti-terrorist duties after September 2001.

Most of the areas where police required a completed risk assessment prior to going out also asked for at least 24 hours notice. ASWs were expected to use 999 if the situation could not wait. One anonymous responder told of police not responding to repeated 999 calls, leaving ASWs and other professionals in dangerous situations. In some local authorities (Luton, Camden, Westminster, Haringey, West London Mental Health Trust, Oxleas) police require a substantial level of risk before they will respond to a request for assistance. This can lead to assessments being carried out without adequate backup.

Good practice example

In Hackney there is a dedicated police mental health team which responds to requests from ASWs

Local authority liaison with the police (continued)

In five local authorities police required a section 135(1) warrant before they would attend an assessment. This has resulted in ASWs applying for warrants at a lower threshold than would be normal in order to secure police attendance. In Coventry, Camden and an anonymous local authority, police have erroneously stated to social services that ASWs have the power of a police constable under Section 135, so that police presence is not required. This is an incorrect reading of section 135, which only permits a constable to enter premises by force if necessary and remove a person.

Good practice example

In Newham, an enhanced Public Protection Unit will respond to requests from ASWs. This is hoped to aid in developing levels of knowledge and expertise, and fostering good working relationships.

Some police forces appear to show insufficient flexibility of response when attending assessments. The Commission has heard of police units attending in number and in full riot gear, when this has been considered inappropriate by social services. Some police forces use videoing equipment at such incidents. Services should beware of overzealous responses, which can greatly increase patients' distress, social isolation and later rehabilitative problems.

Frail elderly patients

Twenty-two local authorities said that sometimes police and ambulance services would refuse to help in the conveyance of a frail elderly person who refuses admission to hospital. In some cases ASWs had been unable to persuade police to attend, even though the patient required detention in hospital and was extremely at risk in the community.

Some respondees said that force was never used, as the patient usually responded to a policeman's status. On occasion ASWs have found that the ambulance crew can be more helpful than police, others report that the presence of a doctor or nurse is helpful.

Conclusions

There is a need to ensure that ASWs understand police requirements for risk assessments and the way in which these can differ from social services' assessments. Ideally, joint policies should establish mutually acceptable assessment criteria.

In some, mainly urban, areas there appear to be problems in persuading police to attend assessments. The causes appear to be police staffing levels and other demands on police time. ASWs need to know when police in their area are unlikely to be available to assist with Mental Health Act assessments.

In a few areas, police appear to be re-interpreting the Mental Health Act and the Code of Practice in order to justify their difficulty in responding to requests for assistance from ASWs. As a result some vulnerable people are being left at risk in the community. There is a need for joint agreements and more creative ways of managing these difficulties.

Medical recommendations for detention under sections 2 and 3

8.63   The Act requires that applications for detention under sections 2 or 3 shall be supported by two medical recommendations, one of which must be from a doctor approved "as having special experience in the diagnosis or treatment of mental disorder". The Act requires that at least one of the medical recommendations shall, if practicable, be given by a doctor who has "previous acquaintance" with the patient. Chapter 2 of the Code of Practice provides guidance on the assessment procedure.

Previous acquaintance in medical recommendations

8.64 The Code of Practice states that, unless there are exceptional circumstances, the second recommendation for an admission under the Act should be provided by a doctor whose "previous acquaintance" with the patient amounts to knowing the patient personally in a professional capacity[196]. The Code even appears to require that this should be the case where the section 12 approved doctor providing the other recommendation also has 'previous acquaintance' with the patient. In this way the Code attempts to preserve the Act's apparent intention of ensuring that a patient's General Practitioner is involved in any decision over the use of its powers to detain that patient in hospital.

8.65 The Code's expectation is increasingly difficult to fulfill, due to the changing patterns of primary care provision, where patients are frequently registered with GP practices rather than a particular doctor and 'out of hours' services are contracted to deal with emergencies when surgeries are closed. The Department of Health informed the Commission that 'previous acquaintance' is not provided simply by having access to a patient's records[197], but this advice must be read in the light of *A.R. (by her litigation friend J.T.) v Bronglais Hospital Pembrokeshire and Derwen NHS Trust* [2001], in which Scott Baker J. held that the Code's conflation of previous acquaintance and personal knowledge does not reflect the true legal position. His Lordship held that the requirement of section 12(2) over "previous acquaintance" means that the doctor should have "some previous knowledge of the patient and must not be coming to him or her cold, as it were [but that] there is no indication as to the extent of the previous acquaintance that is necessary" so that the meaning of the phrase 'previous acquaintance' would "have to be interpreted according to the circumstances of the particular case". The Court allowed that a doctor who had attended a previous case-conference, and had scanned through the medical notes and met the patient briefly immediately before an assessment, did have 'previous acquaintance" with the patient.

8.66 The Commission continues to encourage services to have regard to the Code's advice on the matter of 'previous acquaintance' as good practice guidance, notwithstanding the above clarification of the law. Where it is not practicable to involve a doctor who has genuine 'previous acquaintance' of a patient, ASWs should perhaps seek to follow the Code in locating a second doctor who is approved under section 12, rather than colluding with the manufacture of previous acquaintance to little purpose.

8.67 In their examination of detention documentation on Commission visits during this reporting period, Commissioners found that neither doctor had 'previous acquaintance' with the patient in 28% of section 2 papers, and 8% of section 3 papers examined and available for analysis[198].

Section 12 doctors

8.68 In December 2002 the Department of Health issued guidance clarifying that responsibilities for the approval of doctors under section 12(2) of the 1983 Act had fallen, from October of

---

[196] Mental Health Act Code of Practice, Chapter 2.29. This is not a legal requirement, however: see Chapter 8.65-66 above.

[197] Mental Health Act Commission (1995) *Sixth Biennial Report 1993-5*, London: Stationery Office, Chapter 8.1

[198] CVQ data from 2002-03: percentages relate to 65 of 233 section 2 detentions and 124 of 1,655 section 3 detentions. See Chapter 19.11(c) below for discussion of the CVQ exercise.

that year, to the 28 new Strategic Health Authorities that replaced the health authorities previously responsible[199]. Arrangements set in place for health authority approval (including funding arrangements) could nevertheless carry on basically unchanged. The consortia arrangements whereby certain health authorities took on the responsibility for a number of authorities have also continued in many instances. Although Primary Care Trusts have no responsibilities for the approval of doctors under section 12(2), they are held accountable for the maintenance of lists of available doctors who are so appointed. The Departmental guidance reminded PCTs that social services and other agencies, including the police, require access to the lists of available approved doctors.

8.69   Practitioners, particularly Approved Social Workers who are responsible for co-ordinating Mental Health Act assessments, frequently express their concern at the difficulty in locating available section 12 approved doctors. It is likely that locating available medical practitioners will always be a challenge, but it does seem as though there is a great shortage of such doctors in some regions of England and Wales. Our Ninth Biennial Report listed suggested measures for the Department of Health to consider, which we have summarised at Figure 14 below.

Suggested actions to address shortages of section 12 approved doctors

* Inclusion of a clause in the contract of consultant psychiatrists requiring them to seek section 12 approval.

* Ensuring that all medical students involved in training in psychiatry are made aware of the need for and importance of more section 12 doctors.

* Making entry requirements for approval more flexible so that GPs who can demonstrate that they have sufficient knowledge and experience in treating mental disorder are eligible to apply.

* Making section 12 approval training available to any interested GP without committing them to become approved.

* Encouraging Primary Care Trusts to try to increase the number of their GPs seeking section 12 approval.

* Encouraging Primary Care Trusts to require co-operatives providing out-of-hours services in their area to guarantee the availability of at least one section 12 approved doctor at all times.

* Streamlining payment systems to ensure prompt payment of fees.

* Inviting Chief Constables to require forensic medical examiners to become approved.

Fig 14: Suggested actions to address shortages of section 12 approved doctors[200]

Recommendation 24: The Commission urges Government to ensure that action to increase availability of section 12 approved doctors is undertaken by appropriate authorities.

Monitoring Mental Health Act Assessments

8.70   The remit of the Mental Health Act Commission is restricted to patients who are detained under the 1983 Act and therefore, for example, we would be unable to undertake investigation

---

[199] Department of Health (2002) *Arrangements for approving doctors under section 12(2) of the Mental Health Act 1983 post April 1 2002.* www.doh.gov.uk/mentalhealth/approvingdoctors.htm. See Code of Practice Chapter 2.40 for the duties of Health Authorities in regard to section 12(2).

[200] Adapted from Mental Health Act Commission (2001) *Ninth Biennial Report 1999-01,* London: Stationery Office, Ch 2.61.

of a complaint lodged by someone who had been subject to a Mental Health Act assessment without this leading to detention[201]. The Commission does not monitor Mental Health Act Assessments at present, although it does meet with social services authorities and takes great interest in their own arrangements in this respect. We believe that a future monitoring body should have explicit powers to monitor and investigate matters relating to assessments of the need to use compulsory powers, whether or not those assessments lead to the imposition of compulsion.

8.71   The Commission commends the Mental Health Act Monitoring System established by the University of Manchester Mental Health Social Work Research Unit. The monitoring system has been collecting data from anonymised standard returns from local authorities in the Northwest of England for over ten years. Data is recorded about the individuals assessed in terms of:

* gender;
* age;
* marital status;
* ethnicity;
* housing and living group;
* employment status;
* psychiatric diagnosis;
* alcohol and drug misuse;
* whether cases are known to services (including legal status at referral, whether CPA arrangements are already in place, etc);
* whether assessments are 'out of hours'; and
* what the outcome of the assessment is in terms of number and type of detentions.

8.72   Figures supplied to the Commission by the Research Unit show the following general demographic information for all nine authorities covered by their study between 1998 and 2002[202]. These figures therefore summarise over 13,000 Mental Health Act assessments.

* Whereas women make up 52% of the population of all nine authorities, men were the subject of 50.6% of all Mental Health Act assessments.

* Roughly half of all people assessed were single people; a further quarter were widowed, separated or divorced.

* White people formed 85.7% of all assessments, thus reflecting over-representation of other ethnic groups in some localities (see Chapter 16.12 *et seq* below on ethnicity and assessments)

* Less than a quarter (23%) of all assessments were of people living in owner-occupied accommodation. In each authority the proportion of persons living in owner-occupied accommodation who were assessed was consistently and markedly lower than the proportion of persons with such housing arrangements in the general population.

---

[201] Although section 120 provides the Secretary of State with a duty to monitor the use of the Act "relating to the detention of patients or to patients liable to be detained" the practical remit of the Commission as established at sections 120 and 121 restricts its monitoring role to patients who are or have been made subject to powers of the Act.

[202] Authorities covered are Bolton, Bury, Manchester, Rochdale, Salford, Stockport, Tameside, Warrington and Wigan.

* On average only 6.8% of assessments involved people with full or part-time employment. This proportion was consistent across the five years. Retired people accounted for 18.7% of the total; students for 2.4%.

* Two-thirds of assessments involved patients diagnosed with one of the psychoses; 9% involved persons diagnosed with depression. Only 10% of diagnoses were classed as unknown at the time of assessment.

* Two-thirds of assessments involved persons known to services. On average, 13.6% involved patients already detained under section 5; and around 5% patients held under section 136. The proportion of patients assessed whilst held under section 136, considered annually, has risen slightly from 4.9% in 1998 to 6.4% in 2002.

* In 1998, 34.2% of assessments were if persons receiving services under CPA; by 2002 this had risen to 41.1%.

* Consistently over the five years, roughly a quarter of assessments took place out of hours.

* The overall number of detentions has "levelled off" over the five years, reflecting national trends (see Figure 6, Chapter 8.25 above). The average proportion of detentions has remained consistent in this period: 44.7% for section 2; 47.3% for section 3; and 8% for section 4.

The role of social workers

8.73 The role of social workers in the care and treatment of psychiatric patients under compulsion has altered radically over the last half-century[203]. Responsibilities for arranging admission and aftercare of psychiatric patients have rested with social workers (as "mental welfare officers") from the establishment of the NHS in 1948, and became especially relevant with the abolition of judicial involvement in compulsory admissions by the Mental Health Act 1959. The 1957 Percy Commission's view that "no responsible mental welfare officer would lightly disregard or dissent from [a doctor's] advice" was reflected in the limited professional independence of social workers expected and, according to many accounts, provided under the 1959 Act. It was not until the passing of the 1983 Act that social work was given a powerful independent role in determining the suitability of compulsory admission.

8.74 Many social workers have expressed fears to the Commission that this role may be diminished under the next Mental Health Act. The combination in the draft legislative proposals of quasi-judicial certification of long-term compulsion and the diminution of the centrality of social workers' views could, indeed, give rise to concern that the history of mental health law in this respect is being re-enacted backwards.

8.75 Social workers who are approved under section 114 of the 1983 Act to make applications for the admission of patients undergo what is probably the most thorough training on the provisions of that Act currently available to any mental health professional. Social workers provide a safeguard against unnecessary use of compulsory powers by bringing a balancing, non-medical view of the best interests of the patient and the need to use the least restrictive option available to provide necessary care.

---

[203] see Hoggett B (1996) *Mental Health Law*, Fourth Edition, London: Sweet & Maxwell p52-3, whose presentation and arguments we follow in this paragraph.

8.76 The Commission is concerned that proposals to widen the ASW role to other professionals (such as community psychiatric nurses) under new legislation should not be allowed to diminish the non-medical contribution to decision-making over issues of compulsion[204]. It is essential that the highest degree of confidence is maintained in professionals' objectivity and fairness in taking decisions relating to the deprivation of liberties. The Commission is of the view that, to maintain such confidence, the decisions should be continue to be taken by a multi-disciplinary group of professionals. There is real danger that teams consisting of nursing staff and doctors will be perceived as operating in collusion or from a particular viewpoint without appropriate checks and balances. The Commission has also pointed to the important benefits to be had from ensuring social work involvement from the start of any episode of compulsion, particularly in respect of the timely initiation of aftercare arrangements. Furthermore, the process of compulsory admission can involve the police, ambulance services, GPs, locksmiths, general community liaison, and the protection of property: the co-ordination of which would seem best suited to a social work role[205].

> **Recommendation 25:** If the ASW role is to be widened to professionals other than social workers under new legislation, the potential loss of the particular social work perspective must be countered by stringent training requirements for the equivalent of ASW approval. Careful consideration must be given to ensuring the continuation of multi-disciplinary input to decision-making, including, for example, providing Tribunals and their medical advisers with a duty to consider multi-disciplinary views on patients' care and treatment in the course of their decision-making process.

8.77 There is already some blurring of responsibilities between Community Psychiatric Nurses and social workers in some services. The Commission has been contacted for advice on whether, for example, CPNs employed in Integrated Community Mental Health Trusts might take on some of the roles traditionally (but not legally) reserved for ASWs, such as submitting social circumstances reports for the purposes of MHRT hearings, or similar reports for managers' reviews. The Commission has advised that, in our view, there is no reason in law why a CPN might not submit such reports. However, we have expressed concern that CPNs may not be best placed to comment on all of the requirements for such reporting to MHRTs, which includes issues to do with patients' housing, financial and employment circumstances[206]. Where the completion of such a report by a CPN is resultant from a failure of the local authority to assign an ASW to the patient, it is suggested that Tribunals should remind authorities their obligations under the law and Government guidance, if necessary rejecting such reports as inadequate[207]. Although the Commission

---

[204] see also Mental Health Act Commission (2001) *Ninth Biennial Report 1999-01*, London: Stationery Office. Chapter 2.48; (2002) *The Mental Health Act Commission's Response to the Draft Mental Health Bill*, p 7, para xvii

[205] Mental Health Act Commission (2000) *The Mental Health Act Commission's Response to the Green Paper Proposals on the Reform of the Mental Health Act 1983.* Nottingham: MHAC.

[206] Mental Health Tribunal Rules 1983, Rule 6. The Commission commends the MHRT for preparing the guidance paper *Social Circumstances Report by Social Workers for Mental Health Review Tribunals*, July 2002, in relation to these requirements.

[207] see Eldergill, A (1997) *Metal Health Review Tribunals; Law and Practice.* London, Sweet & Maxwell p745-761, 784.

therefore takes the view that it is poor practice not to involve an ASW assigned to a patient's care in the production of social circumstances or other, similar reports, this should not prevent collaborative working between ASWs and other professionals where this is in the interest of both patients and professionals.

8.78   With the emergence of integrated care Trusts that take on both health and social service functions, issues have been raised over the appropriate employment status of ASWs. The 1983 Act states that ASWs will be 'officers' of a local social services authority (section 145(1)) and, in local government law, the term "officer" is used to denote a member of an authority's staff. It would therefore seem to be the case that social workers who are not employees of local social services authorities are technically ineligible for appointment as ASWs[208]. The issue is complicated further by the fact that a number of authorities have, possibly erroneously, approved agency-employed social workers as ASWs. Although a number of social workers have approached the Commission over this issue with concerns that these employment status issues may pertinent to the autonomy of ASWs, we take the view that the primary issue here is one of technical legality[209]. The Commission approached the Department of Health regarding this matter in 1999, inviting it to take a view and consider possible remedies to any problems caused by emerging employment structures. In particular, we suggested that the Department might consider whether it would be appropriate to seek amendment of the law to remove any technical difficulties in relation to the employment status of ASWs. If the Department decided against seeking such amendment, we urged it to ensure that guidance was issued to social service authorities explaining the requirements of the law. We regret that the Department has not taken up our suggestion.

8.79   The Commission has advised authorities contacting us in the meantime that they should seek their own legal guidance to ensure that their arrangements provide for the lawful approval of social workers to operate as ASWs under the 1983 Act. We are not aware of any argument counter to that which states that employees of bodies other than local social services may not be approved as ASWs under the 1983 Act, but also advise authorities that there appears to be reason why employees of local social service authorities might not be seconded to other agencies to fit with the new structures of NHS delivery.

> **Recommendation 26:** The Commission urges the Department of Health to readdress our request that it consider seeking amendment of the Mental Health Act 1983 section 145(1) to remove any technical difficulties in the employment status of ASWs that it considers immaterial to the propriety of their role, or else ensure that guidance is issued to social service authorities explaining the requirements of the law.

---

[207]   see Eldergill, A (1997) *Metal Health Review Tribunals; Law and Practice*. London, Sweet & Maxwell p745-761, 784.

[208]   see, for example, Jones R (2003) *Mental Health Act Manual*, eighth edition. London: Sweet & Maxwell. paras 1-1046 and 1-1233

[209]   The House of Lords debated at committee stage of the Mental Health (Amendment) Bill whether the law should preclude ASWs from making applications for admission to a hospital in which they work, but determined that this should be a matter of good practice rather than legislation (HL Vol 426, col 1167). As more than one hospital may be managed by an NHS Trust, and as not all Trust employees are necessarily employed at a particular hospital site, the Commission considers that it is still appropriate for potential conflicts of interest to be determined by professionals involved.

8.80 Some aspects of social work practice that may have been obscured by the ASW role under the 1983 Act may now be re-emerging. Traditionally, the role of social workers in hospitals had been concerned principally with the families of the mentally ill, but the 1959 Act refocused this social work contribution on the direct treatment situation of the patient. In the annual report of one hospital forty years ago, the social work department noted that the increasing rate of admissions and discharges strained social work resources and had led to neglect of the aspect of social work dealing with relatives, carers and other agencies[210]. Although, of course, resource pressures continue to challenge social services, in recent years the renewal of emphasis on involving relatives and carers in care-planning, and the importance of inter-agency working, have provided at least a policy context to ensure social work involvement with patients and carers from admission to compulsion through to aftercare arrangements (see Chapter 9 below). The Commission is fully supportive of the policy aims of the Care Programme Approach. It remains the case, however, that practice may not yet match policy aspirations. Commissioners visiting services frequently express concerns over timely social work involvement in care planning, particularly in relation to establishing arrangements for meeting the duties of section 117 in respect of aftercare arrangements for patients detained under sections 3 and 37.

Bed pressures and ward environments

8.81 In our Ninth Biennial Report, we dealt at length on the continuing pressures facing many hospitals in relation to bed of overcrowding. Our observations regarding the pressure on beds and their concomitant effects on the service's ability to deal with patients humanely and effectively remain valid. In one London hospital, shortly before this report went to press Commissioners recorded bed-occupancy figures of 200% (see Chapter 9.5 below). Concerns over the pressures on wards are not limited to large urban areas, however.

8.82 We note Government recognition of "the significant pressure on acute psychiatric beds, with services forced to maintain waiting lists, send people home on leave and place users in services outside their area" and the need for a whole-systems approach in tackling the problem[211]. We also recognise that the Department of Health's Policy Implementation Guidance seeks to address the problems of providing a therapeutic experience to patients under circumstances of overcrowding and pressures on services[212]. The Commission will continue to give high priority to monitoring the general conditions into which detained patients are compelled to receive treatment.

---

[210] Annual Report of the Psychiatric Social Work Department, Moorhaven Hospital, South Devon 1962/63. Quoted in Heimler E (1967) *Mental Illness and Social Work.* Middlesex: Penguin. p 67

[211] Department of Health (2002) *Cases For Change, Introduction.* National Institute for Mental Health England. P 6

[212] Department of Health (2002) *Mental Health Policy Implementation Guide: National Minimum Standards for General Adult Services in Psychiatric Intensive Care Units (PICU) and Low Secure Units;* Department of Health (2002) *Mental Health Policy Implementation Guide: Adult Acute Inpatient Care Provision*

9

The Use of the Act in Patients' Hospital Care

Detained patients and the Care Programme Approach

9.1   The Care Programme Approach has now been operative in England for more than a decade, and was updated in 2000[213]. It seeks to ensure that all mental health patients, their carers and the full range of agencies responsible for delivery of services are actively engaged in the decisions and activities relating to mental health treatment and care, and that patients do not lose contact with services. All inpatients subject to the CPA must:

* receive a thorough and systematic assessment of their health and social care needs;

* have in place an individualised, written care plan addressing those needs, which optimises engagement, anticipates or prevents crises and reduces risk;

* have a care-coordinator who will maintain contact with them and monitor the implementation of the care plan; and

* have their care regularly reviewed and modified or changed where necessary, culminating in a written aftercare plan upon discharge from hospital that, amongst other matters, specifies actions to be taken in a crisis.

9.2   The Commission has, over the course of its Biennial Reports, noted increasingly evidence of the effective use of the Care Programme Approach, alongside many examples of poor practice[214]. In our Ninth Biennial Report we highlighted the confluence of effective CPA practice and good practice in section 117 aftercare planning. We highlighted the need for CPA documentation to clearly identify those patients to whom section 117 applies. This continues to be important now that the House of Lords has confirmed that patients may not be charged for aftercare services provided under section 117 (see 9.62 below). Our Ninth Biennial Report also called for a systematised approach to risk management as an integral part of the application of the CPA to patients[215]. The IMHAP Policy Compendium, produced in conjunction with the Commission and published in 2002, outlines a policy for

---

[213]   Department of Health (2000) *Effective Care Co-ordination: Modernising the Care Programme Approach* London, Stationery Office.

[214]   Mental Health Act Commission (1991) *Fifth Biennial Report 1989-91* Chapter 14.2; (1993) *Sixth Biennial Report 1991-3*, Chapter 10.2; (1995) *Seventh Biennial Report 1993-5*, para 8.3; (1997) *Eighth Biennial Report 1997-9*, Chapter 5.48 - 5.68; (2001) *Ninth Biennial Report 1999-01*, Chapter 2.68-2.73. London: Stationery Office

[215]   Mental Health Act Commission (2001) *Ninth Biennial Report 1999-01*, London: Stationery Office paras 2.68-2.73, 4.62 - 4.63

aftercare planning under CPA, an outline risk assessment strategy and model forms for setting out a patient's care plan[216].

Risk assessment

9.3 The risks that need to be considered in any comprehensive risk assessment as a part of a patient's care plan must not be limited to risk behaviour shown by the patient in the past, but should extend to consideration of the risks of interventions designed to meet the patient's healthcare needs. Partly as a result of the polarisation of the debates over the draft Mental Health Bill of 2002, there is a danger of 'risk' being interpreted as relating only to potential harm that a patients might do to themselves or others, with no consideration being given to the harm that interventions might do to the patients they are designed to help. These risks encompass physical risks from, for example, control and restraint interventions or from the side-effects of medication or other treatments, to psychological or social risks, such as the alienation of a patient from services and from seeking help when needed, or the isolation of a patient within their home community through heavy-handed interventions.

> **Recommendation 27:** All authorities concerned with the implementation of powers of compulsion are reminded that the use of such powers entails a number of risks to *patients*, and that risk assessments should consider and balance such risks alongside the risks that patients may be deemed to pose to themselves or others.

Deaths of detained patients and others

9.4 In our Ninth Biennial Report we highlighted the following specific dangers to detained patients:

(a) **Ligature points enabling suicide attempts in hospital premises**

The Ninth Biennial Report highlighted our finding that a considerable proportion of suicides by 'hanging' were, in fact, probably due to strangulation[217]. It is insufficient for hospitals to remove or make unusable only those weight-bearing ligature points that are at a certain height from the ground. Potential ligature points provided by furniture and fittings, including low-level piping, need to be removed or securely 'boxed-in' to ensure a safe hospital environment. Commissioners continue to find and draw the attention of hospital managers to low-level ligature points in many different types of hospital setting. Staff should be trained in resuscitation techniques appropriate to strangulation.

(b) **Leave and absence without leave from hospital as opportunities for suicide**

In our Ninth Biennial Report we stated that one in five detained patient deaths occurs whilst a patient is on authorised leave from hospital. One third of deaths of detained patients by suicide occurred whilst the patient was absent from hospital without leave[218].

---

[216] Institute of Mental Health Act Practitioners (2002) *Mental Health Act 1983 Policy Compendium.* May 2002. pp36 & app.12. See Appendix E below for publication details.

[217] Mental Health Act Commission (2001) *Ninth Biennial Report*, London: Stationery Office Chapter 4.17 - 4.20, Rec. 35.

[218] see Mental Health Act Commission. (2001) *Ninth Biennial Report*, paras 4.23, 4.26 and Appendix B

Patients' care plans should pay particular attention to the risks of leave and absence without leave with regard to every individual patient (see 9.36 below).

9.5   Hospital managers should ensure that Mental Health Act Commission visit reports and other findings of outside organisations who visit their services are fed into their risk assessments:

* During this reporting period, the Commission attended a pre-inquest directions hearing in the case of an informal patient who had hanged himself from a ligature point identified in two consecutive Commission visit reports, but not effectively made safe by hospital managers, despite assurances to the Commission that the matter had been addressed. Following the suicide, and after a further assurance that ligature points had been identified and removed in a risk assessment, a visiting Commissioner identified several remaining ligature points and recommended that the risk-assessments be revisited.

* Commissioners had raised concerns about arrangements for intensive nursing of patients on a hospital ward that is sited over two floors. Although the Trust concurred with the Commission's concern that the ward was unsuited to its task, needing extensive renovation or closure and replacement with a purpose-designed environment, it took no substantive action stating that there were 'no ready answers'. Just over a year later, and despite the Commission repeating its concerns, a nurse who was alone with a particularly disturbed patient on one level of the ward was attacked and killed by that patient without being able to summon help.

* In a visit report issued as we go to press, Commissioners have alerted the hospital managers of one Trust to problems of serious overcrowding, with bed occupancies of up to 200%, low staff morale and the use of excessive force during control and restraint. The Commission has asked that senior Trust staff and service commissioners attend to our concerns urgently before there are serious injuries on the wards concerned.

Involving service users and carers at service level

9.6   As of September 2002, 40% of acute inpatient wards were reported to have a service user and staff forum at least once a week[219]. A further 47% were described as having some kind of user/staff forum at less frequent intervals, or to be establishing such a forum. The mechanisms for responding to service users and carers, as described by Local Implementation Teams, are set out at Figure 15, with an indication of the numbers of LITs that mention each mechanism expressed as a percentage of the total respondents. Almost a quarter of respondents failed to give any indication of mechanisms for recording or responding to service users' concerns and comments.

9.7   In the good practice example below we outline some of the ways in which Mersey Care NHS Trust, one of only three Trusts that provide mental health services from community care to high security care, seeks to involve users and carers at all levels of its organisation. We

---

[219] Data from responses to NIMHE Acute Inpatient Care Programme; LIT Stage IV Themed Review for Adult Mental Health Acute In-Patient Care. Sample size (Local implementation Teams) is 139 from a possible total of 160, although the sample number has been reduced to avoid duplications where LITs share provider Trusts. We understand that only four LITs failed to return questionnaires.

commend the Trust's approach, particularly in relation to the involvement of users in care-planning. If service-users are to be involved in mental health services at a stakeholder level, where they act as true partners in the development of services, their involvement must extend beyond post-facto 'customer-satisfaction' surveys[220].

Mechanisms for responding to service users as reported by Local Implementation Teams, Sept 2002

* NHS complaints procedure (32%)
* minuted staff/user forum meetings (29%)
* informal ward-level discussion and resolution (18%)
* advocacy, PALs or patients' councils (15%)
* suggestion box (5%)
* user survey by questionnaire (4%)
* care plans, ward notice board or 'Talkback' system (1%)

Fig 15: LITs' mechanisms for responding to service users
data source: see footnote 219

9.8   It is important that user-involvement is not marginalised as a matter concerned only with collective consultation. It is one of the guiding principles of the Mental Health Act Code of Practice that patients should be treated and cared for in such a way as to promote to the greatest practicable degree their self-determination and personal responsibility, consistent with their own needs and wishes (para 1.1). User-involvement should therefore reach right down into individual patients' care plans. This is central to considerations of consent to treatment and keeping patients therapeutically engaged with services. We discuss this in relation to consent to treatment at Chapter 10.2 *et seq* below.

Good Practice Example
Mersey Care NHS Trust: Involving Service Carers and Users

The Trust has established:

* a service user and carer on the Trust Board;
* a Board-level Director, Service Users and Carers to provide leadership;
* a network of Lead Officers across the Trust;
* a budget of £50,000;
* a policy on payments to service users and carers as equals;
* a Service User and Carer Forum;
* service user and carer involvement in staff recruitment and induction; and
* a plan, currently being implemented, to employ service users in the Trust.

---

[220] see Simpson, E..L. and House, A.O. (2003) *User and carer involvement in mental health services: from rhetoric to science.* British Journal of Psychiatry (2003) 183, 89-91; Simpson, E.L., House, A.O. & Barkham, M (2002) *A Guide to involving Users, Ex-users and Carers in Mental Health Service Planning, Delivery and Research: A Health Technology Approach.* Leeds: Academic Unit of Psychiatry and Behavioural Sciences, University of Leeds.

Service users and carers within adult mental health services have been involved with:

* a cultural sensitivity audit;

* a Sainsbury Acute Solutions initiative to improve the quality of inpatient environments;

* developing a family room in an inpatient unit in conjunction with Barnardo's Young Carers' Project;

* developing a therapeutic community day service for people with personality disorder; and

* planning the re-provision of the low secure service and a new learning disability service for people with Asperger's Syndrome.

All wards in the high secure services have established community meetings, operating to agreed standards, where policy issues and initiatives are debated and fed back to management. User forums, such as the Women's Service Forum are being established to allow patients to engage directly with service management structures.

Contact Lindsey Dyer, Director, Service Users and Carers, Mersey Care NHS Trust, Hamilton House, 24 Pall Mall, Liverpool L3 6AL. 0151 285 2000

Advocacy

9.9 From the survey discussed at 9.6 above, we know that, as of September 2002, 65% of adult acute inpatient wards are reported to have advocacy input at least on a weekly basis, with many reporting daily attendance of advocates. MIND is the most frequently cited provider of advocacy services. 21% of wards report no advocacy at all, and 14% limited or partially engaged advocacy services.

9.10 We welcome the Government's stated intention to introduce a statutory right of access to advocacy for patients subject to compulsory powers under the next Mental Health Act. In this reporting period the Commission has provided detailed input to the consultation on advocacy organized on the Government's behalf by Durham University[221]. Our full response to this consultation is available on our website[222].

9.11 The Commission welcomed the University report's attention to training, accreditation and supervision and to a paid service. We suggested that such a service be specifically identified as "Independent Mental Health Act Advocacy" (IMHAA) to stress its difference from traditional concepts and structures of advocacy, but also urge caution about over-extending agreed practices of advocacy. In particular, the Commission is concerned to maintain clear boundaries between advocacy and scrutiny by a monitoring body or inspectorate. It is important that advocates are not expected to perform functions at the direction of any party other than the patient, so as not to dilute their role. The Commission will also take great interest in proposals for advocacy in relation to patients who lack mental capacity to make their wishes known, or whose refusal to participate with advocates may be, or may be thought to be, a consequence of their mental state.

[221] Barnes, D & Brandon, T with Webb, T (2002) *Independent Specialist Advocacy in England and Wales: Recommendations for Good Practice.* University of Durham Centre for Applied Social Studies, June 2002. www.doh.gov.uk/mentalhealth/advocacy

[222] www.mhac.trent.nhs.uk

9.12 The Commission understands there to be widespread acceptance that it is unnecessary to agree a single model of advocacy or a 'one model fits all' approach. It is much more important to have appropriate advocacy wherever people are under compulsion. Our preferred way of achieving this is through a service specification with explicit principles and service outcomes built in, and sufficient resources to meet specific local needs. To this end we envisage roles and responsibilities at national level in England and Wales for:

* agreeing and allocating enough funding to commission adequate IMHAA services;

* ensuring that the IMHAA service is available across England and Wales, through monitoring provision (including the offering of and take-up of services for all patients under compulsion) and taking action to ensure that gaps are filled;

* high level monitoring of advocacy performance, including assessing patients' experience of advocacy services; and

* agreeing an advocacy code, service standards, accreditation standards and processes, and criteria for commissioning the service.

IMHAA services could be commissioned and performance-managed at regional level through service-level agreements. Current regional or sub-regional arrangements for Approved Social Workers could provide a model for training and accrediting advocates.

9.13 We discuss advocacy and future arrangements for monitoring the Mental Health Act at Chapter 20.18 below.

Providing information to patients

9.14 The de-institutionalisation of mental health services for detained patients and others (see Chapter 1.4 *et seq*) requires the free passage of information from the care team to the patient, and for the patient's voice to be heard within discussions on care and treatment. More than forty years ago, Goffman described as a characteristic of the total institution the boundaries to communication erected between staff and patients. In the total institution, information exchange from patient to treating doctor is limited, for example by nursing staff being required to act as mediators between the patients and the physician, ostensibly so that the latter is not 'swamped' by the treatment demands of the former. Just as importantly, in the total institution information about the staff's plans for patients are withheld on a number of pretexts, some of which are given medical glosses and some of which are just characteristic of the bureaucratic management of large blocks of people. Such exclusion gives staff a special basis of distance from and control over patients[223].

9.15 Most services would not see themselves reflected in the above description of institutional structures, and indeed most staff working within today's hospital environments do not seek and would resent the idea of a controlling distance between themselves and patients under their care. However, even though the 1983 Act sets legal requirements on the giving of basic information to patients admitted to hospital under its powers of compulsion, all too often these requirements are not met. The fault may be at an institutional level, in that no member of staff has been given responsibility for providing information and no mechanisms exist to check whether anyone has done so, rather than a reflection of individual staff attitudes, but the

---

[223] see Goffman, Erving (1961) *Asylums: Essays on the Social Situation of Mental Patients and Other Inmates.* Middlesex: Penguin, 1968 p19-20

result is the same exclusion of patients from participation in their care, reinforcing the institutionalism of compulsory treatment.

9.16 The duty to "take such steps as are practicable" to ensure that a patient has been given information about his or her legal situation and rights falls to the hospital managers (section 132). It will usually be appropriate for nursing staff to actually provide patients with the information required. This information is, insofar as it is relevant to a patient's individual circumstances:

* the powers of the hospital mangers, RMO and MHRT in relation to discharge;

* the consent to treatment provisions of the Act;

* the existence of the Code of Practice and Mental Health Act Commission; and

* the powers of the Act in relation to patients' correspondence.

In practice, the powers of the Act in relation to patients' correspondence are likely to be relevant only to detained patients who are resident in a High Security Hospital[224], although the Commission recommends that all patients are advised of how they can communicate with family and friends on admission under the Act.

9.17 Article 5 of the ECHR is almost certainly engaged in the performance of the duties under section 132. A failure to inform a patient of his or her rights, including the rights of appeal, could breach ECHR Article 5(4) by depriving a patient if the right to challenge the lawfulness of detention speedily. A failure to explain to a patient *why* he or she has been detained could breach Article 5(2) by depriving him or her of the reasons for detention[225].

9.18 Good practice is often noted where managers have ensured that there are robust recording mechanisms in relation to providing patients with information, and these records are subject to audit and ongoing monitoring. The Commission has recommended to all services that they adopt a locally standardised form for such records, which has space for recording: the name of the person giving the information:

* the date that the information was given;

* whether the patient understood the information;

* subsequent attempts to give the information; and

* the planned date for the next attempt[226].

A sample form for the recording of such information, and advice on establishing a policy on section 132, is given in the IMHAP Policy Compendium, produced in conjunction with the Commission[227].

---

[224] The only power provided by the Act in respect of the correspondence of patients who are detained in services other than High Security Hospitals is that which allows the addressee of any postal packets sent by a patient to ask the hospital managers to intercept and withhold such packets from the post (see section 134(1)(a), MHA 1983). In the Commission's view it is sufficient for this power to be explained if and when such circumstances arise.

[225] This is a requirement of the Code of Practice 14.5b, although not of section 132 of the Act itself, so that the 1983 Act may itself be in violation of the ECHR on this point. See Jones, R (2003) *Mental Health Act Manual*, eighth ed., para 1-1159.

[226] Mental Health Act Commission (2001) *Ninth Biennial Report*, London: Stationery Office. Recommendation 2.

[227] Institute of Mental Health Act Practitioners (2002) *Mental Health Act 1983 Policy Compendium*. May 2002. pp11 & app.3. See Appendix E below for publication details.

9.19   In the following examples, hospital managers have devised visiting arrangements to ensure that a number of the duties delegated by managers to hospital staff are being met, and to check on patients' welfare in a more general sense. Many services might benefit from similar arrangements.

Good Practice example: Bedfordshire and Luton Community NHS Trust
Patient Information Sheets and Hospital Managers' Visit Records

Bedfordshire & Luton Community NHS Trust have developed personalised information sheets to complement MHA leaflets on patients' rights. The local information sheets have spaces for the identification of the starting date of detention and names of the RMO, named nurse and keyworker.

Within a week of a patient's detention in the Trust, a hospital manager will visit the patient and also check detention documentation for evidence that;

* detention papers have been scrutinised by a delegated officer;
* the Nearest Relative has been informed of detention; and
* patients have received statutory information orally and in writing, and are aware of their rights.

The hospital manager can use the form to record comments or concerns, or to request a meeting with any professional involved in the patient's detention. The completed form is returned to the MHA Department.

Contact: Sylvia Jeffreys, MHA Manager, Bedfordshire & Luton Community NHS Trust, Mental Health Act Department, Orchard Unit, Calnwood Road, Luton LU4 OFBH Tel 01582 707601

Good Practice example: Priority Healthcare Wearside NHS Trust
Hospital Managers' Welfare Visits

The Trust's Hospital Managers Group has instigated 'welfare visits' to all patients detained within the Trust. The primary purpose of such visits is to enable the managers to fulfil the requirement of the Code of Practice para 2.2 that they "ensure that patients are detained only as the Act allows; that their treatment and care accord fully with its provisions, and that they are fully informed of and are supported in exercising their statutory rights". Visits also consider patients' general welfare, including the following issues:

* cultural and spiritual needs;
* dietary requirements;
* contact with relatives, advocates, social workers;
* exercise and recreation opportunities;
* privacy, dignity and safety (sleeping arrangements, bathroom facilities, access to quiet areas and smoke-free zones, problems with other patients' behaviour etc); and
* financial matters.

Visits take place 3 months after initial detention, six months after the first renewal and thereafter annually. Patients receive written notification of impending visits and are informed that relatives or carers may also attend. Visits are by two managers, one of whom must be a

Non-Executive Director or Associate Hospital Manager. A team including at least one woman will visit women patients. Discussions are usually in private and issues raised are discussed with staff where a patient consents to this. General matters raised by such visits are discussed at monthly Mental Health Act Managers' meetings and taken up in writing with the Trust Chief Executive by the Trust Chairman.

Contact: Office of Mrs C W Rickett, Chairman, Priority Healthcare Wearside NHS Trust, Cherry Knowle Hospital, Ryhope, Sunderland, SR2 0NB 0191 569 9409 cynthia.rickett@phw-tr.northy.nhs.uk

Patients' contact with their Responsible Medical Officers and other medical staff

9.20   The Department of Health publication *Adult Acute Inpatient Provision* (2002) recognised the dangers of "over-pressurised staff having difficulty maintaining a consistent therapeutic engagement with service users in inpatient settings".[228] One specific danger is that a service under stress will quickly jettison the less easily defined roles of medical staff, such as engaging meaningfully with patients about their treatment and consent, etc, which enable patients to fully participate in their treatment.

9.21   Over fourteen months from December 1999 to January 2001, Commissioners collected data on patients' contact with their Responsible Medical Officers (RMO). We have not previously published the findings, which are shown at Figure 16 below. Of 1,443 patients who had been detained for more than 28 days at the time of their meeting with Commissioners, 816 (57%) had seen their doctor within the last week. 209 of the remainder (14% of the total) had seen their doctor between 7 and 14 days previously, and 182 (13% of the total) had seen their doctor between a 14 and 28 days prior to their meeting with a Commissioner. This leaves a significant minority (236, or 16% of the total) who had no contact with their RMO in the 28 days prior to their meeting with a Commissioner.

9.22   Although other medical staff are more likely than the designated RMO to have significant day-to-day contact with patients, the RMO has a number of non-delegable responsibilities, particularly in relation to discharge, leave and consent to treatment, that makes his or her direct involvement in the patient's care of paramount importance, not least in terms of patients' perceptions of their care and treatment. Hospital managers should monitor patients' perceptions of their contact with their RMO and other medical staff and use monitoring results to ensure a patient-centred service.

Identifying the Responsible Medical Officer

9.23   Many services have difficulty in identifying the appropriate Responsible Medical Officer (RMO) for particular patients. The designation of RMO is important under the 1983 Act as it carries a number of powers and duties, not all of which may be delegated. Difficulties in deciding who is the RMO for particular patients can sometimes be caused by arrangements made to cover vacant consultant posts, which leads to uncertainties about who takes

---

[228] Department of Health (2002) *Mental Health Policy Implementation Guide: Adult Acute Inpatient Care Provision*

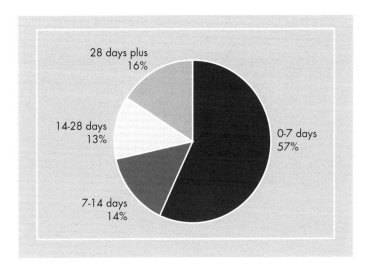

Fig 16: Patients' last contact with RMO prior to MHAC visit (see 9.21 above)

responsibility for particular patients' care. It is sometimes due to the fact that consultants who are nominally in charge of many patients' treatment seek to delegate responsibilities to more junior doctors who have more day-to-day contact with those patients.

9.24   The statutory definition of an RMO is simply "the registered medical practitioner in charge of the treatment of the patient" (section 34(1)(a)). Determining the identity of the RMO is therefore a question of fact: whoever is the registered medical practitioner in charge of the treatment is the RMO, and any doctor answerable to that medical practitioner is not.

9.25   Department of Health guidance now requires each acute adult inpatient ward to have a dedicated lead consultant psychiatrist[229]. This doctor would be the RMO for patients detained on that ward. It may that the reality of service organisation will hamper the meeting of this requirement. Some wards are 'shared' by a number of consultants, each of whose primary responsibilities rest in community practice. In such structures there cannot but be a number of RMOs operating on the same ward.

9.26   A similar problem may be encountered in Psychiatric Intensive Care Units (PICUs), into which patients may be moved for relatively short periods of their detention in hospital. It appears to be quite common practice for patients who are moved into PICUs to remain formally under the care of their consultant outside the PICU. In this way, many patients resident in a PICU will have an RMO who is not actively involved in their care on the ward. In part, this practice appears to be aimed at ensuring that a place remains for patients when they can leave the PICU for less acute forms of medical care. Similar arrangements have been operative in relation to transfers of patients between security levels with the NHS, or between NHS and the independent sector. We recommend that, as far as possible, formal transfers of RMO status should be a feature of all such patient movements, so that the consultant receiving the patient takes on full and acknowledged clinical responsibility for his or her care. Service protocols could be established where there is a need to ensure that patients can return to their previous placements when appropriate.

---

[229] Department of Health (2002) Mental Health Policy Implementation Guide: Adult Acute Inpatient Care Provision, p 32 -4

9.27 In some psychiatric services, the term "RMO" has been adopted as a generic title for any doctor in charge of any patient's treatment, whether or not that patient is subject to a part of the 1983 Act to which the term can be properly applied, and in some case even whether or not the patient is subject to the 1983 Act at all. The Commission is opposed to this inaccurate use of the term, which can cause confusion about patients' legal status and lead to assumptions being made about the powers available to professionals with regard to their treatment. We suggest that doctors in charge of informal patients' treatment are referred to simply as that patient's "consultant" or "treating clinician".

> **Recommendation 28:** The term "Responsible Medical Officer" should not be used to describe the doctor in charge of treating informal patients or patients detained under holding powers of the 1983 Act, as this can cause confusion over that doctor's legal powers over such patients.

9.28 We are frequently asked by patients and professionals for advice over patients' requests to change their Responsible Medical Officer. Patients who are made subject to compulsory powers may have had difficult past relationships with their doctors and may, for example, have experience of changing their GP. We advise patients and services that all patients have a right to request that their doctor is changed, but that patients who are subject to compulsory treatment given under the direction of a particular doctor cannot expect, of right, to remove themselves from that doctor's care upon request. We do, however, expect hospital managers to take such requests seriously, consider whether it is practicable to meet them, and provide the patient with a clear and reasoned response.

Patient activity and access to fresh air

9.29 In our Ninth Biennial Report, we underlined the concerns of the Department of Health's own Standing Nursing and Midwifery Committee that in-patient units were becoming more custodial in atmosphere, with service users feeling deprived of therapeutic activity, contact with professional staff and a sense of security[230]. Our Ninth Report:

* highlighted patients' requests for access to more recreational activities, including access to sports facilities, better reading matter, cooking or craft activities, drama or art therapy workshops, etc[231];

* drew attention to the link between boredom and frustration amongst patients and particular management problems arising from patient behaviour[232];

* suggested that hospital managers

  • ensure patients are aware of activities on offer through individual care-plan discussions and displayed notices, etc;

---

[230] Department of Health (1999) *Addressing Acute Concerns: Report by the Standing Nursing and Midwifery Committee.* London: Stationery Office. June 1999.

[231] Mental Health Act Commission (2001) *Ninth Biennial Report* 1999-2001. London: Stationery Office, para 3.25.

[232] *ibid*, paras 4.3, 4.33

- use monitoring and user-surveys to identify needs and opportunities; considering the use of voluntary and other agencies as well as existing contracted staff;

- employ or designate an activities co-ordinator[233]; and

* recommended that service commissioners and providers should agree specific standards for access to fresh air, recreational, educational and therapeutic activities, and monitor their availability and uptake taking account of patients' views[234].

9.30   We are pleased to find our concerns echoed in the Department of Health's *Mental Health Policy Implementation Guide: Adult Acute Inpatient Care Provision* (2002), which identifies the problem of a 'lack of "something to do", especially activity that is useful and meaningful to recovery' in acute inpatient services, and notes that too often in existing provision, potential activity areas are not made available in the evenings and at weekends and/or they are seen to be exclusively for weekday therapeutic activities[235]. We look forward to the effective implementation of this policy guidance and will continue to monitor patients' activities closely.

9.31   Figure 17 shows the limited progress, even amongst hospitals that responded to a voluntary self-assessment exercise, in relation to the implementation of the Commission's recommendations in relation to patient activity and access to fresh air. It is notable that over a quarter of reporting hospitals could point to no review or audit of patient recreational and therapeutic activities, or access to fresh air. The Commission will be pressing all services to adopt such monitoring in the next two-year period. The Commission's own observations of

Access to fresh air, recreational, educational and therapeutic activities	N/A		Red		Amber		Green	
	n.	%	n	%	n	%	n	%
Are written policies available, understood and followed in practice with adequate staff complement and training ?	1	1.4	13	18	28	38.9	30	41.7
Are there at least annual in-house reviews with Board reporting ?	3	4.2	19	26.4	22	30.5	28	38.9
Is there on-going audit leading to remedial action on issues raised ?	1	1.4	20	27.8	31	43	20	27.8

Fig 17: Self-assessments of 72 hospitals/Trusts in relation to progress in implementing Commission Ninth Biennial Report Recommendations 30 and 32[236]

---

[233]   *ibid*, recommendation 31

[234]   *ibid*, recommendations 30 & 32

[235]   Department of Health (2002) *Mental Health Policy Implementation Guide: Adult Acute Inpatient Care Provision* para 6.1.7

[236]   Based upon a voluntary (and therefore self-selecting) return of 72 self-assessment forms, representing approximately a quarter of all detaining hospitals in England and Wales. Recommendations 30 and 32 of the Ninth Biennial Report called for agreed and monitored standards between service commissioners and providers over access to fresh air, recreational and therapeutic activities,

recreational and therapeutic activities and access to fresh air in the High Security Hospitals is discussed at Chapter 12.46 *et seq* below.

9.32   We welcome the Government's setting of "access to fresh air and secure external space" for "all patients, including those who are acutely disturbed" as a minimum standard for low secure and Psychiatric Intensive Care Units[237] and its recognition that all acute "service users need to be able to leave the ward to attend activities elsewhere in the building and to access usable outdoor space"[238]. Strategic Health Authorities should seek to establish more detailed minimum requirements and monitor their attainment.

9.33   At the end of this reporting period (March 2003) most of England and Wales experienced unseasonably fine weather. The Commission was contacted by patients and advocates who were frustrated at the lack of access to outdoors offered to detained patients during this time: in some units patients had not been outside for over a week. Pressures on staffing levels were suggested as one major cause of this problem. Where patients' access to fresh air is determined by the availability of escorting staff, the Commission expects the staffing establishment of wards to take this into account. Denying patients access to fresh air is not only a denial of a basic rights but is also likely to be causative of a number of management problems that will, in turn, cause much greater pressures on staff and patients alike.

> **Recommendation 29:** Where patients' access to fresh air is determined by the availability of escorting staff, the Commission expects the staffing establishment of wards to take this into account.

Ground–leave

9.34   Many hospitals formalise arrangements to grant patients "ground parole" or "ground leave", enabling them to leave the ward area but remain within the grounds of the hospital. In law, formal leave under section 17 is very rarely required for this[239], and so it is not the case that, for instance, "ground-leave" may only be authorised by the RMO and not a member of nursing staff. Most services who operate "ground leave" recognise this fact in having separate forms and records for "ground-leave" and leave under section 17.

9.35   We have some concerns that arrangements for "ground-leave" may, under the guise of a culture of risk-assessment, be unduly restrictive of patients' movements within the facilities that detain them. In lower-security facilities, we would expect wards to be unlocked on a day-to-day basis and for patients to have free rein over the hospital site. This is not to say that patients' whereabouts cannot be recorded or that care-plans should not discuss appropriate

---

[237]   Department of Health (2002) *Mental Health Policy Implementation Guide: National Minimum Standards for General Adult Services in Psychiatric Intensive Care Units (PICU) and Low Secure Units,* para 2.6.1.

[238]   Department of Health (2002) *Mental Health Policy Implementation Guide: Adult Acute Inpatient Care Provision* para 6.1.6

[239]   Under current arrangements, only patients subject to a court order with restrictions detaining them in a named hospital unit require section 17 leave to leave the unit (see section 45A of the 1983 Act, which was inserted by section 46 of the Crime Sentences Act 1997. If a High Security Hospital had services of lesser security on site, a patient would require section 17 leave to move from level of security to another within that site.

limitations on patients' freedom. Restrictions on individual patient's movements should, in these circumstances, be based upon a risk-assessment finding that such action is warranted. Rather than patients having to demonstrate their suitability to have restrictions lifted, the care team should demonstrate why such restrictions are required.

> **Recommendation 30:** limitations placed upon patients' movements, particularly within hospital grounds, should be operated according to the guiding principles of the Code of Practice, so that all patients are treated and cared for in the least restrictive manner possible and with the greatest practicable promotion of their own self determination and personal responsibility.

Section 17 leave

9.36   The Commission publishes a Guidance Note on good practice and the law in relation to sections 17, 18 and 19[240]. In our last Biennial Report we recommended further practice guidelines on section 17 leave, reproduced as Figure 18 below. These are reflected in IMHAP's section 17 guidance, available in its policy compendium, prepared in conjunction with the Commission in 2002[241].

> Hospital managers should ensure that sole discretion for the granting of authorised section 17 leave is not left to the supervising nurse alone but is approved only:-
>
> * following consultation with involved professionals to ensure that the patient's needs for health and social care are fully assessed and addressed by the care-plan (see Code of Practice, paragraph 27.5), all of which should be recorded in the patient's clinical record;
> * following a detailed risk assessment which is similarly recorded;
> * with carefully considered contingency plans, including contact telephone numbers;
> * with clearly set down parameters, including the time of return;
> * with clearly set down supervision arrangements; and
> * with a copy of the Section 17 leave form given to the patient, and to the carer, if appropriate.

Fig 18: Commission Practice Guidelines – section 17 leave

(Recommendation 36, MHAC (2001) Ninth Biennial Report, Chapter 4.23)

9.37   Figure 19 below shows self-assessment returns describing progress against our Ninth Biennial Report recommendations regarding leave and AWOL policy and practice (Section 18 AWOL procedures are discussed at 9.55 below). Given the Commission's emphasis in recent years on the need for robust policies and procedures, we are pleased to note from our

---

[240] *Mental Health Act Commission Guidance Note: Issues surrounding Sections 17, 18 and 19 of the Mental Health Act 1983.* Available from www.mhac.trent.nhs.uk

[241] Institute of Mental Health Act Practitioners (2002) *Mental Health Act 1983 Policy Compendium.* May 2002. pp22, app.7. See Appendix E below for publication details.

general experience that the majority of units have such policies, although the returns set out below confirm Commissioners' experience from visits that a considerable number of hospitals find that staff shortages inhibit their ability to implement such policies fully. Patients who require escorting by staff on outings from the hospital are most likely to be denied agreed periods of leave by staff shortages (see 9.33 above, 9.43 and Chapter 12.15 below).

Section 17 leave of absence from hospital and section 18 AWOL procedures	Red		Amber		Green	
	n	%	n	%	n	%
Are written policies available, understood and followed in practice ?	3	4.2	7	9.7	62	86.1
Is the staff complement adequate in number and training to implement ?	3	4.2	28	38.9	41	56.9
Are there in-house reviews with Board reporting and on-going audit leading to remedial action on issues raised ?	16	22.2	23	31.9	33	45.8

Fig 19: Self-assessments of 72 hospitals/Trusts in relation to progress against Commission Ninth Biennial Report Recommendations 36 and 37[242]

9.38   We suggest that new legislation should require the completion of statutory documentation in respect of the granting of leave from hospital for detained patients. Such regulation of practice should not aim to fetter clinicians' discretion to grant leave under any particular circumstances. It should aim to ensure that basic planning, risk-assessment, information-sharing and consultation is undertaken in respect of planning and authorizing leave from the patient's entry into detention.

Recommendation 31: Statutory documentation should be developed for use under the next Mental Health Act in recording leave authorisations and the processes leading to such authorisations.

Defining hospitals for the purposes of leave

9.39   The current Mental Health Act predates the establishment of National Health Service Trusts, and in many places refers to a 'hospital', defined broadly by reference to the NHS Act 1977 as any institution for the reception of persons suffering from illness. At the time of drafting the 1983 Act it was not therefore envisaged that a single hospital site might have

---

[242] Based upon a voluntary (and therefore self-selecting) return of 72 self-assessment forms, representing approximately a quarter of all detaining hospitals in England and Wales. Recommendations 36 and 37 are reproduced above as Figures 18 (Chapter 9.36) and 21 (9.55).

more than one set of managers, and this causes some doubts over the use of its powers where this is the case.

9.40   The Commission has suggested that where there are two NHS Trusts comprising a single hospital site (ie a building or set of buildings with attendant grounds surrounded by a curtilage), the whole site should define the 'hospital' for the purposes of detained patients' leave. Therefore, in our view section 17 leave is not required for patients to move freely within a hospital site, even if it is managed by more than one NHS Trust, even though we still recommend that clear protocols over clinical responsibilities should be agreed between the managing Trusts. We recognise, however, that some commentators on the Act do not share our view on this legal question.

9.41   Professor Anselm Eldergill has argued that where two or more NHS Trusts manage a hospital site, each separately managed part of that site should be considered as a hospital for the purposes of the Act[243]. In this case, leave under section 17 would be required for patients to move out of the part of the hospital site that is managed by the detaining Trust. The current edition of the *Mental Health Act Manual* prefers Professor Eldergill's position to that of the Commission, pointing to the fact that staff employed by an NHS Trust sharing a site with a detaining hospital will have no powers over a patient allowed to wander within their facilities, unless such formal leave arrangements are in place[244]. Whilst we accept this specific argument in part, we do not think that this need determine the question.

9.42   Even in a Trust that is a detaining authority, staff employed in capacities that are neither nursing nor medical probably have limited powers of control over detained patients. The Act does allow that any "officer on the staff of the hospital" (the definition of which encompasses any employee of a detaining hospital) may take into custody and return an AWOL patient under section 18(1), and may be authorised by a patient's RMO to act as that patient's escort as a condition of leave (section 17(3)). In general, however, we doubt that non-medical and non-nursing staff should be expected to take an active part in the control of patients.

9.43   By extension, it seems reasonable to us that, where a hospital site is shared between separately managed mental health and general health services, medical and nursing staff employed by the general health service Trust should also not be expected to take on the routine management and control of patients detained by the mental health Trust. It would be possible, however, to designate such staff to take on any specific role in relation to the taking and returning of AWOL patients, or the escorting of patients on leave, using the existing provisions of the Act. This means that, whether or not the general health service Trust's territory is recognised as being a part of the hospital site open to detained patients, the powers of general hospital staff over such patients can and should be a matter for agreement and formal arrangement between the managers of the respective Trusts. It may be, for instance, that the mental health Trust should undertake to provide staff upon request for the retrieval or control of detained patients who have crossed into the general healthcare Trust's site.

---

[243] Eldergill A (1998) *Mental Health Review Tribunals, Law and Practice.* London, Sweet and Maxwell, p144

[244] Jones R (2003) *Mental Health Act Manual*, eighth edition, London: Sweet & Maxwell para 1-208

9.44 We do not insist that Trusts should follow our view in this debate, but rather encourage mental health services who share sites with another Trust to seek formal advice where necessary to determine the boundaries of their hospital, and to make such boundaries known to their patients. Some Trusts provide clearly marked maps for patients so that they are aware of the legal boundaries to their movements on site. However Trusts interpret the law on this question, where the territory managed by a mental health Trust on a combined site has restricted access to outdoors or other facilities, we will encourage that Trust to make arrangements with its neighbours to overcome any unnecessary limitations that this will place on patients. Patients can be particularly confined where isolated mental health wards are sited within large general hospital buildings.

> **Recommendation 32:** The Commission recommends that where more than one Trust shares a single hospital site, clear protocols are agreed between the Trusts and made available to all relevant staff regarding responsibilities for the control and management of detained patients. Such protocols may, for example, cover arrangements for staff of the detaining Trust to attend other parts of the hospital where such control and management is required.
>
> Where two hospital boundaries abut each other, Trusts managing such hospitals should seek to make such arrangements to facilitate detained patients' movement between hospital sites as would be of benefit to patients.

9.45 It is clearly unfortunate that there should be uncertainty over this matter, and advice from the Department of Health would be welcome and may save unnecessary legal expense.

Advance authorisation of leave

9.46 On a number of occasions we have been asked for advice over how best to arrange leave for patients who may require urgent treatment of physical disorders at another hospital to that in which they are detained, either because of general ill-health or because of self-harming behaviour. Such medical emergencies may occur when the RMO is not easily available to authorise leave. We have suggested that there is no reason why leave for patients where such situations may be envisaged might not be authorised in advance by the RMO, to be put into effect at the discretion of nursing staff. Locally-produced leave documentation could have built-in reminders for RMOs to consider these eventualities early in the patient's treatment in hospital. If statutory documentation is developed for use under forthcoming legislation, it could be designed to prompt clinicians into considering such matters as a matter of routine.

Section 17 as a community treatment order?

9.47 Although the 1983 Act uses the language of "treatment in a hospital" (i.e. sections 3(2)(a), 20(4)), the notion of a community treatment order has haunted the Act from its inception. Prior to 1986, some practitioners used the powers of section 17 to grant effectively indefinite leave to patients on the condition that they would continue their treatment or be recalled to hospital. In some cases, patients were being detained under the Act solely for this purpose. In order to renew the authority for detention, patients would be likely to be recalled to hospital for a nominal stay as an inpatient[245].

9.48 The Commission's First Biennial Report (1985) set out our objections to this use of the Act[246]. We argued that it was a misuse of the Act either to detain a patient solely for the purpose of immediately granting leave, or to renew detention whilst a patient was only nominally resident in hospital. This was because a condition of both sections 3 and 20 is that medical treatment received *in a hospital* cannot be provided without detention under the Act. The *Hallstrom* judgment of December 1985[247] confirmed the Commission's contention, noting the similar constructions of the conditions for use of section 3 and for its renewal under section 20. The court held that both constructions implied that inpatient treatment was the core criteria of detention under section 3 and its renewal. Therefore a patient could not be detained under section 3 unless there was a genuine need for detention in hospital, and such a need would not be demonstrated if immediate leave of absence was granted. The detention of a patient could not be renewed if that patient was away from hospital on leave, and such a patient could not be recalled specifically for such a renewal, as section 17(4) only empowers the RMO to recall a patient "in the interests of his health or safety" and not for an administrative reason.

9.49 The *Hallstrom* judgment gave a clear signal that section 17 should not be used as a long-term community treatment order, but it did create some dilemmas for professionals. The point at which an authority for detention comes up for renewal is, after all, an arbitrary point in the course of a patient's treatment. A number of cases highlighted the possible absurdities inherent in determining the lawfulness of renewal on the patient's situation at this arbitrary point.

9.50 The *Barking* case of 1999[248] involved a patient whose treatment plan only required residence in hospital for two days a week, and whose detention was renewed during a period when she was away from hospital. The court overruled the *Hallstrom* judgment in respect of the question of whether a patient who is not physically in hospital may have their detention renewed, arguing that it was sufficient if the treatment plan taken as a whole involved periods of inpatient hospital treatment. Two years later, the courts allowed that a renewal could be lawful even where a patient on leave was receiving no inpatient treatment of any kind, the court allowing that "the prospect of future inpatient treatment" could be sufficient reason for liability to detention to continue, providing that the timing of such future treatment was not too uncertain[249].

---

[245] Until its amendment by the Mental Health (Patients in the Community) Act 1995, section 17(5) expressly stated that a patient shall cease to be liable to detention six months from the day leave was granted, unless recalled to hospital or AWOL at that time. Following amendment in 1995, the effect of section 17(5) was that a patient's liability to detention must cease if s/he remains on leave for a maximum period of twelve months (the longest possible interval between renewals of section 3). As a result of *D.N v Mersey Care NHS Trust* (see para 9.52 below) there no longer appears to be a limit of time that a patient may remain on section 17 leave in the community.

[246] Mental Health Act Commission (1985) *First Biennial Report* London: Stationery Office. Chapter 8.12(d)

[247] *R v Hallstrom ex p W (No.2)*; *R v Gardner, ex p L* [1986].

[248] *B v Barking Havering and Brentwood Community Healthcare NHS Trust* [1999].

[249] *R (on the application of Epsom and St Helier NHS Trust) v the Mental Health Review Tribunal* [2001].

9.51 The basic criteria for lawful renewal were further widened in 2002 by the decision in *R (on the application of D.R.) v Mersey Care NHS Trust*, which held that it was an impermissible and illogical gloss on section 20(4)(c) to read "treatment in hospital" to necessarily mean *inpatient* treatment (i.e. where a patient is admitted to a hospital bed). Thus a renewal was deemed lawful although the patient's only hospital treatment amounted to weekly attendance at a hospital for occupational therapy and a ward round. It was enough that there was a significant component of hospital-based treatment in her care plan, and that there was a clear clinical rationale for that treatment to take place in a hospital rather than any other location.

9.52 The *D.R.* case would seem to have broken the link between inpatient hospital treatment and *continued* liability to detention held in previous judgments. It is ironic that the Courts did so, largely unheeded, at the time of wide and fairly polarised debate over the Draft Mental Health Bill's proposed community treatment orders. The judgment in *D.R.* may even have introduced into current practice a form of community treatment powers that would meet the criticisms of professional bodies over the Government's proposals, given that the power is only available subsequent to detention in hospital.

9.53 Authorities should be wary of interpreting case law to anticipate powers suggested for new legislation. In the absence of formal guidance on the consequences of the *D.R.* case for practitioners and patients[250], we have set out a Commission view at Figure 20 below.

9.54 In the Commission's view, despite the clear parallels between section 20 criteria and the criteria for detention under section 3, and irrespective of certain *obiter* comments in the judgment itself[251], it would be incorrect to read the *D.R.* judgment as having severed the link between inpatient treatment and the initiation of detention of a patient under section 3. The Commission supports the contention of the *Mental Health Act Manual* (Eighth edition, para 1-046) that an application for section 3 admission can only be made if the patient is assessed as requiring a period of hospital *inpatient* treatment for mental disorder. The context of section 3 clearly establishes that it relates to admission to hospital for treatment. In particular, social workers applying for section 3 admissions must state why "detention in hospital" is appropriate, and recommending doctors must state why other forms of treatment, such as outpatient treatment, is not. The Act is clear that a duly completed application for detention provides authority for conveyance to hospital and subsequent admission and detention there, and the Code of Practice requires recommending doctors to identify a bed for patients subject to such applications. Consequently, the admission of a patient under section 3 with the sole purpose of granting immediate leave (or instigating supervised discharge) must remain a misuse of the Act and unlawful treatment of a patient.

---

[250] Extant guidance at paragraphs 96 – 7 of the Mental Health Act Memorandum is no longer valid, and the Code of Practice's statement at paragraph 20.13 that detention may be renewed "…if the RMO thinks that further formal in-patient treatment is necessary…" is no longer a correct reflection of the law.

[251] see *D.R. v Mersey Care NHS Trust*, para 34: "the law…(if my interpretation of it be sound) [is] that the compulsory administration of medication to a patient may be achieved only if a significant component of the plan is for treatment in hospital, and that … the difference between in-patient and out-patient treatment is irrelevant"

On the renewal of detention for patients on leave

(a) As a result of *D.R. v Mersey Care NHS Trust* (2002), "treatment in hospital" at section 20(4)(a) need no longer be read to mean inpatient hospital treatment, but can also apply to outpatient treatment. The *Barking* case established that a patient does not have to be physically present in hospital for their liability to detention there to be renewed under section 20.

(b) It remains a requirement of section 20 that:

* it is necessary for the health or safety of the patient or for the protection of other persons that the patient should receive hospital treatment of some description;

* such treatment must be likely to alleviate or prevent a deterioration of the patient's condition;

* treatment cannot be provided other than in a hospital setting; and

* treatment cannot be provided unless the patient continues to be detained.

(c) The Commission urges practitioners and the Mental Health Review Tribunal hearings to be vigilant in ensuring that the law is operated according to the principles established by the Code of Practice, particularly:

* that patients should receive care in such a way as to promote to the greatest practicable degree their self determination and personal responsibility; and

* be discharged from detention or other powers provided by the Act as soon as it is clear that their application is no longer justified. (Code of Practice 1.1).

(d) Good practice requires that assessment prior to renewal has as its focus the question of whether powers of detention are still necessary, or whether alternative and less restrictive arrangements would meet the patient's medical needs.

(e) In the Commission's view it is not lawful to detain a patient under section 3 for the sole purpose of either granting immediate long-term leave or placing the patient under supervised discharge (see 9.54 above).

Fig 20: Commission Practice Guidelines on the renewal of detention for patients on leave

Section 18 – Patients Absent without Leave

9.55   The Commission has repeatedly pointed to the fact that patients are often at severe risk when absent without leave. Patients' care-plans should involve a risk assessment relating to leave and absence without leave that establishes expected actions of staff and acknowledged risks to the patient. It is a requirement of the Code of Practice (21.5) that services develop and implement policies in relation to absence without leave. The IMHAP policy compendium, produced in conjunction with the Commission, contains advice on establishing such policies[252]. At Figure 21 below we reproduce the recommendation from the Commission's Ninth Biennial Report in relation to absence without leave policies: at Figure 19 above we show hospitals' self-assessments in relation to progress in implementing the recommendation.

---

[252]   Institute of Mental Health Act Practitioners (2002) *Mental Health Act 1983 Policy Compendium.* May 2002. pp25. See Appendix E below for publication details.

Managers' review of detention

The jurisdiction and procedures of Managers' hearings

9.56 Section 23 of the 1983 Act provides managers with the power to discharge unrestricted patients from detention, and specifies that this power can be exercised by any three or more members of that authority or of a committee appointed by it for that purpose. Aside from this, neither the Act itself nor any associated Regulations provide specific legal requirements for the procedures to be followed in holding managers' reviews of detention. Nevertheless, hospital managers engaged in managers' hearings have a general legal duty to exercise their power of discharge fairly and with due regard to human rights requirements.

Hospital managers should ensure that AWOL policies and procedures clearly indicate:

* when the patient should be regarded as AWOL;
* who has responsibility to return the patient;
* which staff are authorised under Sections 137 and 138 to act to take a patient into custody, convey or detain;
* what the expectations are of the police in terms of finding and returning patients; and
* who should take charge of the AWOL procedure, and how they should determine:
* who should undertake a local search and the extent of the local search;
* when a wider search should be undertaken and by whom and what areas should be searched;
* when to contact the police; and
* when to contact the carers or relatives.

Fig 21: Commission Practice Guidelines – section 18 AWOL procedures
(Recommendation 37, MHAC (2001) Ninth Biennial Report, Chapter 4.26)

9.57 Chapter 23 of the Code of Practice provides guidance designed to help ensure that managers exercise their legal powers with due regard to principles of natural justice, but the Code's guidance is not legally binding and therefore creates no specific legal duties. The IMHAP policy compendium, produced in 2002 in conjunction with the Commission, provides further guidance[253]. In *South West London and St George's Mental Health NHS Trust v W* [2002], it was stated that the matters to be considered at a managers' hearing should be the same as those for a Mental Health Review Tribunal. The Code of Practice sets out the basic criteria at paragraphs 23.11 and 23.12, but these are incomplete. Managers' hearings must also take into account 'treatability' criteria at section 3(2)(b) if the patient is detained under section 3 and classified as suffering from psychopathic disorder or mental impairment, and must ensure that the renewal criteria of section 20(4) have been met if the hearing has been triggered by a renewal of detention by the RMO.

9.58 The Commission is sometimes asked for a view on the powers of managers' review hearings. We agree with the contention of the *Mental Health Act Manual* that a reasonable exercise of

---

[253] ibid, pp27

managers' discretion to discharge would enable managers to exercise options broadly similar to those enjoyed by the Mental Health Review Tribunal[254]. Therefore, managers could:

(i) adjourn hearings if an important piece of information has not been provided to them;

(ii) order the discharge of a patient subject to the achievement of a condition, such as obtaining hostel accommodation;

(iii) order the patient to be discharged on a future specified date within this period of detention to allow for preparations for such discharge to be made; and

(iv) make an unenforceable recommendation in respect of the patient, including relating to clinical care.

If a recommendation of the managers is not complied with, the Mental Health Act Manual further suggests that the hearing should reconvene. A reconvened panel would, as the law appears to stand at the time of writing, only have one enforceable power, which would be absolute discharge of the patient. At Chapter 3.16 *et seq* above we discuss the current debate over the powers of Tribunals to require certain actions of doctors. It may be that any decision that gives Tribunals such authority could extend to hospital managers' hearing panels, no doubt to the chagrin of many doctors. At present, hospital managers' hearing panels who find that their recommendations are not implemented could, as representatives of the managers of the hospital, decide that the matter requires to be raised as a clinical governance issue.

Unanimity and majority in decisions of Managers' hearings

9.59　In March 2003 the Court of Appeal provided an interpretation of section 20(4) of the 1983 Act[255]. This section provides that three or more members or appointees of a detaining authority may exercise its power of discharge. The Appeal Court determined that this must be interpreted to mean that, in any such managers' panel, there must be three members willing to discharge a patient for that discharge to be lawful. As managers' hearing panels usually consist of three members, this means that such panels must reach a unanimous decision if they are to exercise their power of discharge. When managers' hearing panels consist of more than three members, and at least three members are willing to exercise the power of discharge, the common-law rule that a body exercising powers of a public nature may do so by majority, as established by *Grindley v Barker* [1798], will prevail.

9.60　The Code of Practice guidance on managers' hearings assumes that the patient's RMO will attend the hearing or at least submit a report to it. In practice, another doctor may attend hearings in the RMO's place, and submitted reports are likely, in some cases, to be compiled by medical or nursing staff other than the RMO. Some managers have therefore sought to require that any doctor standing in for the RMO at a managers' hearing should be section 12 approved. This is, in our view, a reasonable (albeit neither enforceable nor legally binding) requirement, given that the hearing is concerned with the criteria for detention under the Act, which is precisely what section 12 approved doctors are trained to consider. Just as the burden of proof rests with the detaining authority in Tribunal hearings, at a managers' hearing it would seem that it is necessary for the doctor to demonstrate that a patient

---

[254] Jones R (2003) *Mental Health Act Manual*, eighth edition, London: Sweet & Maxwell para 1-294

[255] *R (on the application of Tagoe-Thomspon) v Hospital Managers of the Park Royal Centre* [2003]

requires detention, and so that doctor should be suitably trained to do so. Particularly given the general shortage of section 12 approved doctors, Trusts should perhaps therefore encourage doctors junior to RMOs, such as senior house officers, to gain section 12 approval.

9.61 As well as a duty to ensure that they exercise their specific powers of detention fairly, hospital managers have a general duty to ensure that patients' detentions are kept under constant review by their clinical teams, and that patients are discharged from detention orders as soon as it is apparent that detention is no longer justified. RMOs should be supplied with a suitable local form to record their decisions to discharge patients, a copy of which should be given to the patient.

Section 117 Aftercare

9.62 During this reporting period the question of funding for section 117 aftercare reached the House of Lords. In *R v Manchester City Council, ex p. Stennett and Two Other Actions* [2002], their Lordships confirmed the Government's position from 1998 that "charges cannot be levied for services, residential or non-residential, which are provided as part of the programme of aftercare for a patient … under section 117"[256]. The judgment rejected arguments put by a number of social services authorities that section 117 is only a "gateway" to the provision of services under other statutes (e.g. housing under the National Assistance Act 1948). Instead, the ruling determined that section 117 imposes a free-standing duty jointly on health and social services authorities to provide such aftercare services as the patient is assessed to require.

9.63 In the judgment Lord Steyn rejected arguments described by counsel for the appellant authorities as "the anomaly of the compliant and non-compliant patients in adjacent beds". This argument, which relied on comments in the Mental Health Act Manual[257], contrasts two patients with identical needs who can only be distinguished by the fact that one happened not to be compliant with admission to hospital at the time of his mental health crisis, and was therefore detained under the 1983 Act, whilst the other was admitted informally. The first patient will be entitled to aftercare services without charge, whereas the second can be charged for such services. His Lordship rejected this view as "too simplistic", stated that there may well be a reasonable view that generally patients compulsorily admitted under sections 3 and 37 pose greater risks upon discharge to themselves and others than compliant patients, and agreed with the observation of Buxton LJ in the Court of Appeal that "the statutory provision is not at all anomalous, and not at all surprising. The persons referred to in section 117(1) are an identifiable and exceptionally vulnerable class. To their inherent vulnerability they add the burden, and the responsibility for the medical and social services, of having been compulsorily detained. It is entirely proper that special provision should be made for them to receive after-care and it would be surprising… if they were required to pay…". Lord Steyn added only the observation that the Code of Practice

---

[256] Hansard Written Answers, 28 July 1998, col 172. See also MHAC (1999) *Eighth Biennial Report*, paragraph 4.117

[257] Jones, R (2001) *Mental Health Act Manual*, Seventh ed. 1-967 (this edition used in the HL hearing); see also (2003) *Mental Health Act Manual* 1-1067, which repeats the 'anomaly' examples but reports their Lordships' decision and views.

requires that detention under the 1983 Act "should only be used in the last resort", and the suggestion that "in practice section 117 will in large measure cover patients whose mental illness is such that they pose a risk to themselves or others"[258].

9.64   Social services and health agencies should have joint policies to ensure that s117 duties are met (HSC 2000/003). The apportioning of funding responsibilities continues to cause difficulties between health and social services authorities, as health authorities are only obliged to meet health service costs under section 3(i)(e) of the NHS Act 1977, and social services may only provide services falling within section 21 of the National Assistance Act. The respective responsibilities of the two authorities were determined in part by *R v North & East Devon Health Authority ex parte Coughlan* [2001], and has been the subject of Government guidance[259], but the latter has been criticized as insufficiently explicit by the Health Service Commissioner for England (the Ombudsman)[260]. Even though section 117 of the Mental Health Act protects patients who are discharged from sections 3 or 37 from being involved financially in these funding disputes, their discharge from hospital may be delayed or made problematic by them. One solution is available through new arrangements under the Health Act 1999, which allow for pooling of health and social care budgets where provisions overlap and apportionment of funding responsibilities through local agreements.

> **Recommendation 33:** Government should provide substantive guidance – and consider the provision of additional funding – to enable health and social services authorities to meet fully their responsibilities under section 117 of the 1983 Act.

9.65   Section 117 does create a financial disincentive for authorities to use formal powers of detention. This issue arose in one case investigated by the Health Service Ombudsman and published as a part of her February 2003 report on *NHS Funding for Long-term Care*[261]. The complainant was the son (and closest surviving relative) of Mrs Z, who suffered from dementia. Mrs Z's son alleged that the consultant responsible for Mrs Z's care had been willing to recommend formal admission to hospital under the 1983 Act but had been dissuaded from doing so in order to safeguard the health and social services authorities from any financial liability concerning her continuing care. He also complained that he had not been advised that he had the right, as Mrs Z's Nearest Relative, to apply himself for her formal admission under the 1983 Act. The Ombudsman, aided by her Psychiatric Adviser, did not find in favour of the complainant in respect of these aspects of the complaint (although other aspects of the complaint were upheld), finding "no reason to believe that,

[258] *R v Manchester City Council, ex p. Stennett and Two Other Actions* [2002], para 13-14. Whilst the Act also allows detention in the interests of health, rather than only because of danger to self or others, "Parliament necessarily legislates for the generality of cases" (para 13).

[259] HSC 2001/015, LAC (2001)18 *Continuing Care: NHS and Local Councils' Responsibilities*, 28 June 2001

[260] Health Service Ombudsman (2003) *NHS Funding for Long-Term Care. 2nd Report, Session 2002-03* HC 399. London; the Stationery Office, February 2003, p3-5

[261] *ibid*, Annex D. p 35-48. Case No E814/00-01.

even if Mr Z had attempted to make an application for compulsory admission under the Act, the necessary medical recommendations would have been obtained". The report shows that the Director of the Health Authority had assured the Ombudsman that the consultant in question was firmly of the view that Mrs Z's condition had not necessitated formal admission under the Act. However, the report also shows that Mrs Z's son had had to use force to get her into the ambulance to admit her to hospital; that he stated that she had been very resistant to leaving her house and had said 'I'm not going' three times; and that this account was substantiated by the Ambulance Service records, which stated 'Mrs Z refusing to travel and is very confused'. Even though Mrs Z's admission took place in 1998 (in the midst of changes in the law due to the *Bournewood* case, which are treated, possibly erroneously, as central to the question of admission by the Ombudsman's report), as she does not appear to have been compliant with her admission it is far from clear how, had a Mental Health Act Assessment been underway at that point, the use of the Act could be avoided.

9.66   We have no reason to believe that any authority involved in the above case sought to avoid detention under the Act to avoid financial liabilities. It seems likely, as the Ombudsman acknowledges, that the use of compulsion was rightly considered to be a last resort and, in the view of professionals coming into contact with Mrs Z and her son at the time of the admission, the point at which compulsion could be justified had not been reached. But the case is troubling nevertheless. It would appear that Mrs Z's admission was prearranged, so that, although an ambulance fetched her to hospital, no professional assessment of her attitude towards admission would have been made at that time. Although force was used in her removal from home, it was Mrs Z's son who was placed in the position to use it. We suspect that similar situations, where the coercion of a patient is left by default to their carer or relative, are common, and that underlying the recognised use of formal powers of compulsion there is a much greater incidence of such practice. We discussed our concerns over these hidden incidences of compulsion in Chapter 1.7 above. The fact that admission to hospital under the 1983 Act carries potentially serious financial burdens on health and social services authorities makes an overview of this situation all the more urgent.

Aftercare duties under the next Mental Health Act

9.67   The Commission notes with great concern the lack of an equivalent duty in the draft Mental Health Bill of 2002 to that created by section 117 of the 1983 Act. As such, the draft legislation made no provision that place a duty on health and social service providers to provide adequate aftercare in respect of individual patients who are discharged from compulsion[262]. This would be a retrograde step in that it would remove the reciprocal aspect of compulsion under the 1983 Act that theoretically guarantees patients adequate aftercare services for prompt discharge and continued wellbeing in the community. Furthermore, of course, the abolition of any duty equivalent to section 117 could reverse the recent rulings on funding for aftercare provided under such a duty, making patients liable to pay for aftercare services provided following compulsory treatment. We have had no indication from Government that this is its intention, and therefore trust that the Mental Health Bill that is presented to Parliament will restore this omission from its draft stage.

---

[262]   see Jones, R (2003) *Mental Health Act Manual*, eighth edition, London: Sweet & Maxwell para 1-1060. Jones sets out why the arguments of Government in 1982 that the section 117 would duplicate other legislation, particularly the provisions of the 1977 NHS Act, were incorrect, in that the NHS Act only directs authorities to provide for the generality of mentally disordered persons.

Recommendation 34: Duties equivalent to those placed upon health and social care authorities by section 117 of the 1983 Act should be retained by the legislation that replaces that Act.

Community Care (Delayed Discharges etc) Act 2003

9.68   The Commission followed the debates regarding the above act with great interest. In March 2003 Earl Howe's amendment to the legislation was agreed to in the later stages of the Bill's Parliamentary progress[263]. This amendment excludes mental health services from the scope of the above Act, which will allow penalty charges to be made against local authorities where hospital discharges are delayed due to lack of social support.

9.69   The Commission submitted views on the subsequent drafting of the Delayed Discharges (Mental Health Care) Order 2003 to Government. In our view, the original drafting of the order (which excluded 'psychiatric services or other services ... where the person primarily responsible for arranging those services is a consultant psychiatrist') was too limited, and would certainly seem not to encompass developing personality disorder services or plans for their extension under a new Mental Health Act.

---

[263]   see Lords Hansard, 10 March 2003, Cols 1111- 6

10

Treatment under the 1983 Act

10.1   The great advance of the 1983 Act over previous mental health legislation was that it circumscribed the powers of compulsory treatment over those made subject to detention in hospital. Twenty years later, it is undoubtedly the case that there is more respect and consideration given to questions of patients' consent to treatment and the circumstances when treatment may be justified in the absence of such consent. But the concerns that we have raised in every Biennial Report regarding the prevalence of poor practice in the assessment of, and subsequent respect for, patients' capacity and consent to treatment continue to be a major feature of many Commission visits.

The reality of consent

10.2   There will always be a danger that any "consent" given by a patient who is subject to compulsory powers such as detention in hospital is not given freely or willingly, particularly when a patient may understand that a refusal of consent may be taken as a sign of continued illness and, in any case, is likely to be overridden. The Code of Practice states that "permission given under any unfair or undue pressure is not 'consent'" (chapter 15.13), but in practice the distinction between such agreement and a patient's resigned co-operation with treatment may be very fine indeed. Vigilance and sensitivity to the patient's perception and feelings, as well as thorough administrative systems, are required to ensure that the consent to treatment safeguards of the Act are purposefully applied.

10.3   We constantly urge doctors to make adequate records of their discussions with patients over consent to treatment. Such records are required not only by the Mental Health Act Code of Practice (chapters 16.11, 16.13), but also by the GMC[264]. Good recording of consent discussions should not only allow the Commission, or any other scrutineer of a patient's record, to be assured that undue or unfair pressure has not been exerted, but also act as an impetus to ensure that such discussions are themselves adequate. We continue to find examples where no record of a consent discussion is entered into the patient's notes, although an RMO has completed a statutory form (Form 38) to certify that the patient consents to particular treatments falling within the safeguards of section 58(1).[265]

---

[264] General Medical Council (1998) *Good Medical Practice* . London, GMC

[265] i.e. medication for mental disorder administered after three months have elapsed from the first administration to a detained patient, or ECT at any time to a detained patient.

10.4 At the time of writing, we had available for analysis data from examinations of 1,616 patients' Forms 38 and medical notes from Commisssion visits[266]. Commissioners found evidence of the determination of patients' mental capacity and ability to consent in only 1,099 (68%) of these records, and found evidence of a discussion between doctor and patient about the proposed course of treatment in only 1,012 (63%) of them. Even allowing that the overall number of patients without such records may reflect under-recording rather than a failure to carry out the processes of assessment and discussion, this implies that many patients' "consent" may not be true consent at all.

10.5 Some doctors continue to record no more that "Form 38 signed, has capacity" and argue that this is a record of the discussion. Other records are more exemplary and include an outline of the discussion itself, with reference to patients' attitudes towards certain proposed treatments.

10.6 We continue to be concerned that RMOs may not provide patients with adequate opportunities to discuss their treatment plans on a one-to-one basis. Patients whose only contact with their RMO is on a ward round are not adequately served in this respect.

> **Recommendation 35:** From the start of a patient's detention under the 1983 Act, it is imperative that there is a written record within his or her clinical notes outlining:
>
> * assessments of the patient's mental capacity
> * discussions about proposed treatments; and
> * the patient's consent or refusal of consent to such treatment.

Ensuring the regular review of consent documentation

10.7 The revised Code of Practice (1999, chapter 16.35) incorporated the Commission's suggestions regarding good practice in the review of Forms 38[267]. The Code now requires that a new Form is completed upon any permanent change of RMO or when detention is renewed. According to the Code, no Form 38 should be left extant for more than a year. Most services follow the Code's guidance on renewing Forms 38, although we found, for example, that around 7% of Forms 38 examined on Commission visits during 2002/03 and available for analysis had been completed by someone other than the RMO[268].

10.8 It is the Commission's view that, particularly following the declaration of the Court in *Munjaz* (2003) in relation to the status of the Code of Practice (see Chapter 6.17 *et seq* above), practitioners must make every effort to comply with the guidance of the Code. Failure to follow the Code's guidance without good reason based upon an individual

---

[266] examined as a part of the Commission Visiting Questionnaires (CVQ) exercise on MHAC visits – see paragraphs 10.7 and 10.11 above for further CVQ data and Chapter 19.11(c) for a description of the exercise.

[267] see Mental Health Act Commission (1995) *Sixth Biennial Report.* London, Stationery Office. Para 5.12

[268] i.e. 117 from a total of 1,616 Forms 38, examined as a part of the CVQ exercise (see note 266 above).

patient's best interest not only denies patients the level of safeguard required by the Code, but could leave detaining authorities vulnerable to legal challenge from any patient who subsequently disputes the authority upon which treatment was given.

10.9　We draw particular attention to this here as the current edition of the *Mental Health Act Manual* (2003), which predated the *Munjaz* [2003] judgment, advises against following the Code of Practice guidance in relation to reviewing Forms 38, arguing that "neither this Act nor the Mental Health (Hospital, Guardianship and Consent to Treatment) Regulations 1983 provide for the 'renewal' of Form 38" and "a statutory form should only be completed in response to a statutory requirement: it should not be completed in order to comply with notions of 'good practice'"[269]. The Commission disputed this reading prior to the *Munjaz* [2003] judgment, as we could see no reason in law why such a view should prevail over the Code of Practice's approach to Forms 38 as living records of the patient's consenting status. Following the *Munjaz* [2003] judgment, which provided the Code of Practice's guidance with greater legal authority, we consider the approach of the Manual to be untenable. We strongly advise services not to follow the Mental Health Act Manual's recommendation that the Code of Practice should be ignored.

10.10　The Commission will continue to advise that Forms 38 should, as a matter of good practice, be renewed as suggested in the Code of Practice. We will continue to consider Forms 38 that are over a year old, or signed by a doctor who is no longer the patient's RMO, as *prima facie* evidence of poor consent to treatment practice, which may fall short of ECHR requirements in the event of any legal challenge.

> **Recommendation 36:** The Department of Health should reaffirm its commitment to the advice given in relation to reviewing consent in the current edition of the Code of Practice.

Commission findings on the completion of Forms 38

10.11　Of the 1,616 Forms 38 examined over 2002/03 and available for analysis[270], nearly a quarter (24%, or 394 Forms) were considered by Commissioners to fall short of the requirements of chapter 16.14 of the Code of Practice, which are:

* that they are completed by the RMO;

* that the RMO should indicate all drugs prescribed for mental disorder, including "as required" medication, either by name or by classes described in the British National Formulary (BNF);

* that maximum doses and route of administration should be clearly indicated for each drug or category of drug listed.

---

[269] Jones, R (2003) *Mental Health Act Manual*, Eighth Edition. London, Sweet & Maxwell. Para 4-142.

[270] using Commission Visiting Questionnaires (CVQs). See note 266 above .

10.12 Commissioners found prescribed drugs being administered to patients that were not included on Forms 38 in 316 of these cases, or 20% of all forms examined (see 10.16 below). A common fault in the completion of Forms 38 is lack of clarity in treatment descriptions, particularly in relation to the number or maximum dose of drugs authorised (see our advice regarding pharmacists and other professionals as safeguards at 10.20-23 below).

Commission findings on the completion of Forms 39

10.13 When a patient is administered treatment that falls within the safeguards of section 58(1) without consent, such treatment must be authorised by a Second Opinion Appointed Doctor on a Form 39 (see 10.33 below on incidences and outcomes of the Second Opinion process). Commissioners examine these Forms and the context in which they are used when checking consent documentation on visits.

10.14 Of the 1,460 Forms 39 examined by Commissioners over 2002/03 and available for analysis, 75 (5%) failed to meet the requirements of the Code of Practice paragraph 16.14. These would have been referred back to the Commission to arrange remedial action by SOADs where necessary. Commissioners found a record of the RMO informing the patient of the SOAD's decision, as required following the *Feggetter* judgment of 2002 (see Chapter 3.38 above) in only 207 (14%) of examples. It may be that RMOs are interpreting the *Feggetter* ruling not to apply to incapacitated patients, although, even so, we will expect to find a record in the patient's notes detailed what action has or has not been taken and why.

10.15 Records by statutory consultees only appeared in 626 patients' notes (43% of all Forms 39 examined over this period). Hospital managers should consider introducing a standard form for such records, as described in the practice example at 10.21 below.

10.16 133 Forms 39 (9%) did not cover all the medication that was being given at the time of Commissioners' visit. This is considerably less than for Forms 38 (see 10.12 above). This suggests, as might be expected, that that staff are more vigilant when administering medication on the authority of a Form 39 in the absence of a patient's consent, than when they believe the patient to be consenting and the medication to be covered on a Form 38. However, when Commissioners note this error in relation to either Forms 38 or 39 they will treat it as a serious maladministration of the Act and expect immediate remedial action (see 10.18 below).

10.17 Whilst the majority of extant Forms 38 and 39 were copied and kept alongside patients' medicine cards, 104 Forms 38 (6.7%) and 180 Forms 39 (12.3%) were not. There are great risks of unlawfully administering treatment where medicine cards are not checked against statutory authorisations (see 10.20–23 below).

Notification letters for serious maladministration of consent to treatment provisions

10.18 In the last year the Commission has developed a letter for issue to Chief Executives of NHS Trusts or independent hospitals where it encounters systemic failures of compliance with the consent to treatment provisions of Part IV of the Act. The letter identifies the patients whose treatment is of concern and requires action to be reported back within five working days.

Where a patient has been treated unlawfully, we expect hospital authorities to inform that patient of the fact.

10.19 Commissioners will issue this letter where examination of patients' records show serious incidences of the following failures:

* There is no form 38 or 39 covering medication for mental disorder that is being administered outside of the three month period, or for ECT administered at any time;

* The Form 38 is signed by someone other than an RMO or a SOAD, such as junior doctors, nursing staff etc;

* There are doubts about the validity of a patient's consent although treatment is authorised on Form 38;

* Medication administered is outside of the parameters authorised by either Form 38 or 39.

Commissioners have discretion over the issue of a letter to the Chief Executive, and will usually seek remedy from patients' RMOs for isolated incidents that can be addressed directly on the visit.

Professionals' roles in ensuring lawful treatment

Pharmacists

10.20 In our Ninth Biennial Report we recommended that pharmacists be more involved in ensuring good consent to treatment practice. We are pleased that subsequent guidance from the Department of Health has also advised "regular pharmacy input to inpatient wards to educate staff and service users in medication management skills" and "consistent pharmacy input and membership of the acute care forum"[271]. Implementation of the Commission's recommendation that Forms 38 or 39 be attached to the patient's medicine chart and checked by pharmacists responsible for dispensing medication[272] could be one way for services to meet government requirements.

The nurse in charge's responsibilities

10.21 The Commission welcomes the Government's view that "the role of the nurse in charge of the ward needs to be reviewed and strengthened" and that "there needs to be investment in the development of managerial and leadership competencies of ward managers or sister/charge nurses"[273]. The Commission has suggested to many service managers that they introduce a secondary check by the nurse in charge on all aspects of capacity and consent, just as such nurses are often required to check detention documentation. Such checking already falls within the general remit of the sister/ charge nurse job description and has been enthusiastically and fruitfully taken up in some areas.

---

[271] Department of Health (2002) *Mental Health Policy Implementation Guide: Adult Acute Inpatient Care Provision*, para 4.4.10.

[272] Mental Health Act Commission (2001) *Ninth Biennial Report*. London: Stationery Office, para 4.28, Recommendations 23 & 39

[273] Department of Health (2002) *Mental Health Policy Implementation Guide: Adult Acute Inpatient Care Provision*, para 4.5.5.

Good practice example

Consent monitoring forms in Denbighshire

Conwy & Denbighshire NHS Trust have produced the following forms to encourage good consent to treatment practice:

* Capacity & consent to treatment assessment form. Used to accompany Forms 38, the form requires RMOs to answer a short structured question on the patient's mental capacity (based upon the Code of Practice definition at para 15.10), and has a space for the patient and doctor to both sign a record that the patient has consented to treatment.

* RMO's treatment plan form. Used to accompany Forms 39, the form includes the structured question on the patient's mental capacity mentioned above, with a space for RMOs to record the treatment plan authorised and spaces for statutory consultees to record details of their part in the second opinion procedure (as required by the Code of Practice 16.34).

* Scrutiny of consent to treatment papers form. Used for both Forms 38 and 39, the form provides structured checklists for administrative and clinical scrutiny of statutory consent documentation, to identify any problems for rectification.

* Nurses' checking form. Used for both Forms 38 and 39, the form provides structured questions for nurses to use to check that treatment administered and the patient's consent status is as described on current statutory consent documentation.

Contact: Conwy & Denbighshire NHS Trust, Glan Clwd District General Hospital, Rhyl, Denbighshire, LL18 5UJ www.conwy-denbighshire-nhs.org.uk

The role of the Responsible Medical Officer

10.22 Whilst the Commission recognises the increasing responsibilities placed upon sisters/ charge nurses as a positive trend, the Mental Health Act 1983 places certain responsibilities squarely with the doctor in charge of a patient's treatment, or Responsible Medical Officer (RMO). Therefore, whilst the sister/charge nurse "should be the point of contact for consultation, negotiation and decision-making for all ward organisational matters"[274], the RMO must not seek to delegate key responsibilities, such as those regarding consent to treatment, to staff working under his or her direction. Services should ensure that any doctor who may assume RMO responsibilities receives adequate training in the requirements of the Act. One way in which this could be achieved would be for services to require such doctors to be required to undergo section 12 training and approval. At the very least any doctor who could serve as a patient's RMO should be contractually required to maintain adequate training in and knowledge of the requirements of the Act (see Chapter 9.23 above in relation to identifying the RMO).

The role of technology

10.23 Innovative use of information technology may provide additional safeguards in consent and prescribing practice.

---

[274] Department of Health (2002) *Mental Health Policy Implementation Guide: Adult Acute Inpatient Care Provision*, para 4.5.5.

Good Practice Example
Automated records checking in Somerset

Somerset Partnership NHS and Social Care Trust is establishing an electronic records system that we believe to be the first of its type in the UK. It will have an automatic facilities to assist in ensuring compliance with the Mental Health Act's requirements, so that, for instance, it will warn professional staff if they enter any medication into the Medicine Card that is not shown on the current Form 38 or 39.

Contact: Dr Martin Eales, Director of Clinical Governance, Somerset Partnership NHS Trust. Tel 01460 7877

The role of clinical governance

10.24   Good consent procedures are one of a number of important features within a clinical governance framework. Clinical governance has been defined simply as "accountable care" and is a process driven approach to continuous quality improvement. Audit of consent procedures, for example, would be a critical element in a Trust's clinical governance programme. The regular use of plan-do-study-act cycles within clinical care management linked with effective audit of care processes – especially when related to the views of service users themselves – will identify where processes are failing or where service users feel that their views are not being considered adequately. Most Trusts have clinical audit committees which will be reviewing regularly critical aspects of care such as consent, use of seclusion, communication, side effects of medication, and so on.

Certificates of Consent to Treatment and the next Act

10.25   The draft Mental Health Bill of 2002 appeared not to require any certification of a patient's consent such as is required by the current Act and its Regulations. This could be argued to bring psychiatric patients into line with other types of patient, in that ordinary consent forms would presumably be used in place of a statutory form completed by a patient's doctor. However, it is likely that the lack of an equivalent to Form 38 – which, if nothing else, assures staff and external scrutineers of the reason why there is no need for authority to administer treatment without consent – will erode the protection currently offered to patients. The Commission is concerned that, without a requirement upon doctors of regular certification of a patient's consent status, there would be a real danger of some long-stay patients being treated on aged and long-forgotten signed consent forms.

10.26   The Commission believes that the new Act should require a patient's doctor to complete some form of statutory documentation certifying that patient's consent to treatment for mental disorder whilst subject to compulsion under the powers of the Act. This could, of course, be a matter for Regulations, as now. New statutory regulation would be an opportunity to increase the protection offered by the equivalent of Forms 38 in new legislation, by requiring details of process (such as dates of consent discussions) to be recorded and by setting requirements for regular review of consent status.

Recommendation 37: The Commission urges Government to restore to planned legislation some form of statutory documentation equivalent to Form 38 of the Mental Health (Hospital, Guardianship and Consent to Treatment) Regulations 1983.

Statutory reports on patients' treatment and condition – MHAC1

10.27　When the detention is renewed of a patient who has been treated without consent, section 61 of the Act requires RMOs to submit reports on that patient's treatment and condition to the Secretary of State. The Secretary of State is required by section 121(2)(b) to delegate the role of receiving and scrutinising such reports to the MHAC[275]. The Commission has produced a standard reporting form (MHAC1) for RMOs to use in submitting these reports. It scrutinises every report received, particularly with a view as to whether a further statutory Second Opinion is warranted for any reason. We view this statutory requirement as a valuable if imperfect safeguard for patients that should be retained and strengthened under future legislation. We discuss this further at Chapter 20.26(c) below.

10.28　During checks on patient records over during 2002-03, Commissioners identified 636 patients whose detention had been renewed and who had been treated under a Form 39. Although all of these patients should have been subjects of reports under section 61, there was no record of such a report for a quarter (164) of them. Because the Commission is not notified of individual detentions or renewals of detention, it cannot track those patients for whom it should receive reports under this section (the majority of patients' detentions are not renewed and so quite correctly are not reported on under section 61). Commissioners will continue to draw lapses in submitting reports to the attention of hospital managers on its visits. It will also continue to draw RMOs' attention to the requirement in the Code of Practice (chapter 16.36) that patients should receive a copy of section 61 reports made out on their care and treatment: of our sample, records demonstrated that only a fifth (98) of patients for whom reports had been submitted received a copy.

10.29　It would clearly be helpful for any monitoring body, whether it is charged with only general monitoring duties or with specific duties such as the receipt of reports on certain patients, to have access to an on-going register of patients subject to compulsory powers (see Chapter 20.26(c) below).

Urgent treatment

10.30　Section 62 of the Act allows that treatment otherwise falling within the safeguards of sections 57 or 58 may be given in an emergency under the direction of the RMO. The Act sets out specific conditions of urgency in relation to the risks of treatment that must be followed for the authority to be valid. The Code of Practice requires incidences of emergency treatment under sections 62 to be recorded and monitored[276]. Sample non-statutory forms for monitoring uses of section 62, which may be adapted by services to suit

---

[275]　This delegation is enacted under S.I. 1983 no 892, para 3(2)(b).

[276]　*Mental Health Act Code of Practice* para 16.41

their individual needs, are provided by the Mental Health Act Commission and the Institute of Mental Health Act Practitioner's *Policy Compendium*[277].

10.31 In our evidence to the David Bennett Inquiry[278], the Commission pointed to the fact that emergency medication had been administered to Mr Bennett on the apparent authority of a nurse during the control and restraint episode in which he died. The on-call doctor had not yet arrived at the scene. Medication had therefore been administered outside of the authority of the 1983 Act, which does not allow nursing staff to authorise medication without consent, even in an emergency. We await the findings of the inquiry with interest.

10.32 In the introduction to this report (Chapter 1.6) we noted that emerging structures of service delivery may be creating legal and ethical dilemmas of the kind faced by the Bennett Inquiry and, of course, by the staff involved in the incident during which Mr Bennett died. We raise a similar question at Chapter 11.23 in relation to seclusion. The 1983 Act's and Code of Practice's procedural requirements for some emergency interventions, such as that emergency treatment should be given under the direction of the RMO, or that a doctor must attend seclusion episodes, may be impossible to meet given the staffing of some units. Yet, by definition, in a genuine emergency, some sort of intervention is required and staff may be held accountable for failing to take appropriate action. We recognise this as an issue that requires Government consideration (not least in the formulation of the next Act, which shall, we trust, seek to enhance rather than lessen safeguards for patients). We suggest at Recommendation 44, Chapter 11.23 that limitations on the use of restraint practices and seclusion in non-medical staffed units might be justified on safety grounds. We consider there to be an even stronger case for non-medical staffed units to have strict policies against the giving of medication outside of limits authorised, even in an emergency, given the very great risks to patients that such practices can entail.

Incidences and outcomes of statutory Second Opinions

10.33 Figure 22 below shows the numbers of Second Opinion requests received from 1985 to 2003. Whilst the number of requests for authorisations in relation to ECT have remained relatively constant, the rise in requests for compulsory medication appears to be increasing. It is possible that this rise reflects improved practice, in that patients' capacity or consent status is now much more likely to be appropriately judged, so that patients whose consent is doubtful are now more frequently afforded the protection of a Second Opinion. The increase also suggests, given that Second Opinions for medication are not required for patients who have been detained for less than three months, that the numbers of long-stay detained patients has also risen considerably over the lifetime of the Act.

10.34 Figure 23 shows the year-on-year percentage change for Second Opinion requests over the last six years.

---

[277] Institute of Mental Health Act Practitioners (2002) *Mental Health Act 1983 Policy Compendium.* May 2002. pp14 & app.4. See Appendix E below for publication details.

[278] see also Chapters 11.23 (recommendation 44), 11.29 and 16.18 below.

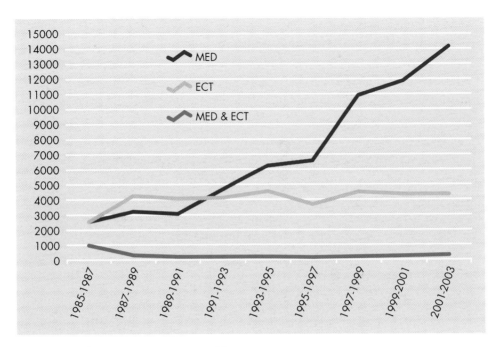

Fig 22: Second Opinion requests received by MHAC, 1985–2003

Source: MHAC Biennial Reports 1-9

	97/98	% change	98/99	% change	99/00	% change	00/01	% change	01/02	% change	02/03
Medication	4,732	29.2	6,116	-5.8	5,761	4.7	6,033	12.4	6,781	8.1	7,331
ECT	2,197	1.5	2,229	-2.7	2,169	-3.0	2,105	3.5	2,179	-7.8	2,008
Med & ECT	74	6.8	79	27.8	101	-12.9	88	35.2	119	-15.1	101
TOTAL	**7,003**	**20.3**	**8,424**	**-4.7**	**8,031**	**2.4**	**8,226**	**11.6**	**9,179**	**2.8**	**9,440**

Fig 23: Second Opinion activity 1997–2003, showing percentage changes

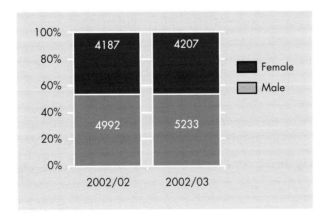

Fig 24: Second Opinion requests by gender of patient, 2001-03

10.35   It is possible that the gender balance of patients receiving Second Opinions, as shown at Figure 24 above, is shifting away from the roughly equal numbers observed in previous reports[279]. This may be a result of the proportionate decline in requests for authority to administer ECT. In past Biennial Reports we have noted that women are more likely to be

---

[279]   see, for example, Mental Health Act Commission (1995) *Seventh Biennial Report* 1993-5 London: Stationery Office p102-103.

referred for ECT treatment than men, and men are more likely to be referred for compulsory medication than women.

10.36　Ethnicity and age profiles of patients for whom Second Opinions were requested in this reporting period are shown at Figures 25 and 26 below.

Ethnic category	2001-02	%	2002-03	%
White	7,029	76.5%	7,036	74.5%
Black-Caribbean	702	7.5%	695	7.5%
Black- African	277	3.0%	310	3.0%
Black-other	57	0.5%	72	0.75%
Indian	154	1.75%	170	2.0%
Pakistani	127	1.5%	141	1.5%
Bangladeshi	39	0.5%	52	05%
Chinese	19	0.25%	24	0.25%
Other	298	3.25%	388	4.0%
Not stated	477	5.25%	552	6.0%
Total	9,179	100%	9,440	100%

Fig 25: Second Opinion requests: ethnicity of patients 2001/02 & 2003/03

Age range	2001-02	%	2002-03	%
Under 16	42	0.5%	43	0.5%
16-18	213	2.5%	129	1.5%
19 – 59	6,42	70.0%	7,133	75.5%
60 – 74	1,504	16.5%	1,296	13.5%
over 75	998	10.5%	839	9.0%
Total	9,179	100%	9,440	100%

Fig 26: Second Opinion requests: age of patients 2001/02 & 2003/03

10.37　The outcomes of completed Second Opinions for the reporting period are given at Figure 27.

Although the figures show that the proportion of RMO decisions changed significantly by the SOAD is small, it should be remembered that the absolute numbers are significant. In 2002-03 there were 261 occasions when SOADs changed the RMO's decision significantly – five patients per week – and over 1,000 occasions when there were slight changes. There are also important benefits in these arrangements. The fact that a relatively small proportion of RMO decisions is challenged may be testament to the success of the process. RMOs know that their treatment decisions can be subject to a Second Opinion. Thus the SOAD provides a check on the RMO's practice, and by the very nature of the oversight provided by the Second Opinion ensures that RMOs give careful thought to their decisions. We believe that if this provision had not been available there would have been no check on the appropriateness of treatment, and many more treatment plans could have been the subject of formal complaint.

Outcome	2001-02	%	2002-03	%
Plan not changed	7,549	87%	7,333	85%
Slight change	972	11%	1,039	12%
Significant Change	199	2%	261	3%
Total	8,720	100%	8,633	100%

Fig 27: Outcomes of completed Second Opinions, 2001-02 & 2003/03[280]

10.38 The courts have considered the nature of SOAD opinions during this period in cases discussed at Chapter 3.32 *et seq* above. These cases have clarified and to some extent reversed positions previously held by the Commission on the purpose of a statutory Second Opinion. In the Wilkinson case, the court determined that, although "it is proper for the SOAD to pay regard to the views of the RMO who has, after all, the most intimate knowledge of the patient's case, that does not relieve him of the responsibility of forming his own independent judgment as to whether or not 'the treatment should be given'" [281]. Therefore a SOAD must reach an independent view of the desirability and propriety of the treatment and is not engaged in merely reviewing the "reasonableness" of treatment proposed by the RMO. This was further emphasised in the first instance decision in the judgment in *N v Doctor M and others* [2002], which invoked the principle of necessity in relation imposition of treatment that may engage ECHR Articles 3 or 8. This is relevant to SOAD practice, as it shows that SOADs should consider whether a treatment is medically necessary before authorising it. *R (on the application of PS) v Drs G & W* [2003] determined that where treatment could be shown to be medically necessary its administration under the Act in the face of a patient's capacitated opposition can be consistent with ECHR rights.

10.39 At Chapter 3.38 *et seq* above we outline the court's determination that SOADs have a duty to give reasons for their decisions.

Advance decisions to refuse treatment (advance directives)

10.40 We are pleased to note the proposals in the Mental Incapacity Bill to codify and clarify the common law rules for England and Wales regarding advance decisions to refuse treatment[282]. It was established in *Re C (Adult Refusal of Medical Treatment)* [1994] that a person with mental capacity to do so could make a valid advance refusal of consent.

---

[280] The totals in this table are smaller than for preceding tables, due to the data set used (completed Second Opinion *reports* received and recorded at the MHAC office, as opposed to Second Opinion *requests*). Over the two years presented, there is an average 6 to 7% margin of potential under-reporting. We consider the available data to have sufficient intrinsic interest to overcome these limitations.

[281] *Wilkinson* [2001], para 33. That "the treatment should be given" having regard to the likelihood of it alleviating or preventing a deterioration of the patient's condition, notwithstanding the patient's incapacity or refusal to consent to that treatment is the statutory criteria for SOAD authorisation set by section 58(3)(b) of the 1983 Act.

[282] Department of Constitutional Affairs (2003) *Draft Mental Incapacity Bill.* June 2003, Cm 5859-I Such legislation has already been passed in Scotland in the form of the Adults with Incapacity (Scotland) Act 2000. Proposals for English legislation would meet the recommendations of the Millan Committee's *Report on the Review of the Mental Health (Scotland) Act 1984* (2001, Chapter 15), which considered but rejected giving statutory force to advance directives that might override Mental Health Act powers of compulsion.

Although such advance refusals may be ineffective under particular circumstances, such as when it is determined that the patient did not appreciate the implications of refusing treatment at the time that they did so, in general such advance statements (which need not be in writing) must be treated as capable refusal of treatment even where the patient subsequently loses mental capacity.

10.41   The proposed Mental Incapacity Bill will enact these common law rules, whilst introducing criteria to circumscribe the validity and applicability of advance directives[283]. These criteria may give rise to problems of evidence first raised by the Law Commission in 1995[284]. Whilst we note that liability will not be incurred by professionals who provide treatment that is subject to an advance refusal that they are unaware of, or who withhold treatment in the reasonable belief of an advance statement's existence, careful consideration may have to be given to how professionals' may reach 'reasonable' views about the existence or non-existence of advance statements.

10.42   The proposals for legislation also reflect the present common-law position that advance refusals are no different to other refusals of psychiatric treatment by patients with mental capacity, in that they may be overridden by the powers of the Mental Health Act 1983 where the criteria for detention under the Act are met. This is not, however, immediately clear from the wording of the draft Mental Incapacity Bill or its explanatory notes[285]. Whilst the wording of the Bill may be adequate for legal purposes, the interface between mental incapacity legislation and the Mental Health Act's powers of compulsion must be clearly explained to potential patients, to avoid false expectations, and to healthcare professionals, to avoid potentially dangerous confusion.

10.43   The Commission believes that the recognition of advance statements under the mental incapacity legislation, even without providing such statements with the legal authority to override compulsion under mental health legislation, cannot but play an important role in encouraging mental health practitioners to give full and proper regard to patients' views about their treatment.

Defining medication for mental disorder

10.44   It is an RMO's responsibility to determine whether a treatment falls within the scope of the 1983 Act as treatment for mental disorder. In some cases, this is not a straightforward matter. The Commission is often asked for advice on what constitutes medication for mental disorder, and therefore falls within the scope of section 58. Fig 28 below sets out our attempt to produce a definitive answer.

---

[283]   Department of Constitutional Affairs (2003) *Draft Mental Incapacity Bill* clauses 24 and 27. Explanatory notes 83 - 85 and 89 refer.

[284]   Law Commission (1995) *Mental Incapacity.* Law Commission Report No 231, para 5.21

[285]   In particular, clause 27 ("Mental Health Act Matters") is phrased to exclude the Mental Incapacity Bill from providing authority to consent to or provide medical treatment under Part IV of the Mental Health Act 1983, but makes no explicit mention of advance refusals of consent made under this Bill.

Medication for mental disorder should include:

i) Medication used to alleviate the symptoms of mental disorder included under BNF categories 4.1, 4.2, 4.3 and 4.11.

ii) Medication that is not included in BNF categories 4.1, 4.2 or 4.3 or is not licensed for such use but is used to alleviate the symptoms of mental disorder. This includes, for example, antiepileptic drugs (BNF category 4.8.1) used as "antimanic drugs" ("mood stabilisers") in bipolar disorder.

iii) Adjuvant medication without which the therapeutic objectives of alleviation of the symptoms of mental disorder set out in i) and ii) could not be achieved. Such medication may include, for example:

a) Drugs used to alleviate the parkinsonian and other motor side effects of antipsychotic agents, such as the antimuscarinic drug, procyclidine (BNF Category 4.9.2) or tetrabenazine (BNF Category 4.9.3), used to alleviate dyskinesia such as tremor, chorea or tardive dyskinesia. Dyskinesia may lead to reduced compliance with treatment for mental disorder and may mask or prevent assessment of the underlying symptoms of mental disorder.

b) Antisialogogic agents (i.e. inhibitors of salivation) such as hyoscine (BNF category 1.2). Excessive salivary secretion, caused by antipsychotic drugs such as clozapine, may reduce the ability of the patient to communicate effectively and / or reduce compliance with treatment.

c) Antiepileptic drugs, in BNF category 4.8.1 may also be used to ameliorate or prevent seizure induction by atypical antipsychotic drugs (clozapine): seizures might otherwise preclude the use of such medication.

Medication for mental disorder should not include:

i) Laxatives, which are not considered to be treatment for mental disorder, even when the antipsychotic medication contributes to the constipation. Similarly, medication to treat general side effects of medication for mental disorder should not be authorised under Section 58, unless it can be shown that not giving such treatment would seriously compromise the purpose of the medication for mental disorder (i.e. that the medication for mental disorder could not be given or would not be effective in ameliorating the symptoms of mental disorder without such adjunctive treatment).

ii) Medication used to treat epilepsy: epilepsy is not considered to be a mental disorder.

iii) Some treatments, such as feeding by naso-gastric tube, which may be considered to be treatments for mental disorder but do not involve medicine. The authority for such treatments may be had from Section 63 of the Act.

iv) Generally, homeopathic and alternative medicines should not be considered as medicines for mental disorder that fall within Section 58.

Fig 28: Commission Practice Guidelines – defining medication for mental disorder[286]

---

[286] Adapted from Mental Health Act Commission (2002) Guidance to Commissioners on consent to treatment and section 58 of the Mental Health Act 1983. July 2002. Available from www.mhac.trent.nhs.uk

Complementary or "alternative" medicine and the Mental Health Act 1983

10.45 Many patients voice a wish for better access to and acceptance of alternative medicines and complementary therapies in their treatment and care. Department of Health guidance now states that "it is desirable that the multi-disciplinary team considers the role of complementary therapies on the unit"[287].

10.46 The Commission is often asked questions over the status of complementary medicine and therapies under Part IV of the Act. Although the final decision as to whether such substances such as fish-oil, homeopathic flower remedies and St John's Wort are "medication for mental disorder" must rest with the RMO who prescribes them, the Commission advises that such treatments should in general not be so described (see Figure 28 above). In the rare cases where it is proposed to prescribe alternative treatments to a detained patient who cannot give informed consent to it, authority under section 63 could then be claimed. Of course, most patients who are prescribed "alternative" treatments are able to provide informed consent, and indeed will often have requested the treatment in question, and so no difficulty arises.

10.47 The factors to be taken into account when the patient is incapable of consent would seem to include:

* the wishes of Nearest Relatives and/or carers (these cannot, of course, provide authority for the treatment, but should be considered nevertheless. Alternative medicines and treatments are frequently considered by the care team at the request of relatives of patients);

* the likelihood of the treatment having any beneficial effect set against the potential side-effects or difficulties in administering the treatment, including whether the patient is likely to resist the administration of treatment; and

* where a patient appears not to benefit greatly from traditional medicine, or has a history of treatment-resistance: the "last resort" factor. Thus a particular treatment might be justified in the last instance when all other approaches have had limited success.

Covert administration of medicine for mental disorder

10.48 The Commission's published view on the covert administration of medication (given in our Sixth Biennial Report of 1995) has been criticised as an equivocation[288], and we take this opportunity to clarify it. The Commission has taken the view that, quite apart aside from obvious and general ethical and safety concerns over the covert administration of medicine in patients' food or drink, such practice is extremely difficult to justify with reference to the expectations of the Act and Code of Practice that patients are given information about their treatment and the opportunity, if they are capable of doing so, to give their consent. If a patient is denied any knowledge of their treatment, or even that they are receiving treatment, then it may be difficult to administer that treatment lawfully under Part IV of the Act, which requires that a patient will have the opportunity for such knowledge. It is clearly impossible for a patient to consent to any treatment administered to them covertly. The Code of Practice suggests that, in discussions with capable patients, "there may be a compelling reason, in the

---

[287] Department of Health (2002) Mental Health Policy Implementation Guide: National Minimum Standards for General Adult Services in Psychiatric Intensive Care Units (PICU) and Low Secure Units. Para 2.7.3

[288] Jones R (2003) *Mental Health Act Manual*, eighth edition, London Sweet & Maxwell para 1-723.

patient's interests, for not disclosing certain information" but that any doctor who chooses not to answer a patient's question for such a reason should not dissemble this "so that the patient knows where he or she stands" and must be prepared to justify the decision (Code of Practice 15.16). The Code expects practitioners to provide explanation of treatments appropriate to the level of incapacitated patients' assessed ability (Code of Practice 15.12). None of these expectations can easily be met in the giving of covert medication.

10.49   However, it is the case that a number of practitioners argue that the best interests of patients should override the considerations of the Code of Practice in this matter. It may be that alternatives to covert medication, such as restraint and forcible medication, would seriously endanger patients who are, for example, elderly and frail. In such circumstances there may be a pressing clinical need to depart from the Code's guidance in an individual, case-by-case basis. Even so, it is doubtful that any such justification could protect practitioners who fail in statutory duties under the Act.

10.50   It is true that this area remains difficult and under-discussed. Whilst we therefore applaud the intention of the UKCC (now the Nursing and Midwifery Council) in publishing a position statement on the covert administration of medicines, we regret that this has not been helpful in clarifying the issues and is misleading in respect of the Mental Health Act 1983[289]. We would welcome further guidance on this troubling aspect of medical and nursing practice based upon dialogue between all the professional colleges, interested parties (including user groups) and the Department of Health. This should not be a matter that is confined to the Commission's relatively specialist scope, as it seems likely that there is a higher numerical incidence of covert medication of informal patients (particularly amongst incapacitated elderly or learning disabled patients in hospitals and care homes: see also Chapter 15.9–10 below) than of detained patients.

> **Recommendation 38:** The Commission proposes the covert administration of psychiatric medication in all mental health services as a possible area of study under future monitoring arrangements.

Placebos

10.51   In our Eighth Biennial Report we suggested that placebos, being inert substances, are likely to fall without the definition of "medicine" and therefore remain outside the provisions of section 58 of the 1983 Act. In our view, therefore, any authority to administer placebos without consent would have to be sought under section 63. However, as with covert medication (see 10.48 above), we have grave concerns that it is difficult to justify the implied deception involved in their administration with reference to the expectations of the Act and Code of Practice over patient information and opportunity to consent.

---

[289] UKCC (2001) *Position Statement on the Covert Administration of Medicines – Disguising medicine in food and drink.* Available at www.nmc-uk.org. The Commission has particular objections to the confusion at para 23, particularly the suggestion that SOADs might be expected to authorise covert medication (which they may well not do on principle) and that such authority might extend to informal patients' treatment.

10.52   Some commentators have provided sensible objections to our suggestion that placebo cannot be classed as medicine, arguing that the definition of medicine is broad enough to encompass inert substances used under certain circumstances[290]. We have always held that our view on this matter is provisional and that, without case-law or statutory interpretation, a definitive legal view is impossible. However, even if placebo is considered to be medicine for mental disorder, so that its administration falls within the provisions of section 58 of the 1983 Act, it remains our view that there are serious legal and ethical obstacles to its use if its nature is not fully disclosed to the patient concerned, and that such disclosure would usually undermine the purpose of administering the substance. In our view, it is self-evident that these problems are not limited to certifying that patients consent to such treatments, but must also extend to certifying that they do not consent, whether by reason or incapacity or refusal[291]. A Second Opinion Appointed Doctor would, in our view, be unable to consider whether or not a patient has the capacity or the inclination to consent to a placebo, and therefore whether to authorize it in the absence of consent, if the patient was not aware of the exact nature of the substance being proposed. For this reason we would expect that SOADs would refuse to consider authorising placebo treatments under Part IV of the Act.

10.53   These concerns clearly would not prevent a detained patient from giving consent to partic-ipate in any clinical trial involving placebos, providing that the purpose of detention (i.e. assessment and/or treatment of mental disorder) was not compromised by such partici-pation. If treatment for mental disorder is suspended or a placebo is used in place of a potentially effective drug, this might however undermine the continued justification to detain the patient under the Act.

Naso-gastric feeding for patients with eating disorders

10.54   In 1997 we suggested to Government that naso-gastric feeding for detained anorectic patients should be included within those treatments falling within section 58(3) of the 1983 Act, which would ensure that such feeding, except in emergencies, was only administered in the absence of consent following the authorisation of a Second Opinion[292]. This suggestion was supported by most organisations canvassed by the Department of Health in the following year, and has been repeated throughout the process of consultations and debate over the reform of legislation since that time. We hope that the opportunity of regulating this area of compulsion under the new Mental Health Act will not be overlooked.

Recommendation 39: The Secretary of State should consider the statutory regulation of naso-gastric feeding in relation to its use as a treatment for mental disorder, providing for safeguards equivalent to those relevant to ECT treatment under the 1983 Act.

---

[290]   Hewitt, D (2001) *The legal implications of the administration of placebo to psychiatric patients*, Journal of Mental Health Law, Northumbria University Press, June 2001, p66-74; Jones R (2003) *Mental Health Act Manual*, eighth edition, London: Sweet & Maxwell para 1-723.

[291]   These concerns are shared by Hewitt (2001), *ibid* note 290 above. *The Mental Health Act Manual* does not address the problem.

[292]   Mental Health Act Commission (1997) *Seventh Biennial Report 1995-7*, London, Stationery Office. Chapter 5.2 p110

10.55 We continue to publish a Guidance Note *The Treatment of Anorexia Nervosa under the Mental Health Act 1983*[293], advising on legal and practice issues under current law.

Medication to reduce male sex drive

10.56 The 1983 Act and its Regulations make provision for the strict regulation of the surgical implantation of hormones to reduce the male sexual drive: such a procedure has the same safeguards as are applied to Neurosurgery for Mental Disorder (see 10.60 below). However, the most common sexual suppressant used in psychiatry today is cyproterone acetate ("Androcur"), which is administered orally. When given as an ancillary treatment for mental disorder this may be classed as "medication for mental disorder" and thus require a Second Opinion under section 58 when given to a patient who cannot or does not consent outside of the three-month period. The Commission concurs with the Millan Committee[294] that such treatment under compulsion is a serious interference with human rights, even if the treatment is easily reversed and difficult to physically force on an unwilling patient, and should require a Second Opinion authorisation at any time when it is to be given without consent, as is now the case with ECT.

> **Recommendation 40:** Medication to reduce male sexual drive should be specified as a special treatment under future legislation, requiring consent or the specific authority of the Tribunal.

Electroconvulsive Therapy (ECT)

10.57 At 10.33 and Figure 22 above we showed that ECT accounts for an increasingly small proportion of all treatments administered without consent under the Act. It is too early to tell whether the marginal decrease in the number of such uses of ECT in recent years is a fluctuation or a trend that will continue. There are some reasons to suspect the latter:

(i) The Department of Health's ECT surveys of 1999 and 2002 suggest a more general decline in ECT use. At Figure 29 below we show some figures from this survey, which suggest that the overall usage of ECT may have declined by as much as a quarter over that three-year period. However, no conclusive trend may be drawn over this timescale.

(ii) Some professionals have suggested that advances in treatment generally but psychopharmacology in particular (including, for instance, the introduction of SSRI antidepressants in the late 1980s) have led to a decline in the use of ECT for people with less severe illness[295]. This view has been challenged by others who suggest that an equally plausible explanation, albeit one that is less palatable, is that ECT may have been given needlessly to large numbers of people in the recent past[296].

---

[293] available from www.mhac.trent.nhs.uk. see appendix D below for a list of MHAC publications.

[294] Scottish Executive (2001) *New Directions. Report on the Review of the Mental Health (Scotland) Act 1984* [the Millan Report]. Edinburgh: the Stationery Office. www.scotland.gov.uk/millan. Chapter 10.24-5, Recommendation 10.7

[295] see Eranti S.V. & McLoughlin, D.M. (2003) *Electroconvulsive Therapy – state of the art.* British Journal of Psychiatry 182:8-9, and subsequent correspondence in British Journal of Psychiatry 183: 173

[296] Kemsley, S (2003) *Changing use of ECT.* British Journal of Psychiatry 183: 72

(iii) Guidance from the National Institute for Clinical Excellence (NICE) on the use of electro-convulsive therapy (April 2003) recommends the treatment only for patients with severe symptoms. This restriction may therefore influence the numbers of referrals for ECT for both detained and informal patients.

It is possible, of course, that all of the above will only effect patients with less severe symptoms, who are less likely to be detained under the Act, leaving the use of ECT for detained patients relatively unchanged.

10.58   We recognise that the NICE decision mentioned at 10.57(iii) above was controversial, being appealed unsuccessfully by the Royal College of Psychiatrists but welcomed by MIND and other groups[297]. The Commission recognises that there is deeply felt opposition to ECT treatment from some user-groups, who claim that potential adverse effects of such treatment do not justify the benefits, and regard NICE's decision as an example of their voice being heard. However, we also recognise doctors' concerns that this authority, or subsequent changes in law, might withhold ECT treatment from patients until their condition deteriorates sufficiently to meet the threshold for its application. We do not consider that the current NICE guidance need necessarily lead to such situations, given that 'seriousness' is a relative concept which, perhaps, encompasses the likelihood of imminent clinical deterioration. It may be that further guidance on this issue is warranted.

10.59   The Commission encounters common misunderstandings over the law in relation to ECT. At Chapter 8.9 above we note the widespread misunderstanding that ECT may not be given under the common law when a patient lacks mental capacity but is compliant with admission to hospital, which may lead to unnecessary and therefore unlawful uses of the 1983 Act. The Commission also frequently encounters the mistaken view that patients who are detained under section 2 of the 1983 Act may not be administered ECT, whether in emergencies under section 62 or following a Second Opinion under section 58. In fact there is no reason in law that precludes ECT for such patients. It may be, especially following the NICE guidance discussed above, that the decision to administer ECT with or without consent to a patient who is detained under section 2 might serve as a prompt that section 3 detention should now be considered. This is because the decision to seek authority to administer a course of ECT implies both that the assessment of the diagnosis and prognosis of a patient's mental disorder has reached at least a provisional conclusion and that the proposed treatment is likely to last beyond the 28 day detention allowed under section 2 (see Code of Practice, 5.3(b)).

Recommendation 41: Future editions of the Code of Practice should advise practitioners on legal constraints and good practice measures in respect of the administration of ECT, to counter the frequently noted confusion over these issues.

---

[297] see NICE Health Technology Appraisal *Electroconvulsive Therapy Appeal Panel Decision*, 24 February 2003. www.nice.org.uk; *Mind* press release: *Psychiatrists' appeal to NICE to drop new restrictions on ECT fails as users' views win respect* 26 March 2003, www.mind.org.uk

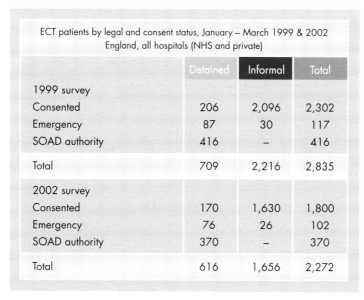

ECT patients by legal and consent status, January – March 1999 & 2002 England, all hospitals (NHS and private)			
	Detained	Informal	Total
1999 survey			
Consented	206	2,096	2,302
Emergency	87	30	117
SOAD authority	416	–	416
Total	709	2,216	2,835
2002 survey			
Consented	170	1,630	1,800
Emergency	76	26	102
SOAD authority	370	–	370
Total	616	1,656	2,272

Fig 29: ECT survey findings, 1999–2002[298] (see 10.57 (i) above)

Neurosurgery for Mental Disorder

10.60 During the reporting period Commission-appointed section 57 panels considered thirteen proposals for neurosurgery for mental disorder (NMD). Seven of these referrals were received in 2001/02, and six in 2002/03. Two patients were referred twice in the period. All the patients were white British, eight were female and three were male. Five patients suffered from severe obsessive compulsive disorder. Others suffered from anxiety and resistant depression.

Six referrals were authorised. Three were declined. Two referrals had to be postponed.

The procedure proposed in all cases was stereotactic bilateral anterior capsulotomy to be performed at the University Hospital of Wales.

Reasons for refusal

10.61 The reasons given by the panel for refusing certification of NMD were:

* Case A: other avenues of treatment had yet to be pursued before NMD could be justified, and the patient had only a superficial understanding of the nature, purpose and likely effects of the procedure.

* Case B: the panel felt there was little evidence of intensive drug treatment; none of the Consultees were convinced that neurosurgery was the only option left and the panel was not confident that the patient would be prepared to follow any proposed treatment plan subsequent to NMD being carried out. This patient was referred again nine months later and a certificate was issued.

* Case C: The panel declined to issue a certificate in this case feeling the treatment was not appropriate. The patient's own doctor had not been convinced of the appropriateness of NMD and had only made the referral at the patient's request.

---

[298] source: adapted from Department of Health (2003) *Statistical Bulletin 2003/08 Electro Convulsive Therapy: Survey covering the period from January 2002 to march 2002, England.* London, National Statistics/Dept of Health, table 7.

10.62 Both cases of postponement were due to problems in accessing the patient's consultant psychiatrist. In the first case the patient had no identified responsible consultant psychiatrist at the time of the referral. In the second case there were problems in arranging for the consultant psychiatrist to attend a panel visit before the operation date. The doctor was also unable to produce reports in time. These problems have been resolved in both cases and the referrals are being reconsidered at the time of writing.

Proposals for NMD under the next Mental Health Act

10.63 The Commission recognises that NMD is a controversial but also frequently misunderstood and misrepresented treatment. We support the continuation of stringent safeguards against its misuse under future legislation. Representations of the dangers of such misuse frequently allude to the long abandoned psychosurgical practices of the mid-twentieth century, but rarely touch upon what we consider to be a more likely danger of unregulated treatment. This is simply that persons who suffer from debilitating obsessive compulsive disorder or refractory depression may view NMD as their best or only hope of overcoming their illness, and may therefore become great proselytizers for the treatment, particularly as many mental health professionals have little or no expertise in it. If society wishes NMD to remain a treatment of last resort, regulation of such referrals which includes consideration of the views of both patients and professionals, and a review of whether treatment may be justified in an individual case, must be retained. Our experience of convening review panels suggests that referrals might easily be accepted despite the misgivings of professionals involved, insufficient understanding by patients or other treatment options not having been exhausted.

10.64 Because current legislation requires that a patient must give informed consent to NMD as a basic criterion of its application, patients who lack mental capacity cannot pass this initial hurdle. The Commission is aware of one case where a patient with learning disability and debilitating obsessive compulsive disorder might benefit greatly from NMD but cannot be considered for it because he could never give valid consent. It is arguable that the law discriminates against patients without capacity in this respect, and that this could be challenged on human rights principles. We therefore welcome the Government's proposals in the draft Mental Health Bill of 2002 to allow the High Court to declare on a case-by-case basis that the administration of NMD to an incapacitated patient would be lawful.

Deep-brain stimulation

10.65 Deep brain stimulation is a procedure involving the implantation of electrodes in the brain that are activated by the patient through an external stimulator. Its use is mainly in Parkinson's Disease, but it has also been applied to some neurological conditions such as severe tremor, dystonia and chronic pain, and it is being used experimentally in the treatment of obsessive compulsive disorder and depression. The Commission has been asked by practitioners to comment on whether the treatment should be considered to fall within the scope of the 1983 Act.

10.66 Clearly any use of the treatment for physical disorders such as Parkinson's Disease or chronic pain would be outside of the Act's scope. Uses for other neurological conditions,

11.4   It is therefore not in the spirit of human rights-based practice to detain a person in surroundings where they might feel threatened or intimidated by the behaviour of other detainees, or at risk from their own actions. Thus the maintenance of orderly and civilised conditions in hospital wards through control and discipline of detained patients is a positive obligation on healthcare providers.

The current legal position

11.5   It should be remembered that action to bring to an end actual or threatened criminal behaviour is permitted under common law, subject to such an action being proportionate to the actual or threatened behaviour. Thus staff should not feel inhibited from intervening to prevent physical or sexual assault, possession or selling of drugs, theft or serious damage to property. Limited legal powers can also be gleaned from existing statute other than the Mental Health Act 1983: for example, section 3(1) of the Criminal Law Act 1967 enables a member of staff in a mental institution to use reasonable force to prevent a patient from committing an assault.

11.6   A patient detained under mental health legislation retains all civil rights that are not taken away expressly or by implication by the detention (*Raymond v Honey* [1982]). The 1983 Act does not provide any formal framework equivalent to that which enables prison staff to discipline inmates. Because of this, some hospital staff may feel vulnerable when enforcing a disciplinary environment, even the relatively innocuous day-to-day 'house rules' of a ward environment. However, case law has determined that there are powers of control and discipline resultant from the detention of patients under the 1983 Act. The leading case of *Poutney v Griffiths* [1976] held that a nurse on duty in a High Security Hospital had the function of controlling detained patients. In *R v Broadmoor Special Hospital and the Secretary of State for the Department of Health ex p S, H and D* [1998], the Court of Appeal confirmed this in deciding that there were "necessary incidents of control flowing from the power of detention for treatment", and hospitals were entitled to give precedence to the interests of the patients as a whole over the interest of individual patients. Upholding the right of Ashworth Hospital to restrict a male patient's freedom to dress as and assume the appearance of a woman, the courts determined that powers of control and discipline implied by the Act can be lawfully applied provided that they are compatible with ECHR rights; reasonable; and for the purposes of detention and/or treatment, rather than for some ulterior purpose (*R (on the application of E) v Ashworth Hospital Authority* [2001]).

11.7   Although all of the leading cases on this issue concern high secure care, the argument that the Act provides associated powers of control and discipline was accepted in a number of cases relating to other security sectors, including *R v MHAC ex p Smith* [1998] and *S v Airedale NHS Trust* [2002]. Powers of control and discipline related to the detention and treatment of patients may therefore be assumed at all security levels, although the reasonableness of any measure of control or discipline may have to be considered as proportionate to the security needs of any particular environment.

11.8   The broad definition of "medical treatment for mental disorder" at section 145 of the Act encompasses "care, habilitation and rehabilitation under medical supervision". This broad definition has been taken by the courts to include many control and discipline measures, including seclusion (see 11.13 below). Such measures can therefore be lawfully imposed upon any patient in the absence of consent under the authority of section 63 of the Act, provided that the measure is taken under the direction of the patient's RMO. It seems unlikely that the decision in *B v Ashworth* [2003] (see Chapter 3.40 *et seq* above) will constrain the uses of such control and discipline measures, unless it can be argued that any such measure is of limited application to certain legal classifications of mental disorder.

11.9   This grounding of the authority for control and discipline measures in section 63 inevitably leads to interventions being couched in therapeutic language. In some cases, this provides a useful reminder to authorities with the power of control and discipline of the purpose of their endowment, and it should also serve as a limit on the application of such powers. However, it can also serve as a euphemism to mask actions that amount to punishment, reinforcing unquestioning attitudes of staff and cutting off patients from any means of appeal or complaint.

11.10   It is doubtful that all aspects of rules and penalties designed to enforce reasonable conduct can be construed honestly as treatment for mental disorder. For instance, it seems evident that the control of noise, smoking, and offensive language on a ward may help to maintain the therapeutic environment and therefore have an overall therapeutic aim, but it is less plausible to describe action taken to stop any particular patient from smoking in a non-smoking area as part of that patient's treatment. It is certainly the case that "patient-contracts" used to set out and agree house rules for informal patients are not generally cloaked in therapeutic terminology.

11.11   Some legal experts have called for the control of patient conduct to be formalised in written, published policies. Such policies would define behaviours calling for sanctions; specify the likely response in terms of loss of privilege or closer confinement; and provide procedures for appeal against penalties imposed[302]. Such an approach no doubt has its own dangers, of which the risk of inflexible responses that are blind to patients' conditions and capacities may be the most obvious. Nevertheless we would welcome a broader debate on these complex issues.

11.12   In our view, issues pertaining to control and discipline in hospitals will continue to be of central concern both to mental health professionals and to the courts. We urge Government to attend to them at a policy level, whether through regulation, Code of Practice guidance or lower-level advice. We explore some specific areas in more detail below.

The legal and ethical basis for seclusion and restraint

11.13   The *Munjaz* judgment of July 2003, which we outline at Chapter 3.2 *et seq* above, confirmed previous findings that a power to seclude may be assumed from the general powers of detention under the 1983 Act[303]. It also allowed that authority to seclude may be found under section 63 of the Act[304]. This is because the broad interpretation of "medical treatment for mental disorder" on which that section relies extends, in essence, "from cure

---

[302]   Richardson, Genevra (1995) Openness, Order and Regulation in a Therapeutic Setting. In J Crichton (ed) *Psychiatric Patient Violence: Risk and Response.* London: Duckworth.

[303]   *R (on the application of Munjaz) v Mersey Care NHS trust & two others; S v Airedale NHS Trust* [2003] para 40

[304]   *ibid.* para 45.

to containment" [305]. Therefore it would seem that the authorities established for seclusion must extend to other forms of control, such as the physical restraint of patients.

11.14   Although the 1983 Act itself provides no particular safeguard or limitation the powers to seclude that it implies, the court in *Munjaz* [2003] ruled that such powers must be operated consistently and transparently within limits set by domestic law to meet the requirements of the European Convention. In particular, seclusion used improperly or without due regard to the welfare of the patient could violate Article 3 of the ECHR (prohibiting degrading treatment or punishment) [306], and Article 8 (determining the right to a private life) may be engaged where treatment, although not so severe as to amount to degradation, does infringe upon a patient's moral or physical integrity without good cause [307]. The court determined that the Code of Practice is the means by which the State undertakes its duty to ensure that public authorities operate powers consistent with the requirements of the ECHR. Seclusion that is not practiced in accordance with the Code's guidance will, unless departure from such guidance can be justified as necessary in an individual patient's case, therefore fail to meet the requirement of legality set by the ECHR.

11.15   The Code of Practice guidance on the use of seclusion and restraint (chapter 19) is grounded in the notion of seclusion or restraint being immediately necessary responses to take control of dangerous situations. For this reason, the Code distinguishes between seclusion and "time out", where the latter is a behaviour modification technique and will, therefore, be a part of a patient's treatment plan. The Code provides guidance on requirements of good practice in seclusion and restraint interventions, and requires hospitals to have operational policies on their use. Sample policies and forms for record keeping in relation to both seclusion and restraint are included within the Institute of Mental Health Act Practitioners' Policy Compendium, produced in 2002 in conjunction with the Commission [308].

11.16   The fact that legal authority for restraint and seclusion stems from a definition of treatment should not disguise the fact that such interventions are only justifiable in practice terms when used as a means of containing severely disturbed behaviour likely to cause harm. Seclusion and restraint are legitimate neither as forms of clinical treatment nor punishment.

Mental Health Act Commission findings and concerns regarding seclusion practice

11.17   We continue to monitor and encourage services' compliance with the guidance given in the Code of Practice. In addition, our last two Biennial Reports provided advice on seclusion, which has been endorsed by the NHS Zero Tolerance Campaign, and listed Commission concerns with the proper use and recording of seclusion [309]. Our concerns remain as follows:

---

[305] *Reid v Secretary of State for Scotland* [1999]. This therefore relates to section 125 of the Mental Health (Scotland) Act 1984, section 125, which is essentially similar to section 63 of the 1983 Act. This case is one of a number that establishes this principle, although it is not actually cited in the *Munjaz* judgment under discussion.

[306] *Munjaz* [2003] para 53-55

[307] *Munjaz* [2003] para 65

[308] Institute of Mental Health Act Practitioners (2002) *Mental Health Act 1983 Policy Compendium*. May 2002. pp20 & app.6. See Appendix E below for publication details.

[309] see Mental Health Act Commission (2001) *Ninth Biennial Report, 1999-2001*, Chapter 4.38 – 4.44. This also includes a summary of the Eighth Biennial Report's advice upon seclusion, originally published in Mental Health Act Commission (1999) *Eight Biennial Report 1997-1999*, Chapter 10.16 – 10.25. London: Stationery Office

* Detention in a small and featureless room is oppressive for anyone, but particularly for a mentally disordered person it may exacerbate feelings of isolation, despair or anger, worsen delusions or hallucinations, or even bring about the behaviour that it is designed to prevent.

* Staff using seclusion may, in some cases, have motivations other than the urgent need to manage a potentially dangerous situation, which is the sole legitimate reason for instigating seclusion. In particular, misplaced therapeutic aims or punitive intent can appear to underlie some episodes. It is important, therefore, that the reasons for seclusion episodes are carefully recorded and monitored by services.

* The physical environments used for seclusion may have poor facilities or be unfit for purpose, whether in terms of dignity and privacy or for more immediate safety considerations. It is common for there to be no washing or toilet facilities in seclusion rooms. Some rooms are badly situated in relation to the wards they serve, so that patients have to be escorted through public spaces or through dangerous environments, such as stairways, to reach seclusion facilities.

* The records of observation and actions during seclusion episodes are not always kept well, either through simple omission or due to illegible, cramped entries on badly designed forms.

Many services have taken up our recommendation in the Ninth Biennial Report that these concerns be addressed in their own monitoring and audit of seclusion episodes. However, even among the services who submitted voluntary self-assessments to the Commission, 40% failed to report any monitoring and audit procedures (see Figure 30 below), and only a quarter of wards that we visited to collect seclusion data could produce any recent audit material[310]. It would seem that safeguards relating to seclusion practice are developing patchily across the country.

> **Recommendation 43:** Minimum standards should be established for seclusion facilities, taking account of physical risks to patients of badly designed or equipped seclusion rooms, and seclusion practice, particularly in relation to record-keeping (see also recommendation 44) and monitoring/audit. Such a requirement should eventually be set by the next Mental Health Act itself, but in the meantime could be established for NHS facilities by Government Directive, and by agreement/contract with the independent sector.

11.18   Over 2002/03 the Commission started a systematic collation of data on seclusion practice.[311] We show some of our detailed findings in Figure 31 below, but wish to particularly draw attention to the rate of failure against the most basic requirements of physical environment set by the Code of Practice, Chapter 19.22. Whilst we make no claim for the statistical significance of these figures in relation to practice across all services, the numbers of services who acknowledge not meeting requirements of the Code of Practice is notable. The Code requires seclusion facilities to:

---

[310] Of 56 wards with seclusion facilities visited over 2002/03, only 15 could produce the results of the most recent audit of seclusion practice. Of these, only six could show that any recommendations arising from this had been actioned.

[311] see Chapter 19.11(c) on the use of Commission Visiting Questionnaires (CVQs).

* provide privacy from other patients   (52% failed)

* enable staff to observe the patient at all times   (46% failed)

* be safe and secure   (68% failed)

* not contain anything which might cause harm to the patient or others   (68% failed)

* be adequately furnished, heated, lit and ventilated; and   (77% failed)

* be quiet but not soundproof with some means of calling for attention.   (39% failed)

Seclusion monitoring and reduction policies								
	N/A		Red		Amber		Green	
	n.	%	n	%	n	%	n	%
Are written policies available, understood and followed in practice ?	19	26.4	3	4.2	8	11.1	42	58.3
Is the staff complement adequate in number and training to implement policy ?	22	30.6	1	1.4	24	33	27	37
Are there at least annual in-house reviews with Board reporting ?	21	29.2	9	12.5	11	15.3	31	43
Is there on-going audit leading to remedial action on issues raised ?	21	29.2	9	12.5	16	22.2	26	36.1

Fig 30: Self-assessments of 72 hospitals/Trusts in relation to progress against Commission Ninth Biennial Report Recommendations 42 and 43[312]

11.19   At the time of writing, we had available for analysis data from 113 individual seclusion records examined by Commissioners over the last year. Of these, 93% (105) recorded clear reasons for the instigation of seclusion, but only about 70–72% (79 – 82) were considered by Commissioners to be 'detailed contemporaneous records' as required by the Code of Practice at chapter 19.23[313]. Compliance with *all* of the requirements of the Code's chapter 19.23 was much rarer: only 53% of records (60) were countersigned by a doctor and senior nurse, and less than half (53, or 47%) were cross-referenced to a special seclusion book or forms giving step-by-step account of the seclusion procedure.

11.20   In a quarter of seclusion episodes monitored (29, or 26%), the need to continue seclusion had not been reviewed according to the requirements of the Code at chapter 19.21. Following the *Munjaz* judgment, failure to follow these requirements of the Code may constitute unlawful practice. We strongly advise hospital managers to review their policies and procedures to ensure that they are operating within the law.

11.21   The Commission's particular concerns about the use of long-term seclusion are discussed at Chapter 12.23 *et seq* below.

[312] Based upon a voluntary (and therefore self-selecting) return of 72 self-assessment forms, representing approximately a quarter of all detaining hospitals in England and Wales. The Commission's Ninth Biennial Report Recommendations 42 & 43 state that hospital managers should audit the use of seclusion regularly to ensure proper use, taking account of Commission concerns. When seclusion use is high, a monitoring plan should be introduced which includes monitoring the effects of any change in management regime on the attitude and behaviour of patients.

[313] 81 records (72%) showed a report on the patient's condition and behaviour every fifteen minutes, as required by the Code of Practice paragraph 19.20, although Commissioners reported only 79 of these to meet their expectation of a record as described by the Code at chapter 19.23.

Physical aspects of seclusion facilities

	Red		Amber		Green	
	n	%	n	%	n	%
Privacy and dignity						
Is the facility located in a quiet area of the ward?	36	64.3	18	32.1	2	3.6
Is it isolated from living and sleeping areas on the ward?	25	44.6	29	51.8	2	3.6
Does it offer privacy from other patients, visitors and other passers-by?	26	29.2	29	51.8	1	1.8
Is the facility clean?	50	89.3	1	1.8	5	8.9
Can staff regulate room temperature?	12	21.4	43	76.8	1	1.8
Can staff regulate room ventilation?	27	48.2	26	46.4	3	5.4
Are there separate shower / bathing facilities for a secluded patient?	10	17.8	45	80.4	1	1.8
Are there separate lavatory facilities for secluded patients?	24	42.9	32	57.1	-	-
Are disposable urine bottles and bed-pans available in case of need?	50	89.2	3	5.4	3	5.4
Safety and security						
Can all the room be seen from outside through an observation panel?	28	50	26	46.4	2	3.6
Can staff observe the patient without being obtrusive?	45	80.4	9	16	2	3.6
Does the seclusion room door open outwards?	55	98.2	-	-	1	1.8
Are there any sharp corners within the seclusion room?	15	26.7	38	67.9	3	5.4
Is there anything in the room that may be used as a weapon?	8	14.3	47	83.9	1	1.8
Are the light fittings out of reach, even if patient stands on the bed?	37	66	16	28.6	3	5.4
Are the light fittings made of unbreakable materials?	35	62.5	14	25	7	12.5
Is the bed-frame suitably secured to the floor?	33	58.9	9	16.1	14	25
Is the bedding tear-resistant?	29	51.8	16	28.6	11	19.6
Is the mattress thick and firm enough to prevent suffocation?	45	80.4	6	10.7	5	8.9
Does the mattress have a tear-resistant, waterproof cover?	46	82.2	4	7.1	6	10.7
Are the furniture and fittings in the seclusion room suitable?	48	85.7	7	12.5	1	1.8
Can the patient call for attention by some means (e.g. buzzer /intercom)?	32	57.1	22	39.3	2	3.6

Fig 31: Data collected by the Commission on physical aspects of seclusion facilities, England and Wales, 2002–03

11.22 Patients should have access to quiet space and opportunity to be alone without seclusion procedures being instigated, as there should be no need for them to be locked into or in any way "confined" in a room. In our Sixth Biennial Report we reported the policy decision to terminate the need for "self-seclusion" in high secure hospitals, as patients' rights to privacy and opportunity for time alone was to be respected, for instance by the installation of privacy locks on patients' rooms[314]. The recognition of patients' right to privacy and time alone has been slow to spread across all psychiatric services. The Commission will be undertaking further work in this area in the coming year (see Chapter 19.19 below).

---

[314] Mental Health Act Commission (1995) *Sixth Biennial Report 1993-5*. London: Stationery Office p120

Seclusion and medical staffing

11.23 The fact that seclusion procedures must now comply with guidance of the Code of Practice to be lawful (see 11.14 above) may cause difficulties in some smaller units where, for example, 24-hour medical cover is not provided on-site. Unless arrangements can be made for the immediate attendance of a doctor when seclusion episodes last for more than five minutes, and for four-hourly medical reviews of the need to continue seclusion, it may not be practicable for such units to use seclusion as an intervention. It seems highly possible to the Commission that resource limitations would not be judged to be an acceptable reason for systematic departure from the Code's guidance in this area in the face of a legal challenge. Units whose medical staffing will not provide 24-hour cover following implementation of the Working Time Directive in regard to junior doctors' contracted hours may experience similar difficulties. Whilst we appreciate that this may be inconvenient for the managers of such units, limitations on the use of restraint practices and seclusion in non-medical staffed units may justified on safety grounds as well as because of this possible change in the law[315].

> **Recommendation 44:** The Commission urges Government to consider the practical problems faced by services without 24 hour medical staffing in meeting basic safety requirements and the requirements of the Code of Practice when operating the powers provided by the Act, particularly in emergency interventions. The Commission particularly urges Government to consider:
>
> * what additional resources may be needed by such services, whether in terms of staffing, training or facilities;
>
> * to consider whether certain types of response to emergency situations (such as seclusion) should be permissible to such services; and
>
> * what guidance might be offered to services on these issues.

The need for statutory regulation

11.24 The Commission has argued for the passing of new legislation to be taken as an opportunity to reconsider and strengthen advice and practice requirements relating to seclusion and restraint. Notwithstanding the fact that the Court in *Munjaz* [2003] has given the Code of Practice greater legal weight (a move that was opposed by the Department of Health at first instance hearing), we believe that it is now appropriate to provide a framework of statutory regulation around these important issues. We have therefore suggested, in our responses to the consultations over the next Mental Health Act, that the following should be considered in the formulation of new mental health legislation:

* Statutory requirements/limitations in relation to the institution, recording and monitoring of seclusion (including its duration) and time-out;

* Statutory requirements in relation to the environment used for the purposes of seclusion;

---

[315] The Commission is particularly concerned about the practice of seclusion without medical supervision following the death of David Bennett (see Chapter 16.18 below). In relation to medical staffing and emergency measures, see also the introduction to this report (Chapter 1.6); and, on urgent treatment under section 62, Chapter 10.32 above.

* Statutory requirements in relation to the provision of food and drinks and other basic amenities to patients subject to seclusion;

* Statutory requirements/limitations in relation to the removal of clothing and/or bedding from patients subject to seclusion, and in relation to "protective" clothing/bedding;

* Statutory requirements/limitations on the use, recording and monitoring of physical restraints and in the training of staff in such procedures;

* Statutory requirements in relation to the locking of wards;

* Statutory requirements as to the qualifications of staff who institute the above; and

* Statutory requirements in relation to observation and care of patients who are at risk of self-harm or of harm to others.

11.25 Regulations could introduce statutory documentation for episodes of seclusion and serious restraint, both as a means of ensuring that actions and their justifications are considered and recorded, and to direct that certain actions be undertaken through requirements to record their having taken place.

> **Recommendation 45:** Statutory documentation should be introduced under the next Mental Health Act to require records of specific actions in relation to seclusion and certain forms of restraint.

11.26 The Commission is aware of ongoing work by the National Institute for Clinical Excellence (NICE) in reviewing research relating to the use of seclusion and restraint so as to develop practice guidelines. We look forward to the publication of NICE's draft guidelines and good practice points and to participating in the ensuing discussion over their final form. NICE's consideration of good practice guidelines will be able to draw a raft of existing and previously issued guidelines, including:

* the current Mental Health Act Code of Practice, Chapter 19;

* the Mental Health Act Commission Ninth Biennial Report recommendations 42 – 45;

* the IMHAP Policy Compendium guidance on seclusion and restraint policies;

* the Police Complaint Authority's *Policing Acute Behavioural Disturbance*, (revised March 2002)[316];

* guidance on restrictive physical interventions in relation to people with learning disabilities and autistic spectrum disorder, issued by the Department of Health and Department for Education and Skills in July 2002[317];

* the resource sheets made available by the Department of Health as a part of its Zero Tolerance campaign on managing violence in health services[318];

---

[316] available from www.pca.gov.uk

[317] Department of Health & Department for Education and Skills (2002) *Guidance for Restrictive Physical Interventions – How to provide safe services for people with Learning Disabilities and Autistic Spectrum Disorder.* London: Department of Health July 2002. www.doh.gov.uk/learningdisabilities

[318] www.nhs.uk/zerotolerance

* the Royal College of Psychiatrists' 1998 report, *The management of imminent violence: Clinical practice guidelines to support mental health services guidance*; and

* the UKCC (now the Nursing and Midwifery Council) report, *The recognition, prevention and therapeutic management of violence in mental health care, published in February 2002*[319].

In the Commission's view, this raft of guidance requires consolidation and official sanction, so that detailed guidance with formal status and legal weight underlies statutory regulation.

Safety and restraint

11.27   Restraint is widely practiced across mental health services that detain patients under the 1983 Act. The varied forms that restraint may take are alluded to at Chapter 19.6 of the Code of Practice, which suggests that restraint must be seen as a continuum from verbal instruction to physical intervention designed to take control of and diffuse a dangerous situation by limiting a patient's freedom for as short a time as is possible.

11.28   Chapter 19.5 of the Code of Practice provides a substantial list of general preventive measures that hospital managers and staff can take to reduce problem behaviour on wards and thus reduce incidences of control and restraint. Although managers must attend to issues of safety in using restraint, it is also imperative that they consider these issues so as to avoid aggressively coercive practice where possible[320].

11.29   In Chapter 16.18 below we highlight the case of David Bennett, the inquiry into whose death is is expected to report as we go to press. The restraint episode that was ongoing at the time of his death was sparked by behaviour resulting from racial abuse directed at Mr Bennett. The Commission continues to emphasise the need for good operational policies that deal promptly with patient to patient racial or other abuse, bullying or goading, and avoid singling out the victims of such actions for special treatment that make them feel doubly victimised.

11.30   There are clear dangers inherent in the use of restraint, as evidenced by the unlawful killing of Roger Sylvester as a result of a restraint episode in 1999. The particular dangers of positional asphyxiation in psychiatric patients may be enhanced by side effects of medication; excited delirium, prolonged struggle or exhaustion; and obesity or underlying ill health[321]. It is important that patients' previous histories are well established when they are deemed at risk of requiring restraint.

11.31   Patients will often react to restraint episodes with anger and a sense of injustice, often refusing to accept the justification of the intervention after the event. Restraint episodes can be particularly distressing for patients who have suffered sexual or physical abuse and staff should be aware of such issues through patients' care-plans regarding restraint practice. It is important that patients are told as much as possible of the reasons for their restraint during

---

[319]   available on www.nmc-uk.org

[320]   The Commission acknowledges the Government guidance already is available, although this has limited application to the care of the majority of detained patients: see Department of Health and Department of Education & Skills (2002) *Guidance for restrictive physical interventions: how to provide safe services for people with learning disability & Autistic Spectrum Disorder*. Available from the website www.doh.gov.uk/qualityprotects/index.htm.

[321]   see also Police Complaints Authority (2003) *Safer Restraint: Report of the conference held in April 2002 at Church House, Westminster*. London: PCA. www.pca.gov.uk. p10-12. The Roger Sylvester inquest verdict was reported widely in October 2003: see, for example, Rebecca Allison & Vickram Dodd *Council Worker Unlawfully Killed by Police* Guardian, 4 October 2003; Stephanie Marsh *Black Man Unlawfully Killed in Custody* Times, 4 October 2003.

the intervention itself, provided with care and support immediately after an incident[322], and that the requirements of the Code of Practice regarding post-incident visits to the patient to talk about the incident and ascertain any complaints are met.

11.32 The Code of Practice requires the use of restraint to be recorded in various ways: individual patients' care-plans should state under what circumstances physical restraint should be used, what form it will take and how it will be reviewed. All episodes of such restraint should be carefully documented and reviewed. Reasons for decisions to allow physical restraint in any care-plan, and for each episode of physical restraint that takes place, should be carefully recorded in the patient's notes. The Commission recommends that policies dealing with practice issues where restraint may be used, such as policies on holding powers under sections 4, 5 or 136, should explicitly state the need for records to be made of any physical restraint. Of 69 section 5(2) policies examined on Commission visits in 2001/02, less than half (32) instructed staff on recording requirements if restraint had been used[323].

11.33 In our Ninth Biennial Report we recommended that all services should ensure that each use of Control & Restraint is immediately reviewed, with regular audits to ensure that management and training lessons are learnt. Figure 32 below, taken from the voluntary returns on progress against such recommendations in 2002, provides an indication that this recommendation has yet to be universally adopted.

Maintenance and monitoring of control and restraint procedures	N/A		Red		Amber		Green	
	n.	%	n	%	n	%	n	%
Are written policies available, understood and followed in practice ?	2	2.8	5	6.9	12	16.7	53	73.6
Is the staff complement adequate in number and training to implement policy ?	1	1.4	0	0	26	36.1	45	62.5
Are there at least annual in-house reviews with Board reporting ?	2	2.8	14	19.4	15	20.8	41	56.9
Is there on-going audit leading to remedial action on issues raised ?	2	2.8	11	15.2	22	30.6	37	51.4

Fig 32: Self-assessments of 72 hospitals/Trusts in relation to progress in implementing Commission Ninth Biennial Report Recommendations 44 and 45[324]

[322] Mental Health Act Commission (2001) *Ninth Biennial Report 1999-01*. London: Stationery Office, Recommendation 44.

[323] Research conducted for the Department of Health concluded that, as well as having little specific human rights focus, available C&R training gave no specific training in report writing, statement making and the linking of physical skills training to reporting process and post-facto evaluation of interventions. Such recorded evaluation would be important as a demonstration of the reasonableness and necessity of an action in the light of subsequent legal challenge, as well as a basic element of good practice. (see Bleetman, A and Boatman P (2001) An *Overview of control and restraint issues for the health service*. DOH commissioned report).

[324] Based upon a voluntary (and therefore self-selecting) return of 72 self-assessment forms, representing approximately a quarter of all detaining hospitals in England and Wales. The Commission's Ninth Biennial Report Recommendations 44 and 45 state that each use of control and restraint should be reviewed, with post-incident care and support, including a visit by a senior officer, arranged for the patient concerned. Regular audits should aim to eliminate poor practice and highlight training needs.

11.34   The apparent slow take-up of the Commission suggestions appear to us to indicate further the need for statutory regulation as discussed at 11.24 above.

Mechanical Restraint

11.35   Few subjects in psychiatry have darker or more reviled histories than the use of mechanical restraints. The founding moment of enlightened psychiatry is regarded as Phillippe Pinel's striking off the chains from the inmates of the Bicêtre asylum in the 1790s[325]. Many lay persons and even clinicians would be shocked to think that mechanical restraint has any part in psychiatric practice in the UK today.

11.36   It is widely assumed that the Code of Practice states an absolute prohibition on the use of mechanical restraints. In fact, paragraph 19.10 of the Code only states that "restraint which involves tying (whether by means of tape or by using a part of the patient's garments) to some part of a building or to its fixtures or fittings should never be used". The Code also provides general guidance that staff, in taking decisions about methods of restraining behaviour, must make a balanced judgment between the need to promote a patient's autonomy to move freely and the duty to protect that person from harm.

11.37   The Code makes no specific reference to forms of restraint used in other countries, particularly the United States, such as belts to which wrist or ankle cuffs may be attached to limit the movement of a patient's arms. An ambulatory device of this type, especially obtained from abroad, was in use in recent years to protect a patient in a High Security Hospital from harming himself or others by restricting the full movement of his arms. The decision to use the device was taken by the clinical team who were concerned that the only alternative was for constant physical restraint by two or more members of staff. The device was employed with the agreement of the patient concerned, and is no longer in use as the patient's mental condition has considerably improved.

11.38   It is also the case that standard handcuffs are widely used, particularly in the transport outside of hospital of patients detained in secure facilities. The Commission has been approached for advice on this matter on a number of occasions. We accept that there is nothing in law that would seem to prohibit the use of handcuffs in certain circumstances, and urge authorities to ensure the Code of Practice principles are adhered to in making risk-assessment decisions about their use. The policy of one Trust which contacted the Commission on this matter required the use of handcuffs to be assessed as necessary by the clinical team prior to use, and reviewed by post-incident analysis, with both processes being recorded in the patient's medical record. This would appear to be a good standard for other Trusts that use handcuffs on their patients in any circumstances. We discuss the police and their use of handcuffs at 11.45 below.

11.39   Acutely disturbed patients who present a danger to self or others are, perhaps surprisingly, probably not the patient group that is most frequently exposed to forms of 'mechanical

---

[325]   see Gordon H, Hindley N, Marsden A and Shivayogi M (1999) *The use of mechanical restraint in the treatment of psychiatric patients: is it ever appropriate?* Journal of Forensic Psychiatry Vol 10 No 1 April 1999 173-186. Gordon *et al* point to the element of romantic myth in the accounts of Pinel and other psychiatric pioneers of non-restraint. As now, certain practices continued even if they were no longer recognised as restraint.

restraint'. Frail elderly patients, or patients with severe learning disabilities, may require bodily support at certain times to prevent dangerous falls or to provide basic mobility. Some apparatus that is probably fairly widely used, such as chairs with harness-style straps, may appear to breach the Code of Practice's prohibition on the fastening of patients to fixtures or fittings. The examples of outright abuse that the Code's prohibition seeks to guard against, such as patients being left tied to lavatories, overshadows a more complex ethical area of the day-to-day care of patients who, in the main, are not formally detained and are thus not subject to safeguards including oversight of the Commission[326].

11.40   In this reporting period the Commission received a complaint from a third party who was concerned at the use of harnessed and fixed chairs for specific elderly patients who were very prone to falling. Although, by chance, the patients concerned were not detained under the Mental Health Act and therefore outside our remit, the Commission did inquire about practices at the unit. We were reassured by the explanations given, and by the clear evidence that staff had considered whether the use of such harnesses was necessary and ethical. As the complainant was not so reassured, we have corresponded further through his MP and drawn the general issues to the attention of the Department of Health. We understand that the use of harness arrangements such as this is not uncommon across the country.

11.41   The Commission is not advocating the use of mechanical restraint, but it does seem to us that this difficult area needs to be openly discussed with a view to practice guidelines and statutory regulation if possible. We commend this issue as an area of study under future monitoring arrangements, which should be restricted neither by our limited remit nor, indeed, resources.

> **Recommendation 46:** The Commission proposes the use of mechanical restraint in all mental health services as a possible area of study under future monitoring arrangements.

Requesting police intervention

11.42   Liaison between social services and the police is discussed at Chapter 8.60 *et seq* above. It is also conceivable that situations may arise where nursing staff require the help of the police to control or resolve incidents in hospital environments. In our Fifth Biennial Report (1993) we expressed our concern at police involvement in clinical situations, following reports of police being called to assist in giving forcible medication[327]. Ward policies should set out when it is appropriate to request the help of police and should generally discourage their use in the day to day clinical management of patients. The Commission has heard of

---

[326] Gordon *et al* (see note 325 above) describe a straw-poll taken at a Learning Disability section meeting of a conference of the Royal College of Psychiatrists, where half of an audience of about 70 psychiatrists admitted to having used some form of mechanical restraint for their patients at some time. "Chairs whose construction immobilises clients" are listed as a form of restraint in Royal College of Nursing Guidance from 1999: *Restraint Revisited – Rights, Risk and Responsibility. Guidance for Nurses Working with Older People* (now under review), although this guidance also recognises that "the most ordinary piece of equipment or the most routine procedure – for example, catheterisation – could, in some circumstances, be regarded as restraint" (p3). The Department of Health/DES publication *Guidance for Restrictive Physical Interventions* (July 2002, see note 320 above) describes the use of arm-cuffs or splints to prevent self-harm in learning disability or autistic spectrum disordered patients as a "low-risk" intervention (p11).

[327] Mental Health Act Commission (1993) *Fifth Biennial Report 1991-3.* London: Stationery Office, Chapter 3.5(f)

some hospitals requesting police assistance on a regular basis for the administration of psychiatric medication to refusing patients. This is an inappropriate use of police resources, may raise questions of law (some police forces are concerned as to their legal powers in such circumstances), and is surely an indictment of staffing and staff-training levels on the hospital wards concerned.

11.43   In past reports, and following Chapter 8.62 above, we have also expressed our concern at some police forces' apparent heavy-handedness in assisting Mental Health Act assessments. In our Fifth Report we warned that sending a number of police officers in riot-gear in response to requests for assistance may worsen rather than help any situation likely to arise. It is important that policies regarding contact with the police set out what kind of assistance may be requested and expected.

11.44   Hospitals should have readily available policies on police involvement in incidents where crime is concerned. Such policies should provide advice on the need to consider reporting such incidents to the police, with a view to investigation and possible prosecution. Matters to take account of may include the needs and wishes of victims (perhaps including requirements for potential criminal injuries compensation claims); the need for special investigative expertise in relation to areas such as drugs concealment; and the making of an effective record of any incident for legal and future risk-assessment purposes. However, hospital staff must be cautious of involving the police in relatively minor incidents. The police may resent being asked to take charge of a situation where nursing skills should suffice. Where incidents are dealt with internally, full records of what happened and what actions were taken must be made.

Use of police or private security firms in transporting patients

11.45   Where the police are required to help with the transport of patients, they will usually consider handcuffing the patient. We recommend that this be taken into account when requesting police assistance, if possible through a clinical risk-assessment prior to the request being made (see 11.38 above). Similar consideration should be given when involving private security firms to transport patients, as well as careful review of the procedures and modes of transport used by such firms. We are aware of some detained patients having been transported between hospitals, sometimes for considerable distances, inside vans fitted with security cages and barely adequate seating. In one case a patient was driven from Bristol to London (120 miles), in another from Aintree to Darlington (140 miles). In the latter case, the van had no windows and the driver was unable to see the patient, who had no access to toilet facilities or drinking water during the non-stop journey. Prior to the journey the patient had been given a high dose of Acuphase for sedation. There were clear risks to the patient's life in such circumstances. The patient was reported to be traumatised and tearful upon arrival at the receiving hospital, and to have talked of "being a monkey in a cage". The Commission wrote a letter expressing our concern to the NHS Trust responsible for making the transfer arrangements within a fortnight of the events described. The Trust have subsequently accepted that the arrangements, which had also been used for other patients' transportation, were unacceptable, and agreed that future transfers would be facilitated using transport facilities from another part of the Trust with appropriate escorting staff.

11.46 The Commission advises all authorities that are responsible for detaining patients to be wary of delegating transport arrangements to other bodies without careful oversight of the procedures and practical means employed. Practices that fall short of the requirements of Chapter 11 of the Code of Practice may be found unlawful at legal challenge. We will draw the attention of authorities, including purchasing authorities, to arrangements that are inadequate in our view.

> **Recommendation 47:** All authorities responsible for the use of the Mental Health Act in the detention and treatment of patients should review their arrangements for the conveyance of patients, ensuring in particular that such arrangements meet the standards suggested by Chapter 11 of the Code of Practice.

Searching and confiscation of patients' property

11.47 Where the 1983 Act specifically deals with a control and discipline issue – the withholding of patient's mail[328] – it is quite exacting about when the use of such a power is justifiable and the procedures that are to be followed in doing so. In the formulation of new mental health legislation similar attention could be given to wider aspects of interference with patient's property, from searching to confiscation.

11.48 Chapter 25 of the Code of Practice provides guidance on personal searches under current legislation and requires hospitals to have a policy covering searching patients and their belongings. Advice on policies is contained in the IMHAP policy compendium, produced in conjunction with the Commission[329]. Hospitals should comply with the Code of Practice's guidance and ensure that:

* permission is sought prior to searches, with searches without consent being instigated only after consultation with the RMO;

* searches are undertaken with due regard to patient's dignity and privacy, with minimum force and by a member of the same sex; and

* the patient is kept informed of what is happening and why.

There may be circumstances where necessity dictates that all of the above conditions cannot be met. Where this is the case, it is important that a full record of the intervention and its justification, with reference to individual risk-assessments, is made in the notes of every patient involved. In the absence of such justification, the lawfulness of searching procedures may be compromised (see Chapter 6.17 *et seq* above).

11.49 Chapter 25.3 of the Code of Practice causes some concern to hospital managers. Whilst allowing that policies may extend to routine or random searching without cause, its example of such a cause, taken from *R v Broadmoor Special Hospital Authority ex parte S and others* [1998], is the definition of "special hospital" patients and as such could only apply within high security services. This is unfortunate, as the judgment relied upon has wider

---

328 Mental Health Act 1983, section 134

329 Institute of Mental Health Act Practitioners (2002) *Mental Health Act 1983 Policy Compendium.* May 2002. pp30 & app. 11. See Appendix E below for publication details.

scope. In the Commission's view, case law has established that random searching of detained patients may be proportionate and therefore legitimate response where there is a pressing social need, including, for example, where there is a chronic problem of drug-abuse on wards of any security level. Lord Justice Judge in the above-mentioned case used as an example a patient admitted to Broadmoor under section 3 of the Act, where

> an essential ground for the application and admission is that it is "necessary for the health and safety of the patient or for the protection of other persons that he should receive such treatment…". It would be absurd, if having been admitted on the basis that either of these two requirements had been established prior to his admission, the criteria of the health and safety of the patient himself or the protection of other persons were minimised during detention…the risk does not evaporate on admission[330]

It would appear that this particular argument relies more on the fact and purpose of civil admission under the Act for the justification for random searching than it relies on the level of security to which such a patient is admitted. It seems to be a logical extension of this argument that, if the actual risk presents a need for random searching in any type of establishment other than a High Security Hospital, then this argument still holds in respect of powers in relation to detained patients. We are aware, however, that our suggested reading of the judgment relies on conjecture. It would be helpful for Government to provide more substantive guidance in the next revision of the Code of Practice or by any other means.

Recommendation 48: The question of the lawful authority for random searches at all levels of psychiatric provision should be re-addressed by Government and the present guidance at chapter 25.3 of the Code of Practice expanded.

11.50   The Commission recommends that policies consider when it would be appropriate for post-incident reviews following searches. Such reviews could include involve advocacy services, or hospital managers visiting patients who have been subject to searches, in part to ensure that patients feel they have a form of appeal and redress where they feel that they have been subject to unnecessary, arbitrary or extreme measures. Such appeals could be directed, in the first instance, through the NHS complaints procedure or its equivalent in the independent sector.

Management of drug & alcohol abuse

11.51   From 1995 the Commission has been calling for better guidance in relation to the control and management of substance misuse amongst detained mental health patients[331]. Over this time the problems associated with drug and alcohol misuse on inpatient mental health units have been growing and are now major concerns for many services. We are aware that some

---

[330] Judge LJ in *R v Broadmoor Special Hospital Authority ex parte S and others* [1998]

[331] see Mental Health Act Commission (1995) *Sixth Biennial Report 1993-5* p105-107; MHAC (1997) *Seventh Biennial Report 1995-7*, p166-167; MHAC (1999) *Eighth Biennial Report 1997-9*, p 231-4, MHAC (2001) *Ninth Biennial Report 1999-01* p 49-51. London, Stationery Office.

services are adopting quite extensive security arrangements in an effort to address the problems of illicit drug-dealing on and around mental health units, including the use of CCTV, locked units, and regular police presence, sometimes with police dogs.

11.52   In our Ninth Biennial Report we recommended that all hospitals should provide their staff with policy-level advice on managing incidents or suspicions of drug and alcohol abuse. Our guidance has been highlighted in the IMHAP Policy Compendium published in 2002[332]. We highlighted some good practice in this area but called for central guidance to help hospital managers and staff provide a consistent and effective response to the challenge of substance misuse amongst their most vulnerable patients.

11.53   In the Ninth Biennial Report we suggested the following safety measures could be considered where an individual patient is suspected or known to be abusing substances:

* increasing observation levels;
* restricting leave;
* searching property;
* limiting or supervising visits; and
* transfer to higher security.

We highlighted that such measures should only be taken as a result of objective, multi-disciplinary risk-assessment on the basis of clinical need, and never as punitive sanctions.

11.54   In relation to ward-level actions, our Ninth Biennial Report recommended that policies should cover the areas listed below, in relation to which we called for Department of Health guidance on:

* expected actions where there is a suspicion of illicit drug use or supply, or of alcohol consumption, whether by patients or visitors;
* expected action where there is knowledge of such illicit drug use or supply;
* powers of staff to search for and confiscate illicit drugs or alcohol;
* reassurance on the powers of staff to handle and dispose of illicit drugs that come into their possession;
* expected arrangements with police services; and
* expectations of service agreements between mental health services and drug and alcohol services in relation to patients presenting with dual diagnosis.

11.55   The Department of Health's *Dual Diagnosis Good Practice Guide* (2002) introduced the policy of 'mainstreaming', bringing specialist drug and alcohol services together with mental health services to provide integrated care for patients with a diagnosis of both mental disorder who misuse substances[333]. The Commission is pleased to note this policy-level action, especially as the publication promised guidance on dealing with drug misuse on wards[334]. At the time of writing (October 2003), this guidance had yet to be issued.

---

[332] Institute of Mental Health Act Practitioners (2002) *Mental Health Act 1983 Policy Compendium.* May 2002. pp45. See Appendix E below for publication details

[333] Department of Heath (2002) *Dual Diagnosis Good Practice Guide.* April 2002. Page 6

Sexual relations

11.56   Few issues relating to the care of detained patients are as difficult, and in the main part avoided, as those relating to the sexual life of patients. Persaud and Hewitt have warned that, in the absence of a professional consensus as to the kind of circumstances in which it will be permissible to prohibit or permit conjugal relations, the domestic courts, influenced by the ECHR, might impose practices which are prejudicial to psychiatric institutions and those working within them[335]

11.57   Some boundaries are being established in law. In particular, *R v Ashworth Hospital Authority ex p RH* (2001) held a High Security Hospital policy that does not permit patients to engage in sexual activity for security reasons to be reasonable and that any infringement of human rights arising from the application of that policy was justified. The hospital's refusal to supply condoms had been challenged on human rights grounds by a patient who was a practising homosexual infected with hepatitis C.

11.58   The Sexual Offences Bill, which is likely to receive royal assent this year, will create new offences of sexual activity with any person whose mental disorder incapacitates them from giving consent, and offences where a care-worker engages in sexual activity with any mentally disordered person in their care[336]. This should fill the serious gaps in current offences specific to the sexual abuse of psychiatric patients. The present law (section 128 of the 1959 Mental Health Act, which was not repealed by the passing of the 1983 Act), makes it an offence for any man who is on the staff of a hospital to have extra-marital sexual intercourse with a woman who is receiving treatment for mental disorder from that hospital, or for any man who is the guardian, custodian or carer of a mentally disordered woman to have extra-marital sexual intercourse with her. Consequently, a number of other situations, such as those involving the abuse of male patients, can at the time of writing only be construed under mental health legislation as the lesser offences of ill-treatment (section 127 of the Mental Health Act 1983)[337].

11.59   It has been argued by some legal commentators that enabling prosecution of persons engaging in sexual activity with mentally disordered persons is not necessarily the best way to protect the latter[338]. The law at present criminalises heterosexual or homosexual activity where at least one partner is severely mentally impaired, even where that partner is capable of giving real consent to such activity and does so. Furthermore, even when a relationship is of an exploitative nature, criminal conviction would be hampered by the victim's perceived ability to give evidence in court. One of the Law Commission's original proposals for a Mental Incapacity Bill was that it could provide a framework within which civil procedures giving powers of entry to property, investigation and removal of mentally incapacitated

---

[334]   *ibid*, p 31.

[335]   Persaud A, Hewitt D (2001) *European Convention on Human Rights: effects on psychiatric care* Nursing Standard, 15, 44, 33-37

[336]   see Sexual Offences Bill, clauses 33-51.

[337]   Although at the time of writing (August 2003), the extant Sexual Offences Acts (1956, 1967) render unlawful homosexual acts with a severely mentally impaired man.

[338]   Hoggett, B (1996) *Mental Health Law* Fourth Edition, London: Sweet & Maxwell, p229

persons subsequently deemed to be at risk might be applied in urgent situations to protect a particular mentally incapacitated persons[339]. No such powers are provided by the draft Mental Incapacity Bill published in 2003. However, the 2003 Bill does appear to retain a mechanism whereby the expanded Court of Protection would be able to grant declarations over a mentally incapacitated patient's personal welfare that could restrict or prevent their contact with abusive persons[340]. The exact scope of such declarations will perhaps be clarified as the Bill is debated in Parliament.

11.60   Although the law has been slow to recognise forms of sexual abuse as offences, in general detaining authorities have had little difficulty in setting appropriate boundaries in relation to staff and patient relationships, and reflecting these boundaries in disciplinary measures. Similarly, detaining authorities are generally aware that their duty of care towards detained patients extends to protecting patients from undertaking harmful activity under the influence of mental disorder. Most health providers will be prepared to prevent sexual relationships that appear exploitative or coercive, or where patients appear not to be in control of their sexual behaviour. Whilst most detained patients are not in conditions of high security, there will also be security and safety considerations to take account of.

11.61   The day-to-day issues around patients' sexual expression are much more problematic. Patients are often not recognised as having sexual identities and needs. Sexual relationships between patients or patients and their visitors may therefore be prevented, discouraged or ignored, particularly by a lack of private space or access to contraceptive/disease prevention products[341]. It may be that the raft of new offences created by the Sexual Offences Bill, which includes offences of incitement and inducement to sexual activity, will further discourage mental health workers from tolerant and permissive attitudes unless these are addressed at policy level and sensible frameworks encouraged. Some mental health users and organisations have been opposed to the Sexual Offences Bill on the grounds that it could criminalise the sexual expression of patients. We trust that Government will address such concerns by ensuring that public authorities can and will apply new law in a way compatible with the Human Rights Act and anti-discriminatory practice.

11.62   The vulnerability of detained women patients to sexual exploitation and abuse was demonstrated in this reporting period by widely reported events at Broadmoor Hospital, where it was discovered that many women patients had experienced sexual harassment and abuse at the hands of male patients. We discuss general issues arising from this at Chapter 12.56 *et seq* below. Although we appreciate that the safety of women patients must be given priority, we are concerned that moves towards total gender segregation in hospitals may deny women, who are often in the minority in hospital environments, from access to the full range of therapeutic and recreational activities.

---

[339] Law Commission (1995) *Mental Incapacity: Item 9 of the Fourth Programme of Law Reform: Mentally Incapacitated Adults.* Law Commission No 231 London: HMSO.

[340] Department of Constitutional Affairs (2003) *Draft Mental Incapacity Bill.* Cm 5859-I, clause 17. London: Stationery Office. This must be read against exclusions in clause 26.

[341] Payne, A (1993) *Sexual activity among psychiatric inpatients: international perpectives* in Journal of Forensic Psychiatry, Vol 4 No 1 109-129.

Patients' physical health

11.63 We welcome the Government's minimum standard that "all patients in Psychiatric Intensive Care Units & Low Secure Units will have core care underpinned by health promotion activities (diet, exercise, substance abuse & smoking cessation)" [342] and trust that this standard will extend to all psychiatric inpatient facilities. It remains the case that some patients have limited access to medical facilities for the care of their physical health needs.

11.64 The Commission is frequently approached for advice as to what measures might be taken to preserve or restore long-term detained patients' physical health. Whilst it is clear that the Act cannot be used to compel patients to undergo medical treatment that is not related to their mental disorder, clinicians sometimes wish to know the extent to which aspects of the hospital regime may be tailored to encourage certain health choices and discourage others. Particular concerns are often patients' nutrition choices, obesity, exercise and smoking. For some patients, these lifestyle choices may be life-threatening.

11.65 It is conceivable that behaviour deleterious to physical health, even such as over-eating or excessive smoking, may in some circumstances be derivative of mental disorder. In some cases, patients may lose their mental capacity to the extent that they are not in control of their actions. For other patients, who are not necessarily incapacitated by their mental disorder, such behaviour can be a form of self-harming, or a means of "self-medication" against the distressing symptoms of mental disorder and the side effects of its pharmaco-logical treatment.

11.66 Mental health professionals should, of course, start from a position of respect for the lifestyle choices made by patients. The fact of detention under the Act should not automat-ically deprive a patient of their autonomy to make such choices. However, section 63 of the Act does provide the RMO with the authority to direct the imposition of nursing care, habilitation and rehabilitation for the treatment of mental disorder. If such nursing care cannot be considered as treatment for the mental disorder as classified by the patient's detention papers, it must at least be a necessary prerequisite to such treatment[343]. For patients lacking capacity, this provides a statutory authority for providing whatever nursing care is in that patient's best interests. For patients who retain capacity, the authority of section 63 should be balanced by a careful consideration of the patient's motives and beliefs regarding their health and lifestyle choices.

Patients' access to telephones

11.67 In 2001 the Commission issued a questionnaire concerning detained patients' access to telephones to all detaining authorities (NHS Trusts and independent hospitals). We received 229 responses from slightly under a third of all such authorities. Many respondent author-

---

[342] Department of Health (2002) *Mental Health Policy Implementation Guide: National Minimum Standards for General Adult Services in Psychiatric Intensive Care Units (PICU) and Low Secure Units.*

[343] *B v Ashworth*, [2003] para 46–7. The court confirmed the *B v Croydon Health Authority* [1995] decision that that treatments ancillary to the core treatment for mental disorder (in that case naso-gastric feeding of a patient with borderline personality disorder whose refusal to eat was a form of self-harm) fell under section 63 of the Act.

ities returned more than one questionnaire to reflect different practices operative across the various units and security levels that make up their service.

11.68   The findings of our survey were as follows:

* The majority of services returning questionnaires (84%, or 193 questionnaires) reported that they did not have policies relating to patients' access to telephones.

* Overall, 54% (124) reported the imposition of some restrictions on patients' access to telephones.

* Ninety questionnaires (or nearly 40% of the total questionnaires returned) reported restrictions on patients' access to telephones in the absence of any operational policy. Of these, 26 banned patients from accessing mobile phones completely.

* Of those questionnaires that indicated the existence of operational policies (36 question-naires, or 14% of total returns) two indicated no restrictions to telephone access at all, and two reported that restrictions were only imposed where individual risk assessments determined them necessary. Ten questionnaires indicated that mobile telephones were banned completely under operational policy guidance.

11.67   Given the high level of restrictions in evidence, it would clearly be better for all services to establish operational policies in relation to patients' access to telephones. Such policies should aim to provide unfettered access insofar as this is consistent with patients' care and safety and the safety of other persons. Therefore, all restrictions on patients' access to telephones should ideally be imposed on an individual basis following a clinical risk assessment.

11.68   The supervision of patients using telephones should be minimal and consistent with ECHR Article 8 requirements to respect private and family life. All telephone policies should identify those organisations and individuals to whom patients' calls will be neither prevented nor monitored, such as the Commission or a patient's legal representative[344].

11.69   We accept that certain units in the secure sector may need to impose blanket restrictions on patients' access to or use of mobile telephones for reasons of physical security. Similarly, house-rules may govern when mobile telephones should be switched off, such as during therapeutic sessions and specific activities. If units detaining patients are in hospital environments where mobile telephone use is restricted to protect sensitive equipment, an area where patients may go within the hospital site to use their telephones should be identified and designated for use.

11.70   Risk-assessment may identify situations where concern for the safety of the patient or his or her property suggests that a patient's mobile telephone should be looked after by staff, although telephones should not be confiscated solely because patients are denied any safe place to keep or use them.

11.71   Special consideration should be given to children and adolescents. Minors may be subject to restrictions imposed by their parents or carers, which staff should take into account.

---

[344] Services may find the list of organisations at section 134(3) useful, although we do not suggest that patients must have an unfettered right to telephone, for example, the House of Lords.

Overall, however, staff (particularly staff caring for minors on adult wards) should recognise that mobile telephones may play an important part in young people's social lives. We are aware of very different approaches to young persons' access to mobile telephones even within the CAMHS sector, and have encountered some practices that seem unduly restrictive.

Recommendation 40: Issues relating to patients' access to telephones should be included in future editions of the Code of Practice, whether in relation to this Act or its successor.

Part 3

Forensic and secure mental health services

12

High Security Hospitals

Structural tensions in High Security Care

12.1 The historical isolation of the High Security Hospitals (HSHs) from mainstream psychiatric provision has had a deleterious effect on their accessibility, culture and overall effectiveness. We believe that this has long been recognised by Government and by the managers of Ashworth, Broadmoor and Rampton Hospitals, and we welcomed this recognition in our Ninth Biennial Report[345].

12.2 Since at least 1996, when the three hospitals were designated special health authorities responsible for providing services in much the same way as NHS Trusts, the Government's policy has aimed to end this isolation. This has been consolidated over the last four years with the merging of all three High Security Hospitals with their respective local NHS Trusts. The Government's policy proposals published in 2002[346] are clearly influenced by recommendations of the Fallon inquiry that high secure services must be mainstreamed through the creation of a regionally organised forensic network covering all levels of security[347]. Performance management of High Security Hospitals has been devolved to Strategic Health Authorities, who have received additional funding and a framework of performance indicators. Initial steps to devolve commissioning responsibilities have been taken, overseen at present by "relatively prescriptive" National Oversight arrangements[348], and further devolution looks likely. Social services provision within the hospitals have been reconfigured on the recommendations of the Lewis Report into 'social care services', that may involve probation officers and those skilled in disciplines such as child protection, learning disabilities, welfare rights and rehabilitation. The first national standards for the provision of such services in the High Security Hospitals were published in August 2001[349]. The Government has stated that the hospitals are at a critical point in their development and that a significant change agenda remains for their future[350].

---

[345] Mental Health Act Commission (2001) *Ninth Biennial Report 1999-01*, London: Stationery Office. Chapter 5.1.

[346] Department of Health (2002) *New Arrangements for the Performance Management and Commissioning of High Security Psychiatric Services.* London: Stationery Office

[347] Department of Health (1999) *Report of the Committee of Enquiry into the Personality Disorder Unit, Ashworth Special Hospital.* Cm 4149-11 London: Stationery Office para 7.3.1.

[348] *ibid*, note 346, para 5.3.

[349] Social Services Inspectorate (2001) *National Standards for the Provision of Social Care Services in the High Security Hospitals.* CI(2001)16 London: SSI, August 2001. www.doh.gov.uk/scg/highsecurity.htm

[350] *ibid.* para 5.4

12.3   We do not doubt that Government intends to break down the institutional isolation of High Security Hospitals, but fear that this aim may yet be frustrated by competing concerns, especially in relation to security matters. In our Ninth Biennial Report we questioned whether the High Security Hospitals were taking on an increasingly custodial focus as a result of the implementation of the November 2001 Security Directions[351]. The Commission recognises the distinctive service provided by High Security Hospitals[352], and our Ninth Report acknowledged the need for an increased focus on security in the light of the Fallon Inquiry report, but overall we remain concerned that the application of some aspects of the Security Directions have continued to be unnecessarily damaging to patient care. We are especially concerned that where Security Directions constrain High Security Hospital managers' autonomy to take decisions about the day to day running of their establishments without good cause, this can only reinforce the isolation of such services from mainstream psychiatric practice. This is a particular concern as we recognise that hospital managers are sensitive to and willing to confront the worst aspects, considered from the viewpoint of therapeutics, of their hospitals' culture.

12.4   There has been some controversy over whether the 2000 *Report on the Review of Security at the High Security Hospitals* (the Tilt Report)[353] gave a sufficient focus to issues of 'relational security' (i.e. those aspects of security that are based in the treatment of patients, whether this is medical treatment given under a treatment plan or wider therapeutic relationships and activities)[354]. The Tilt report *did* conclude that physical and procedural security (i.e. the physical barriers to escape and operational policies on searching, etc) must be attended to alongside an increase in therapy and activity. However, the Security Directions issued in response to the Tilt report, perhaps unsurprisingly, have focused on the more tangible aspects of security implementation. We focus on some specific aspects of concern at 12.18 *et seq* below.

12.5   It is a sad reflection that current policy directives on security appear to be less humane than those produced over a decade ago. In 1992 the Director of Security of the Special Hospital Service Authority (SHSA) stated as a guiding principle that "the most effective form of security and, indeed, safety lies in the treatment of the patient". This dynamic relational security "begins with the patient and is essentially concerned with detailed knowledge of the patients and their situation…it will extend to relationships and professional agencies outside the hospital, so that although the institutional boundaries are very definite, effective security can often have its roots in the community. The provision of education, rehabilitation and pastoral facilities as well as leisure and social activities all have an important part to play…"[355]. This is, indeed, the security approach of mainstream psychiatry, and insofar as the High Secure Hospitals fail to adapt this approach to their needs they will remain outside of that mainstream to the disadvantage of their patients.

---

[351] see Mental Health Act Commission (2001) *Ninth Biennial Report 1999-01*, London: Stationery Office. Chapter 5.23 – 5.34

[352] see, for example, Mental Health Act Commission (1997) *Seventh Biennial Report 1995-7*. London: Stationery Office. Chapter 4.5.1

[353] Department of Health (2000) *Report on the Review of Security at the High Security Hospitals.* London, Stationery Office

[354] see Exworthy T & Gunn, J (2003) *Taking another tilt at high secure hospitals: the Tilt Report and its consequences for secure psychiatric services* in British Journal of Psychiatry 182:469-471 and correspondence from Sir Richard Tilt, ibid. p548.

[355] Kinsley, J (1992) *Security in the Special Hospitals – a Special Task.* Published as Annex F of Department of Health (1994) *Report of the Working Group on High Security and Related Psychiatric Provision* [the Reed report]. London, Department of Health.

Recommendation 50: Government should confirm its commitment to relational security as the core security aspect of mental health services by ensuring a focus on the relational security and treatment shortfalls within the High Security Hospitals that are discussed in this chapter.

The physical estate of the High Security Hospitals

12.6 Both Ashworth and Broadmoor Hospitals require considerable investment in the overall fabric of the hospitals to bring all the wards up to the basic standard expected elsewhere in the NHS[356]. Commissioners have noted structural limitations of the hospitals' environment, in terms of ensuring a pleasant living environment for all patients and in relation to such issues as safety of seclusion facilities or access to fresh air (see 12.46 below), etc. In Broadmoor Hospital, for example, it is not possible to deliver a safe and therapeutic environment within the antiquated and sometimes listed Victorian facilities that make up parts of the hospital. Hospital managers are unable to create appropriately sized wards without hazards such as blind spots and ligature points. We are concerned at the message provided to both patients and staff of the High Security Hospitals by high-profile investment in physical security that is not matched by investment in improving these conditions. There is a danger of creating cynicism amongst both patients and staff over the therapeutic aims of the hospital regime, and thus engendering a 'prison' mentality amongst both groups. We touch upon this in relation to the justifications for seclusion practice at 12.23 *et seq* below.

The stigmatisation of High Security Hospitals and their patients

12.7 We are very aware of the difficulties faced by the High Security Hospitals in providing healthcare to a patient group that is popularly maligned and feared. Whatever gains are made by anti-stigma campaigns such as those promoted by the Royal College of Psychiatrists and Department of Health in encouraging better overall media presentation of mental health issues (see Chapter 6.34 *et seq* above), much media coverage of the high secure sector relies entirely on caricature, inaccuracy and cliché. One recent tabloid newspaper's attack on the humanity of patients in Broadmoor Hospital had a markedly detrimental effect on the morale of the patient population[357]. We are also disappointed at the behaviour of those tabloids that pay for personal health records that are leaked from the hospital. Whilst we acknowledge the difficulties that the hospital management have in identifying who is responsible for such leaks of personal information, we assume that the theft and sale of a health record is a criminal offence and will be treated as such should the opportunity for disciplinary and legal action arise. We recognise that media vilification of this group of patients presents a challenging environment for Government policy makers and hospital managers alike.

---

[356] The Commission has far fewer concerns about the physical state of Rampton Hospital, where considerable updating and rebuilding work has taken place and continues.

[357] *News of the World*, May 11 2003 "Britain's Most Notorious Asylum, Broadmoor: Madness". Then Commission deplores this and similar articles which present patients in high security hospitals as somehow undeserving of decent healthcare, rehabilitation or recreation facilities, etc.

Recommendation 51: We urge Government to consider ways in which patients in the High Security Hospitals and other establishments can be protected from the theft or publication of their personal health records and details of their hospital treatment published. Consideration could be given to creating specific offences under mental health legislation that would apply to persons responsible for the unauthorised disclosure of personal medical records, and any persons involved in their publication. There would be no reason why such offences should criminalise responsible whistleblowing, which need not involve the disclosure of identifiable personal health records.

12.8　In our response to the draft Mental Health Bill, we suggested to Government that it might take the opportunity to reconsider and amend section 4 of NHS Act 1977 as a further indication of its commitment to bringing high secure care into the mainstream of psychiatric services. Section 4 of the NHS Act 1977 establishes a duty to provide "Special Hospitals" as places with "conditions of special security on account of [patients'] dangerous, violent or criminal propensities". This terminology hinders the setting of high secure care within the mainstream, both as a reinforcement of the separate "special" nature of the hospital service and in its reinforcing of patient stereotypes. The language of the NHS Act 1977 continues to have practical effect on services, particularly through citation in court depositions.

Recommendation 52: The Secretary of State should consider emendation of the language of section 4 of the NHS Act 1977 to further the integration of high secure care into mainstream psychiatry.

Continuing inappropriate placements in high secure care

12.9　It is now three years since the Tilt Report recognised that roughly a third of the patient population in the three High Security Hospitals did not require conditions of security equivalent to category 2 in the penal system and should be transferred to less secure facilities. The report stated that it was inappropriate from a civil liberties viewpoint and in terms of the efficient use of resources for these patients to remain in the hospitals[358]. We are unable to provide an equivalent figure for today, given that patients are not routinely assessed according to the criteria used by the Tilt review, but there continue to be a substantial minority of patients who are ready for transfer or discharge, but are waiting for Home Office approval, the identification of placements outside the hospital or an available bed in such a placement.

12.10　Underlying this issue is a possible lack of clarity over the purpose of high secure care. Following the Tilt review, the purpose of High Security Hospitals has been defined as providing psychiatric care for those patients who need the equivalent of category B prison

---

[358] Department of Health (2000) *Report on the Review of Security at the High Security Hospitals* p.12.

security. The hospitals themselves now see their purpose as diminishing the dangerousness of their patients to a point where they can be transferred to conditions of lesser security. A firm commitment to the category B definition would diminish radically the size of the High Security Hospitals. However, the hospitals have continued to contain patients who cannot possibly require such conditions of security, including patients with reduced mobility and frail, elderly patients, many of whom have needed ground-floor accommodation because they are unable to use stairs. The Commission continues to take the view that progress in transferring this population out of the hospitals has been slow overall, although some acceleration in arranging transfers has been noted in the last two years. However, it should be remembered that, even since the Tilt Report's publication, patients discharged from high secure care have included a 94 year old woman, a teenager in a wheelchair and a blind person with severely restricted mobility.

12.11 The implementation of the Security Directions whilst patients await transfer out of the hospitals has intensified the need for patients' transfers to be expedited. Increasing the conditions of security for patients who do not require high secure care but are stuck in the system can only make their inappropriate treatment worse. The reduction in rehabilitation programmes resulting from the refocussing of the purpose of high secure care following the security reviews may actually hamper such patients' chances of being moved on, as many medium secure units require High Security Hospital patients to have completed treatments before transfer. It may be that the expectations of medium secure units need to be adjusted to take account of the emerging role of high secure services, if the latter are to become the equivalent of an acute service for the mainstream secure services provided by the medium secure sector. For instance, medium secure units may have to accept patients whose rehabilitative needs have not been substantially addressed in high secure care, and provide such treatment programmes in their less secure surroundings.

12.12 The main difficulties reported in relation to delayed transfers of patients out of the High Security Hospitals are:

∗ **Obtaining purchaser funding for patients' care after transfer from high security.**

Some purchasing authorities have appeared reluctant to fund patients' care on their transfer from high security. In some cases there are disputes over which purchasing authority is responsible for patients who may have entered the psychiatric system at high security level without previous service contact, or even a fixed place of residence. However, not all disputes centre on complex cases. Some authorities simply do not seem to want to take back the responsibility of a patient who has been within the high secure system for a lengthy period of time. The Commission has attempted to help High Security Hospital managers by raising particular cases of concern itself with the regional authorities responsible for funding, and has noted some subsequent progress for some Broadmoor patients.

∗ **Finding suitable placements outside of the High Security Hospitals**

In some case it is not funding but the identification of a suitable bed to receive patients transferred from the High Security Hospitals that is the problem. This is especially a problem in relation to the continued shortage of medium secure beds, as reported in our last Biennial Report[359]

✻ **Delays in obtaining Home Office permission for the movement of restricted patients.**

Delays in receiving Home Office permission for trial leave or transfer of restricted patients have been reported by all three hospitals during this reporting period, although there are indications that the situation has improved in recent months. The Home Office has undertaken to respond to all requests within eight weeks, but this timescale excludes time spent "waiting for further information". Delays in accessing further information are not caused by the Home Office, but these can add considerably to the process of receiving permission.

12.13   Internal transfers are also subject to delays and a source of frustration to patients and staff in all three hospitals. Delays are caused largely by high bed occupancies across all levels of the hospitals, from admission and intensive care wards to pre-discharge rehabilitation wards. Patients who are identified as suitable to move from one level of nursing care to another may become stuck because no spaces are available. In Rampton Hospital, for example, some patients have been resident on "admission wards" for over three years. Although, in some cases, patients have been transferred out of the high security system directly from such wards, difficulties in moving patients across security or intensive nursing levels within the hospitals probably impedes patients' progress and is especially demoralising for patients. Patients almost inevitably measure their own therapeutic progress by their movement through the hospital structure. We discussed the problem of internal transfer delays in our Ninth Biennial Report, and suggested the maintenance of a number of vacant places upon the discharge of patients from the High Security Hospitals to free up other patients' movement within the system. We continue to suggest that, despite the pressure for high security places, this may be the best use of resources in the interests of patient care.

12.14   Patients' placement within specific wards in the High Security Hospitals may determine their access to specific therapeutic programmes or activities, although such access is also under pressure across all facilities in the hospitals due to limited resources, including staffing shortages (see 12.15 below). Outside transfers can be dependent upon the completion of therapeutic work in hospital and delays in accessing therapies may therefore not only be detrimental to individual patients' care, but contributive towards the silting-up of the high secure system and excessive transfer delays. In our last Biennial Report we highlighted specifically the need for specialist services dealing with issues of addiction, given the high incidences of drug and alcohol abuse in patients' histories[360]. Even though we suggest at 12.11 above that some rehabilitation treatment programmes could be provided to patients outside of high secure care, it is important that programmes dealing with issues that may lie at the root of patients' mental health problems and index offences are available to patients who cannot address past dangerous behaviour without such treatment.

Staffing

12.15   Over this period we have seen evidence in all three High Security Hospitals of staffing vacancies affecting services adversely. Staffing shortages inevitably lead to less therapeutic staff-patient contact and fewer opportunities for patient activities. In one case, for example,

---

[359] Mental Health Act Commission (2001) *Ninth Biennial Report 1999-01.* London: Stationery Office. Chapter 5.8 – 5.11

[360] *ibid*, Chapter 5.14, 5.19 – 5.21

a patient who had been granted Home Office permission for twelve escorted trips was only able to go out of the hospital once over a period of several months, with the CPA record stating this was "due to ward changes and staffing resources directed elsewhere". Such frustrations, and more minor daily problems, can easily lead to patient behaviour that is met with controlling or disciplinary responses.

12.16   Hospital managers have attempted to address staffing shortages in this period with some measures of success. Broadmoor's staffing vacancies, for example, dropped from 20% to 11% in 2002, following the recruitment of new staff. Ashworth Hospital's medical staffing establishment has been improved, so that patients report consistent Responsible Medical Officer (RMO) cover, although we remain concerned at the frequency of patients' one-to-one contact with their RMOs. Patients in all three hospitals have previously expressed concern that frequent changes in their RMO due to shortages of medical cover or other reasons, may have an inhibiting effect on the actual and perceived progress in their treatment[361].

12.17   At Rampton Hospital, whilst we have welcomed the improvements in the staffing establishment, Commissioners have raised concerns about training of new staff. As with all three hospitals, Commissioners visiting Rampton Hospital meet with many highly motivated, patient-centred and professional staff who offer highly skilled and respectful care to patients in sometimes challenging circumstances. However, on some units, the proportion of new staff has been unsettling for patients and may have led to difficulties in maintaining standards. One Commissioner reported witnessing staff interactions ranging from patronising to, on one occasion, wholly inappropriate (where staff action reinforced one patient's bullying attitude towards another patient). Whilst we are confident that these issues will be addressed through staff training, it highlights the problems that can persist even with the recruitment of staff to outstanding vacancies.

The Safety and Security Directions and patient care

12.18   In our Ninth Biennial Report (2001), we reported and underlined concerns expressed by staff and patients in the High Security Hospitals in relation to some aspects of the implementation of the Safety and Security in Ashworth, Broadmoor and Rampton Hospitals Directions 2000[362].

12.19   The Commission recognises that hospital staff of all grades and professions are continuing to work hard to maintain a treatment-focussed service at the same time as implementing the increased security requirements. The Commision's primary concerns over the Security Directions are:

---

[361]   see, however, Dell/Robertson (1988) *Sentenced to Hospital: Offenders in Broadmoor* Oxford, p 45-46, 107: 'A change of doctor carries with it potential advantages as well as disadvantages for patients hoping to be discharged. Changes in consultant account for 1/5 of discharge cases of non-psychotic patients, and the study showed marked differences between individual psychiatrists in discharge rates for psychotic patients, although the doctors "tended to resist the notion that discharge was in any way dependent on them as individuals".'

[362]   Mental Health Act Commission (2001) *Ninth Biennial Report 1999-01*, London: Stationery Office. Chapter 5.23 - 34

* that their implementation should not impose overly time-consuming and restrictive practices in the hospitals at the expense of therapeutic interactions; and

* over the depersonalising and institutionalising effects of some of the measures taken, particularly given blanket application of measures so as to impose restrictions on some patients that could not be justified on through clinical risk-assessment.

12.20   From the introduction of the Security Directions in November 2000, the Secretary of State has issued four Amendment Directions, and it remains in the gift of the Secretary of State to amend or add to the Directions as he sees fit. The Commission has not been consulted in the amendment process. While most of the effects of amendments made in the last two years have been concerned with technicalities of drafting in the Directions[363], the amendments made this year[364] have increased some restrictions and made some security requirements more robust:

* **The ban on computer ownership is extended to games consoles that can be adapted as a computer.**

    The Commission reminds hospital mangers that there is no theoretical restriction on patients' access to computers owned and controlled by the hospital, and of our past recommendation that they should consider ways to improve patients' access to these, particularly during leisure time[365].

* **The requirements regarding testing for illicit substances are expanded to breath testing for alcohol and the taking of mouth swabs or hair samples for drug-tests;**

    The requirement that samples should not be taken by a member of the opposite sex to a patient extends to these new measures.

* **The locking up of patients at night is extended as a blanket practice across all "dangerous and severe personality disorder facilities" within the High Security Hospitals.**

    The Directions allow that hospitals will need to develop mechanisms to review this requirement "on any occasion if there are circumstances, for example the risk of suicide or self-harm, which would indicate that the locking up of the patient in his room on that occasion would be unsafe". The Commission will be taking a close interest in how this requirement is met. The original Directions required the hospitals to have a policy on the locking up at night of any patient who is identified as being at high-risk of harming others, escape, or subverting the safety and security of the hospital in collaboration with others, and have not led to widespread locking in of patients (see 12.68 below on this in relation to the definition of seclusion and human rights).

* **The requirement that risk-assessments determine whether a patient presents a risk of "organising in collaboration with others to subvert security and safety" in the hospitals is extended to individual actions of such subversion.**

    The Commission regrets the language of this amendment, particularly as the Direction already allows that immediate harm to others, suicide or self-harm, escaping and being assaulted are the remaining risks to take account of. These appear comprehensive for a healthcare establishment. The phrase "subverting security and safety", especially when applied to an individual patient, is in our view too ill-defined to prevent abusive or

---

[363] i.e. to reflect the changing authorities responsible for the management of the High Security Hospitals.

[364] see *The Ashworth, Broadmoor and Rampton Hospitals Amendment Directions 2003*, 4 April 2003. Website address: www.doh.gov.uk/hospitaldirections

repressive interpretation. We look to the hospital management to ensure against this, and we will be taking particular interest in risk assessments and their consequences where this concept is engaged.

12.21 The 2003 amendments to the Security Directions relax the restrictions on persons bringing food into the hospital so that the hospital's own catering and supply staff, if authorised by the Chief Executive, may now do so. This amendment could provide hospital managers with more scope to meet the Commission's previous recommendation that the implementation of the Directions regarding the purchase and importation of foodstuffs from outside the hospital should avoid undesirable and unintended consequences, such as, for example, preventing Occupational Therapists from bringing special foodstuffs for cooking activities[366]. During this reporting period the Commission has continued to hear of difficulties caused in patient activities by blanket approaches to this and similar requirements of the Security Directions. In one hospital the popular practice of buying in a shared take-away meal was abandoned at this time, although ostensibly for food safety reasons. Although the hospital offered the services of its own catering department to meet the shortfall, this met none of the underlying reasons the popularity of previous arrangements. In another instance rehabilitative shopping trips were curtailed because of the ban on patients' bringing back foodstuffs purchased outside of the hospital. As a security measure designed to meet the recommendations of the Tilt Report, the latter restriction was doubly counter-productive in that it undermined relational security by establishing unnecessary restrictions on patients' activities, and curtailed activities designed to progress patients towards semi-independent living and eventual discharge.

12.22 In many respects, Commissioners remain as concerned over the implementation of the Security Directions now as they were two years ago, but we can report some mitigating developments. In particular, many managers and staff have responded positively to the Commission's recommendations that they take responsibility for the implementation of the Directions in as sensitive a manner as possible[367]. As might be expected, patients now raise fewer complaints about the Security Directions than when they were first implemented. Although this may be a result of patients' resignation as rules and regulations become established (or of anxiety over the reorganisation of high secure services overshadowing more quotidian concerns, particularly for women patients and patients diagnosed with personality disorder), there is also some evidence that patients' care teams are taking up and resolving some concerns over security matters at an early stage.

Recommendation 53: Government should be prepared to use its directive power to prevent unintended consequences of the Security Directions and to help High Security Hospital managers preserve humane and rational rules within the hospitals.

---

[365] Mental Health Act Commission (2001) *Ninth Biennial Report* 1999-01, London: Stationery Office Chapter 5.28, Recommendation 56.

[366] *ibid*, Chapter 5.29, Recommendation 57

[367] Although the Commission has not had a universally welcoming response, with representation against our Ninth Biennial Report recommendations being received from the Ashworth Hospital Branch of the Prison Officers' Association.

Long-term seclusion and the hospital culture

12.23   The Commission has outstanding concerns about the practice of keeping patients in long-term seclusion. This is mainly a problem of high secure services, as any patient who cannot be managed outside of seclusion in medium or low secure environments will usually be transferred to a more appropriate facility[368].

12.24   The use of extended seclusion in psychiatry has a long and ignominious history. It is now a century since Emil Kraeplin, one of the founders of modern psychiatry, discontinued the use in his practice of 'long confinement' in isolation. Kraeplin believed that such confinement was often the cause of the dangerous behaviour that it sought to manage. He noted, furthermore, that "the practice, once it had been initiated, was always easy to extend and hard to retrench. It would be a mistake to assume that isolation normally eliminates unhealthy symptoms; it merely conceals them and rules out careful supervision and treatment."[369]

12.25   In July 2003 the Court of Appeal in *Munjaz* determined that the seclusion policy of Ashworth Hospital was unlawful insofar as it allowed for long-term seclusion involving review procedures other than those required by the Code of Practice. This policy, and the practice emanating from it, had been the subject of a long-running dispute between the Commission and the hospital managers. We discuss the *Munjaz* judgment in detail at Chapter 3.2 *et seq* above. The Commission was joined as a party to the first instance hearing of the case and submitted a position statement to the Court of Appeal for the July 2003 hearing. Our submission, which remained valid for both hearings, suggested a position that was adopted by the Court of Appeal in its judgment overturning the first-instance decision. We argued that deviations from the Code's guidance should only occur in exceptional circumstances, with full documentation of the reasons for such deviation, and never as a matter of policy or standard practice.

12.26   Ashworth Hospital had taken the view that particular problems in implementing the Code's guidance occur when patients are in seclusion for over 72 hours, and that the Code did not envisage such lengthy periods of seclusion and therefore failed to take account of them. It is, perhaps, true that the Code was written on the assumption that seclusion, as a last resort response to dangerous behaviour, should not normally still be in place after three days, no matter how disturbed the patient may be at the time of its implementation. It is arguable, for instance, that, by the time a patient has been secluded for three days, arrangements should have been considered for alternative management of the patient, such as a trial period of one- to-one (or more intensive) nursing, etc. In principle, the Commission would wish to see such alternatives implemented.

12.27   The Commission's emphasis on alternative management to seclusion, and compliance with the Code of Practice guidelines when seclusion is used, was echoed a decade ago by the Special Hospital Service Authority (SHSA) *Policy Statement The Use of Seclusion and the*

---

[368]   It is true that the *Airedale* case (see Chapter 3.3 above) revolved around the seclusion of a patient for nearly two-weeks in a low-secure unit, but this was in part because of complications in accessing a bed in a more secure establishment. The long-term seclusion of the patient in the *Airedale* case was declared unlawful by the Court of Appeal in *Munjaz*, July 2003.

[369]   Kraeplin, E (1917) *One Hundred Years of Psychiatry*. Translated by Wade Baskin. New York: Citadel Press, 1962 p 141.

Alternative Management of Disturbed Behaviour within the Special Hospitals (October 1993). The SHSA clearly identified that alternative management strategies should be employed for those patients with special needs who are frequently disturbed over a long period of time and suggested the development of specialist units for such patients with demanding behaviour. Our Sixth Biennial report welcomed this policy approach[370]. The Commission's Ninth Biennial Report (Chapter 4.43) commented favourably upon Rampton Hospital's success in reducing episodes of seclusion on their men's intensive care ward through alternative management strategies.

12.28   The SHSA policy statement of 1993 noted that a very small number of patients were considered to be in long-term or "continuous" seclusion in the High Security Hospitals but actually spent some, or even most, of their time in the ward community rather than in conditions of seclusion. These patients were classed to be in permanent seclusion because such periods of association were viewed as being brief respites from seclusion, to which they would be returned once such association periods were over. In reality, such patients were secluded (as the term is defined in the Code of Practice) for relatively short periods on numerous occasions, sometimes several times each day. The SHSA required that the practice of considering such patients to be in "continuous" seclusion must cease and each episode of seclusion be identified and monitored as required by the Code of Practice. Following the *Munjaz* judgment, this requirement must at last be met. This requirement, although emphasised and restated by Commissioners who visited Ashworth Hospital over the next decade, had not been met at the time of the *Munjaz* Appeal Court hearing.

12.29   Commissioners have held many discussions with managers and staff in the High Security Hospitals over the reasons for high seclusion use. The most frequently cited justification for past seclusion practices has related to the nature of the patients being cared for, and it is certainly true that some patients within the High Security Hospitals have posed extremely difficult challenges to hospital managers and staff. One hospital has suggested that a particular problem stems from the management of patients who have been transferred from the prison system, where they may have been held in isolation for long periods and be very disturbed upon admission, although we have seen no direct evidence that such patients are those most at risk of seclusion. It has also been suggested to the Commission that the decreased sedative effect of newer antipsychotic drugs may play a part.

12.30   The Commission holds that, in fact, seclusion is all too often used in the High Secure Hospitals as a preventive or punitive measure. If the former, it may be a substitute for adequate nursing intervention. If the latter, it is a aspect of prison-culture that has no place in a hospital environment and is expressly in contravention of the Code of Practice's guidance. Even in Rampton Hospital, whose seclusion practices we have had occasion to praise in our last Biennial Report (see 12.27 above), Commissioners have noted records of patients kept in seclusion until they are ready to 'apologise'.

12.31   The importance of thorough, frequent and clinically based review of seclusion episodes is illustrated by an allegation concerning one patient's long-term seclusion that has arisen in the context of a wider Commission investigation. It has been suggested that, immediately

---

[370] Mental Health Act Commission (1995) *Sixth Biennial Report 1993-95*. London: Stationery Office p120

prior to one long-term secluded patient's weekly review, some staff members would goad that patient into a reaction that would ensure that his presentation to the clinical team indicated that seclusion continued to be warranted. Whether or not this allegation is true, the infrequency of review and the inadequate record-keeping make it difficult to disprove, and raise the possibility for such abuse in similar situations.

12.32   By the time this report is published, the Commission will have hosted a seminar involving key staff from all three High Security Hospitals to discuss the implications of the legal requirements post-*Munjaz*, and to air continuing concerns held by all parties involved.

The provision of information under section 132

12.33   At Chapter 9.14 above we discussed hospitals' performance of their duties in providing information to patients in the context of Goffman's suggestion that the withholding of such information is a characteristic of the total institution. It is perhaps not surprising that practice in giving patients information has traditionally been quite poor in the High Security Hospitals, which continue to be the most recognisably 'institutional' mental health services.

12.34   Commissioners visiting the High Security Hospitals have noted some serious gaps in practice. There are, of course, some pronounced difficulties in providing some High Security Hospital patients with information on admission, when they may be acutely disturbed, but this is all the more reason to have robust mechanisms in place for ensuring that repeated attempts are made at later stages. The Commission advises sensitivity in giving information to disturbed patients whilst respecting their right to such information: it may be appropriate, for example, to stagger the delivery of information about different aspects of patients' legal position etc to ensure that patients are able to take the information in.

12.35   It is unacceptable that there are patients in High Security Hospitals who do not know what the Code of Practice is, or are unaware of impending Commission visits, etc. This may foster a situation where some patients are relying on other patients for information that they have a statutory right to receive from their detaining authority. Aside from the clear failure of that authority to perform its duties in respect of such patients, this may also contribute to the creation of a hospital subculture where some patients are provided with power over others.

12.36   Following comment and suggestions by Commissioners, senior staff at Broadmoor Hospital have led attempts to address practice in providing patients with information. The hospital's section 132 recording documentation has been redesigned and clinical improvement groups used to train and promote good practice. Although practice is still variable across the hospital, the Commission welcomes the staff initiatives to address this. The Commission is preparing a specific report for all High Security Hospital managers on our audit of their compliance with section 132 as we go to press. We consider that some cultural change is required within the High Security Hospitals, not least so that they meet the requirements and principles of the Freedom of Information Act 2001. Whereas, for example, all policies at Broadmoor Hospital are marked as to whether they may be made available to patients, most patients are unaware that they may ask to see policies. The Commission would wish to see a culture where the assumption is made that information is automatically available to patients unless there is a good reason for withholding it, whereas we frequently encounter the opposite approach.

Patients' activities in the High Security Hospitals

12.37   Over recent years patients have frequently reported boredom and under-stimulation in their lives on the wards of High Security Hospitals. Commissioners visiting wards frequently see patients sitting unoccupied. When asked how they spend their day, some such patients have responded with, for example, 'I make tea, I read the papers, look at television or just do nothing'.

12.38   High Security Hospital patients are frequently detained in secure conditions for many years. We believe that an active therapeutic regime is an essential element of high secure care. Without such a regime the mental state of patients will deteriorate. We believe that there is a clear link between the lack of structured programmes of activities and aggressive behaviour, malaise and patients' complaints.

12.39   Patients have told Commissioners in interviews that they would like to have more structured ward activities, and they have voiced their concerns of the loss of patient-run clubs, the loss of mixed-sex activities, the length of time it takes to arrange and get treatments to happen, and, in particular, the very long psychology waiting lists. Commissioners still report waiting lists of four months to nine months for some therapies at Broadmoor Hospital, despite the development of facilities at Newbury House which have improved matters for those patients able to benefit from a structured group-work approach. We will continue to monitor this vital aspect of patient care and will support patients who speak with Commissioners of their frustration and boredom.

The Commission's Broadmoor study of patient activities

12.40   In November and December 2002 we carried out a systematic study of patients' engagement in "purposeful activity" in Broadmoor Hospital, culminating in a report provided to the hospital managers[371]. The study took place before the opening of the excellent new sports and leisure centre, which has had a positive effect on the lives on many of the younger patients and is applauded by all who make use of it, although both the Commission and the Trust management recognise ongoing concerns about general levels of patient activity.

12.41   For the purpose of this study 'purposeful activity' was defined as including work, therapy, leisure and social activities, and was measured in programmed "sessions". A "session" equates to approximately $2^1/2$ hours of activity time.

12.42   Our study found that each patient had an average of 3.4 programmed sessions per week. This equates with the Trust's own findings, which showed a slow improvement in the amount of activity per patient, although the average time spent in purposeful activities by each patient was only about eight hours per week. While both our study and the hospital's own occupational therapy department use averages to measure patient activities, this can disguise the real experience of some patients. While the averages for most patients may be around four or five sessions per week of activity, these figures are distorted by a few 'outliers'

---

[371] Full report, including methodology, available on www.mhac.trent.nhs.uk

who thus distort the picture. Of the 69 patients randomly picked in our study, 16 had more than six sessions per week and 34 had two or less sessions per week.

12.43 We noted inconsistencies in the management of patients' activity across the hospital. On some wards patients held and could produce a timetable of their own activities, which they used as a reference point and as an element of their care plans, but on others patients claimed to have lost or never had such a timetable. On certain wards where an air of defeatism appeared to prevail, refusals by patients to attend activities appeared to be expected and the follow-up arrangements were less energetic than might be appropriate. The average number of sessions of particular activities evident in patients' ward programmes is shown at Figure 33.

Activity	Average number of sessions
Therapy	1.16
Sport	0.12
Education	0.99
Work	1.68
Leisure Pursuits	0.40
Ward work - cookery	0.07
Ward work - cleaning	0.10
Other	0.71

Fig 33: Activities by average number of sessions per week

Legal Category	Average number of sessions
Mental Illness (MI)	2.1
Personality Disorder (PD)	5.3
MI & PD	5.7
Not known	2.75

Fig 34: Weekly activity by legal category

12.44 Figure 34 shows that while the whole patient population has a relatively unstimulating life, patients who are mentally ill are particularly disadvantaged. We recognise that Broadmoor is working with a patient population who are extremely damaged by their mental illnesses. In particular they experience the negative symptoms of their illness to a considerably degree. These symptoms make it particularly hard to motivate them into activity. Moreover, unlike the personality disordered patients they are less likely to make formal demands on their carers to provide them with treatment and work. As a consequence the challenge facing the Trust is to develop programmes for providing both structure and motivation in a way focused on their needs. Commissioners continue to be concerned at the large numbers of patients remaining in bed until late morning.

12.45 We have made a number of recommendations to the Hospital Managers as a result of our survey, which are summarised at Figure 35 below. Other services, and not just those in the secure sector, should consider whether these recommendations might help their own service improvement programmes.

Summary of recommendations from the Commission's Broadmoor study of patient activity

✳ A target should be set for the average level of purposeful activity appropriate across the whole hospital. The target should recognise that each ward and each patient has different needs and abilities, but that a benchmark can help in reviewing the effectiveness of the hospital's strategy

✳ When monitoring patients' activities, data should distinguish between patients' legal categories of mental disorder to provide a check on whether activities are provided or taken up equitably.

✳ Staff should prepare a strategy for motivating patients with a severe and enduring mental illness who struggle to have a structure and direction in their lives.

✳ Data should be produced so that extremes as well as averages are noted, to ensure vigilance over the experience and needs of the least motivated or most unwell patients.

Fig 35: Summary of recommendations from the MHAC study of patient activity in Broadmoor Hospital

Patients' access to fresh air

12.46 At Chapter 9.29 we highlight problems pertaining to many hospitals in respect of patients' access to fresh air. This issue has long been a concern within the High Security Hospitals, and has once again been an issue over this reporting period, both through lack of appropriate facilities and staff to escort patients who require accompanying off ward environments. At Broadmoor Hospital work was undertaken in 2002 to provide improved access to outdoor facilities and, although this is now complete, limited outdoor spaces provided by airing courts continue to be shared by as many as sixty patients. Access to some outdoor areas at Broadmoor Hospital has been diminished by the building work for the security fence for the new personality disorder units within the hospital confines (see also 12.53 below). All three hospitals should continue to strive to improve patients' access to outdoors: it is unlikely that the ten-year old standard of ten hours per week in summer and four hours per week in winter has yet been met by the hospitals for the majority of their patients[372].

The provision of therapeutic interventions

12.47 The Commission carried out an analysis of psychological service provision at Broadmoor and Rampton Hospitals in 2001, and continues to monitor the provision of therapeutic interventions in the three High Security Hospitals. Psychology services appear not to have been adequately resourced in the history of the hospitals and, as a result, considerable work and investment is still needed despite work undertaken in the reporting period.

---

[372] see Mental Health Act Commission (2001) *Ninth Biennial Report 1999-01*, London: Stationery Office. Chapter 3.20

12.48 The Commission has suggested the following categorisation of of psychology and psychotherapy interventions[373] in the High Secure Hospitals (or anywhere else) as a basis for audit and monitoring of service provision:

> **Type A** interventions include low-key approaches such as craft-work, current affairs discussions, etc.

> **Type B** interventions describe the majority of eclectic therapies carried out by psychology departments and clinical nurse specialists. It comprises interventions that have a defined therapeutic purpose, such as social skills training, relaxation therapy and less intensive forms of group therapy.

> **Type C** interventions have a predefined therapeutic methodology and specific targeted therapeutic goals such as victim empathy group, or individual dynamic psychotherapy.

The Commission has recommended that each hospital should maintain a central database of non-pharmacological interventions with analysis and retrieval capability.

12.49 Because of the different methods used in assigning patients to psychology services within each hospital, it is not possible to provide a simple measurement of the number patients waiting for services or the average length of wait. Neither, given the need to provide patients with proper therapeutic engagement within a limited resource, can waiting lists be automatically assumed to be a mark of failures in service provision. However, the following case-studies perhaps best illustrate the Commission's concerns:

> ∗ Patient J has a diagnosis falling within the legal category of psychopathic disorder and was detained in a High Security Hospital under section 45A of the Act (which allows for the Crown Court to pass sentence and direct that the accused be admitted directly to hospital for treatment as if transferred from prison). He explained to Commissioners that he was committed to addressing his problems and to change, and had therefore welcomed the opportunity of admission to a psychiatric hospital. He was aware that an alternative option would have been admission to HMP Grendon Underwood, where there is a therapeutic community. When he spoke to Commissioners he had been waiting 11 months to commence a course of psychotherapy. Had he been imprisoned in Grendon he would have started attending therapeutic groups from his admission.

> ∗ A young patient within the High Security Hospitals, P, disclosed that he had been the victim of abuse in children's homes. He was supported on the ward in the aftermath of this disclosure but there was recognition from all involved that he required psychotherapeutic assistance. Psychologists recognised that he required long-term treatment and that thus was dependent on the commitment of a skilled professional who could provide continuing therapy for several months. All such staff had full caseloads and, one year later, the hospital was still unable to meet his significant needs.

> ∗ The Home Office refused permission for the transfer to conditions of lesser security of patient C, who had been resident in a High Security Hospital for eight years, because he had not acknowledged or addressed the nature of the behaviour which had contributed to his index offence.

---

[373] Mental Health Act Commission (2001 *Ninth Biennial Report 1999-01*, London: Stationery Office. Chapter 3.26

The hospitals are seeking to address the problems in providing psychological interventions and have, over this reporting period, invested considerable effort into increasing the psychology provision, including through the recruitment of additional staff.

12.50   In Summer 2001 Broadmoor Hospital opened a dedicated unit for the development and delivery of group therapies at Newbury House, where a complete team with its own escort service and nursing support provide a high volume and intensive range of therapies for patients across the hospital. The Commission commends this approach as a constructive way of dealing with the large numbers of patients awaiting therapy, which could be emulated to address a common problem faced in the other hospitals where the physical limitations of wards, pressures on available appropriate accommodation and escorting staff, can restrict group therapy activities. However, the Commission is mindful of the danger that increased emphasis on group therapies may detract from the provision of individual therapy. Some patients will find offence-related behaviour difficult to discuss in a group situation may not be able to profit from or cope with the level of intimacy developed in a therapeutic group. The hospital's psychology department designates any patient who has been on a waiting list for over a year as an emergency case. We find this standard to be insufficiently ambitious.

12.51   There is, in the Commission's view, a danger that the continuing development of specialist personality disorder units within the High Security Hospital and prison system may be to the detriment of psychological therapy provision for patients remaining within the mainstream High Security Hospital services. The Commission expects the hospital managers and the Department of Health to ensure that psychology input to mainstream services continues to remain a focus of the improvement agenda in terms of attention and resources.

Women in the High Security Hospitals

Closure of women's facilities at Ashworth and Broadmoor Hospitals

12.52   In 2003 the intention to cease women's services at Ashworth and Broadmoor Hospitals was announced. The Commission is sympathetic to the need to centralise high secure services for women, especially given the large number of women patients who are to be transferred to other security levels.

12.53   The potential for detriment to the care and quality of life for those women patients who remain in the closing directorates at Broadmoor and Ashworth Hospitals until the end is already apparent. At Broadmoor Hospital, for example, women patients lost a considerable part of their garden and their view to the security fence for the new personality disorder unit over the first six months of 2003. The Commission recognises that it would be increasingly difficult to maintain the already limited range of activities and opportunities available to a dwindling number of women patients on these sites. Perhaps on this basis, we understand that a decision has been made to transfer those women for whom alternative arrangements cannot be made outside of high secure provision to temporary placements within Rampton Hospital.

12.54   This decision, however, has had a notable effect on the morale of many women concerned. Many of the women are anxious about the move, especially those that have been expecting to move to local secure facilities. Some women have been told that the move to Rampton

Hospital is temporary, but that this may mean anything from one or two to five years. Such long periods of time are unacceptable and may have seriously detrimental effects on the lives of the women.

12.55   The Commission's own concerns at the arrangements are as follows:

*   It appears that at least some of the women due for transfer to Rampton Hospital would be transferred out of high secure care if suitable facilities could be identified. Given that a number of the women concerned will have expected their next move within mental health service to be out of the high secure sector, this 'sideways' move may be distressing. The Commission has sought assurances from the National Oversight Group that authorities responsible for each patient will be expected to provide suitable arrangements for their reception as soon as possible, so that patients suitable for placements outside high secure service will be able to tale up such placements within months rather than years of their move to Rampton Hospital. The Commission will monitor carefully the situation of women moved to Rampton Hospital under these circumstances and will be watchful against any detrimental effects of the transfer.

*   It is unclear whether suitable facilities exist at Rampton to care for the women likely to be moved there in an appropriate environment. The draft strategy for women's mental health in England, *Into the Mainstream*, provides a specification for secure units which includes the need for the physical design of units to take into account the primary need for relational security, and that, wherever possible, environmental security should be provided by the built environment rather than perimeter fences. Unit layouts should be such that zonal observation is a realistic alternative to high levels of one-to-one nursing, and that 'crisis suites' can be separated off as alternatives to seclusion. There are also statements about the need for appropriate quiet areas and the importance of small scale, with no more than twelve beds in a unit[374]. Existing facilities at Rampton Hospital cannot meet such standards and provide spaces for an influx of new patients.

The cessation of mixed-sex activities in the High Security Hospitals

12.56   In the summer of 2001, the Commission was made aware of staff concerns that had already been raised with the hospital management regarding the vulnerability of some women during mixed-gender activities at Broadmoor Hospital. The Commission gave evidence to the external enquiry undertaken by the Trust in January 2002 and has been kept informed of hospital actions throughout this period, including the decisions to suspend all mixed-gender social and therapeutic activities and subsequently not to reintroduce them.

12.57   The Commission recognised that the hospital's cessation of mixed-gender activities in November 2001 was prompt and decisive action to deal with perceived risks posed to women patients. We continue to offer constructively critical support to the hospital's action, as we recognise the difficulties in ensuring the safety of women patients given the infrastructure of the hospital.

12.58   The Commission continues to draw to the attention of Broadmoor Hospital management the concerns of women patients and the Commission's own concerns at some effects of the cessation of mixed gender activities. At a time when the lack of purposeful and therapeutic

---

[374] Department of Health (2002) *Women's Mental Health: Into the Mainstream. Strategic Development of Mental Health Care for Women.* Department of Health, October 2002.

activity is a major problem at Broadmoor Hospital, the cessation of mixed gender activities had an immediate and detrimental effect on access to such activities. We recognise the hospital management's considerable efforts to mitigate these effects and to provide a full and appropriate women's service ensuring proper protection of women patients whilst they remain at the hospital.

12.59 However, we remain concerned that all High Security Hospital patients' lives are increasingly circumscribed by blanket rules applied to all regardless of their individual circumstances. The Commission is committed to the view that mental health care must, as far as possible, be based on a sophisticated understanding of the needs (including of course, the need for safety) of individual patients together with an individual risk assessment rather than on institutional requirements. We will continue to urge the managers of Rampton Hospital, who will take on responsibility for all women patients in high secure care (see 12.53 above), to consider this carefully when accommodating and treating their women patients. As we go to press, the Commission is undertaking a further review of women's opportunities for activity in the hospital, where mixed-gender activity is currently suspended pending the hospital managers' own consideration of service structure and delivery. In the meantime, women patients continue to raise concerns with the Commission over their access to activities and facilities in the hospital.

Recommendation 54: Rampton Hospital managers must seek to provide a full range of activities and therapy for women patients who are accommodated within their hospital. We urge the hospital to adopt as flexible an approach to mixed-sex activity as is commensurate with women's safety and security based upon individual risk-assessment.

Children's visiting

12.60 In our last Biennial Report we were critical of the blanket application of measures required of and undertaken by the High Security Hospitals in relation to the visits of children to patients, particularly as these had effected women patients. We noted delays in social services' approval for such visits; restricted opportunities for visits to take place due to limitations in accommodation and staffing; visiting time spent waiting for escorting staff to become available; and distress over the searching of children by hospital security staff.

12.61 We are pleased to report considerable improvements in the situation over the last two years. Rampton and Broadmoor hospitals both have new visitors' centres. The Broadmoor centre opened in February 2003, and has received largely positive responses from patients' families. Separate visiting slots for visitors with children are allocated twice daily, and take place in pleasant surroundings with comfortable seating; facilities for making hot drinks; television, video and games; nappy-changing facilities, etc. Searching arrangements are reported to be sensitively handled. Previously reported delays in getting social services' permission for such visits seem much less prevalent. Broadmoor Hospital is also preparing brochures and a video for relatives and friends of patients who are visiting the hospital for the first time, to make the experience less intimidating.

12.62 The Commission welcomes these positive improvements in services and commends the hospitals on their efforts. In our view there remains a lesson for Government in this issue. We can see no reason why the requirements regarding children visiting should have been applied regardless of known risks or past experience to all patients, and particularly women patients, before the appropriate facilities were in place to avoid purposeless detriment to patients' quality of life. We have no doubt that some women patients' initial experiences of arrangements introduced in 1999 will have been damaging to their general welfare and treatment progress.

> **Recommendation 55:** Particular care should be taken when imposing policy measures that will effect patients' quality of life, so that a balance is achieved between the necessity of intervention against the actual risks and detriment to patients' welfare involved. Where the aims of intervention will not be served by blanket applications, or where services need to develop supporting infrastructures to implement policies effectively or humanely, services should be enabled to make a staggered implementation based upon individual risk assessments.

Personality disorder services in the high secure sector and elsewhere

12.63 Under current arrangements, a considerable proportion of patients with a primary diagnosis of personality disorder who are made subject to the Act (under the legal category of "psychopathic disorder") are admitted to the High Security Hospitals. Figure 36 below shows placements of "psychopathic disorder" patients in 2002, comparing admissions to high security with those to other NHS facilities and independent hospitals.

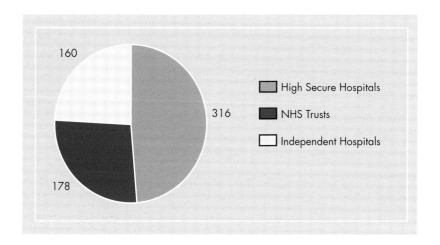

Fig 36 : Placement of "Psychopathic Disorder" patients 31/03/2002

Data Source: DOH (2002) Statistical Bulletin In-patients formally detained in hospitals under the MHA 1983 and other legislation, England: 1991-92 to 2001-02 (Bulletin 2002/26)

12.64 Considerable improvements in existing services for personality disordered patients within the High Security Hospitals have been noted by Commissioners over this reporting period.

Patient care standards have continued to improve on the Ashworth personality disorder units in relation to the medical staffing establishment; provision of therapeutic group work; and the knowledge amongst staff of the requirements of the Act and Code of Practice, particularly in relation to consent to treatment issues. Rampton Hospital's existing personality disorder wards, which house around 120 patients, are highly regarded by the Commissioners who visit them. Commissioners note the high staff/patient ratios; levels of activity and therapeutic input; and clear division between assessment and treatment wards with minimal levels of medication and seclusion evident in the latter. Indeed, the levels of investment and attention given to these services are generally very good, and will hopefully serve as models for similar initiatives across all services within the hospitals.

12.65   Continued inappropriate placements of patients within high security personality disorder services have been recognised by Government. NIMHE have stated this year that:

> there are clearly patients with psychopathic disorder within the current system who could move directly from high secure hospitals to supervised accommodation in the community, with the right level of support. Research indicates that direct transition to a supported community setting may be associated with a better eventual outcome for those whose risk is assessed to be low, than a move to an interim setting of a medium secure unit. [375]

The difficulty is that, as yet, the infrastructure to support such patient movement is not in place:

> There is currently very little dedicated provision for people with personality disorder within regional forensic mental health services. However, there is a widely acknowledged need to move on a number of personality disordered patients from high secure hospitals, and a need to take some personality disordered patients direct from the courts into [medium secure and community settings]…. We are committed to contributing to the development of service infrastructure in order to create resources and facilities that can be used by clinicians to develop expertise in the care and treatment of people who are personality disordered. In time, these facilities will be used for people on the DSPD programme assessed as safe to move on from high security …[376].

12.66   There is, of course, considerable anxiety amongst patients regarding the proposed changes in the law and the provision of services relating to personality disorder (see Chapter 7.10 – 7.32 above). However, most of the patients resident in existing personality disorder facilities are not destined to be moved into the new and unfortunately named "DSPD units" (see Chapter 7.13 and Recommendation 14 above). The new units will take patients from a wide range of services, including directly from the courts and from the transfer of existing inmates of prisons. Whilst staff in the units will have attempted to continue discussions about the future and allowed individual patients to express and discuss their fears about future provision, these are additional challenges in the treatment of this patient group. In Ashworth Hospital in particular, there is a constant change culture which effects both staff and patients' feelings of

---

[375]   Department of Health (2003) *Personality Disorder – No Longer a Diagnosis of Exclusion; Policy implementation guidance for the development of services for people with personality disorder.* NIMHE, April 2003. Para 110

[376]   Home Office (2001) *DSPD Programme Progress Report – a joint initiative between Department of Health, Home Office and Prison Service.* Nov 2001

stability and security. Patients in Rampton Hospital's personality disorder wards, many of whom look forward to progression to lower secure care (and many of whom may already be suitable for such progression) are bound to view the establishment of a purpose-built 70 bedded "DPSD Unit", surrounded by its own perimeter security even within the new hospital walls, with some trepidation.

> **Recommendation 56:** The Commission is concerned that development of services for personality disordered must not be allowed to become asymmetric across levels of security, or between hospital and community-based services, as this can only contribute to the already notable problems in moving patients from secure services when they no longer require care at this level.

12.67   Given our concerns over the possible extent of co-morbidity between personality disorders and other forms of mental disorder, particularly the psychoses (see chapter 7.29-30 above), the Commission trusts that the development of specialist personality disorder units will not create artificial distinctions in treatment opportunity for patients dependent on their primary diagnoses.

Locking patients' rooms at night in new personality disorder units

12.68   As discussed at 12.20 above, the Secretary of State requires all patients in the new High Security Hospital specialist personality disorder units (excepting those at risk of suicide or self-harm) to be locked into their rooms at night. The Commission's concerns at how this Directive would fit with the Code of Practice requirements regarding seclusion practice were answered by the *Munjaz* judgment of 2003, discussed at 3.2-8 and 6.17-23 above. The Court determined that locking patients in their rooms at night is not to be considered as seclusion, but rather that "seclusion is keeping a person under regular, frequent observation, while he is prevented from having contact with anyone in the world outside the room where he is confined" (paragraph 75). The hospital managers must now determine their own protocols and procedures for risk-assessment prior to locking patients down for the night, and any checks and security measures to be taken in respect of patients who are locked into their rooms.

12.69   In directing the hospitals to lock patients' rooms at night in the new units as a blanket measure, with exceptions to be made only for patients who are at risk of suicide or self-harm, Government has overridden clinical discretion on any grounds other than safety. We view this blanket imposition of practices that potentially engage ECHR principles as contrary to the spirit of the recent *Munjaz* ruling. We share the concerns raised by some managers and clinicians from within the hospitals themselves over the potential effects of this on patients transferred into the new units from existing mental health services, on the role of clinical teams in caring for patients and on the culture of high secure care as a whole.

13

The Mental Health Act 1983 and the criminal justice system

Section 35 and dual detention

13.1 Section 35 of the Act allows a court to remand a patient to hospital for a psychiatric report. The data available to the Commission (Figure 37) suggests that its use has declined in recent years, although as this only counts admissions to NHS facilities, increased use of the independent sector to provide medium secure beds could account for some of this apparent decline.

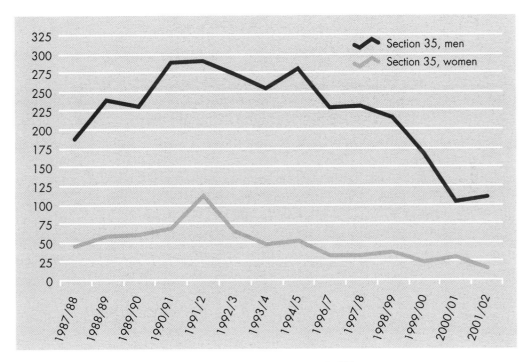

Fig 37: Use of section 35, NHS facilities, 1996 – 2002, by gender[377]

13.2 Like section 48, which is discussed at Chapter 14.5-8 below, Section 35 is sometimes used in conjunction with a civil power of detention. In *R v North West London Mental Health NHS Trust ex parte Stewart* [1997], it was determined that civil powers of detention may coexist with and operate independently from these criminal justice powers of detention. In the case of section 35, under which patients are not subject to the consent to treatment provisions of

---

[377] Data sources: 1987/8-92/3: table 2,DOH statistical Bulletin 1995/4; 1993/4-94/5: table 3, DOH Statistical Bulletin 1996/10996/7-2001/02: table 3, DOH Statistical Bulletin 2002/26.

Part IV of the Act, this legitimised the practice of "dual detention", where a patient would be concurrently detained under section 2 or 3 in order to extend powers of compulsory treatment over their care. In the case of section 48, dual detention may be considered simply as a safety net in case the patient's remand status, and subsequent liability to detention under that power, changes.

13.3   The illogicalities of dual detention are ably presented in the *Mental Health Act Manual*, Eighth Edition (para 1-495). Foremost among these is the fact that certain powers available under civil sections, such as those relating to leave of absence or discharge from detention, are contradicted and in practice cancelled by the patient's status as a prisoner on remand. In this sense it is difficult to see how the detaining power of section 3 and either section 35 or 48 can, in fact, coexist and operate independently of each other. The judgment in the *Stewart* case is also difficult to reconcile with the presumption that Parliament does not enact legislation that interferes with personal liberty without making its intention clear. Notwithstanding these difficulties, the *Stewart* case describes the current state of the law.

13.4   The difficulties and contradictions thrown up by the practice of dual detention under the 1983 Act are undoubtedly due to the fact that the legislation was not drafted with this use in mind. Nevertheless, the concept of some form of dual detention, or flexibility between civil and criminal justice powers, may serve as a useful precedent to Parliament in its scrutiny of the Mental Health Bill. We can see no reason why, instead of the controversial proposal to grant courts the power to detain persons who have not been charged with imprisonable offences[378], the next Mental Health Act should not facilitate the instigation of civil detention where appropriate, even where a person has come to the attention of authorities through the criminal justice system.

Section 37 hospital orders

13.5   The total numbers of patients admitted to NHS and independent facilities under section 37 is shown at Figure 38 below. A notable change is the increased use of the independent sector in providing facilities for the admission of unrestricted patients under this section, shown at Figures 39 and 40 below. There appears to have been an overall decline in uses of section 37 from the start of the Act's implementation, although we advise caution over the accuracy of statistics for 1984-6 in Figure 38. It may be, if these figures are correct, that more accused persons are now receiving custodial sentences. The increased use of the Criminal Procedures Insanity Acts (see 13.8 *et seq* below) does not account for the difference.

13.6   During this reporting period, the case of *R v Galfetti* [2002] highlighted how mentally disordered offenders who are being made subject to a hospital order under this power may be especially disadvantaged by problems in locating an available hospital bed. Section 37(4) precludes a hospital order being made unless the court is satisfied that arrangements have been made for the patient's reception into hospital within 28 days. When, in the *Galfetti* case, no bed could be found, the court repeatedly adjourned sentencing until, nine months after conviction, a bed was available and the order was finally made. The patient appeared to have no right of appeal against the adjournment. Even though this situation surely

---

[378] Adam James *Government powers plan 'shameful'* <u>Guardian</u> 11 June 2003.

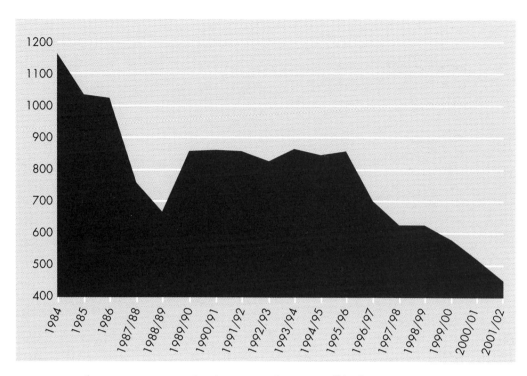

Fig 38: Uses of section 37, (restricted and unrestricted patients), all facilities, England 1987–2002[379]

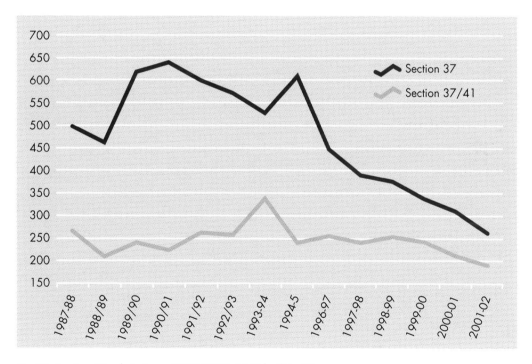

Fig 39: Section 37 admissions, 1987–2002, NHS facilities[380]

---

[379] Data sources: 1984-86: table D1, DHSS Mental Health Statistics for England 1986: 1987/8-92/3: table 2,DOH statistical Bulletin 1995/4; 1993/4-94/5: table 3, DOH Statistical Bulletin 1996/10996/7-2001/02: table 3, DOH Statistical Bulletin 2002/26.

[380] Data sources: DOH statistical Bulletin 1995/4, table 2; DOH Statistical Bulletin 1999/25, table 3. DOH Statistical Bulletin 2002/26, table 3.

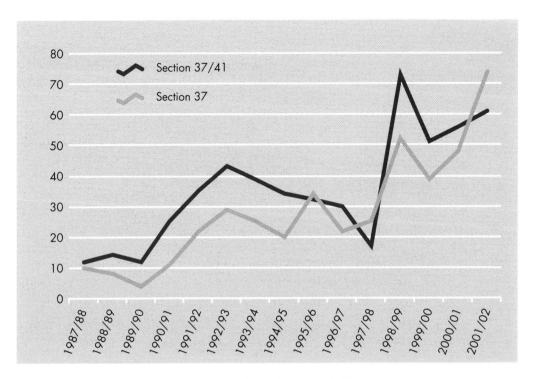

Fig 40: Section 37 admissions, 1987–2002, independent hospitals[381]

curtailed the patient's human rights, the court concluded that "whenever a hospital place is not available within a reasonable time… the court is disabled from affording justice in the way in which Parliament has provided".

13.7   There would seem to be no easy remedy to the *Galfetti* dilemma. Twenty-eight days to arrange hospital admission is a considerable length of time, and should probably not be extended. Any change in the law that allowed an order to be made without first having secured a hospital place could simply place the patient into a legal and clinical limbo after sentencing rather than before it. This can happen now with the Criminal Procedures (Insanity and Unfitness to Plead) Act 1991, which can raise a number of other problems (see 13.13 below).

13.8   We note that no change was proposed in the draft Mental Health Bill of 2002[382], and it therefore seems that the only solution is to ensure that delays in locating appropriate placements are avoided. Section 39 of the 1983 Act provides a power for the court to require information on available placements from any authority. This useful lever for judges in persuading hospital authorities to locate a suitable bed did not appear to be preserved in the draft Mental Health Bill of 2002, although we can see no reason why it should be omitted from the final legislation.

---

[381] Data sources: as above: tables 5, 9 and 9 respectively.

[382] Department of Health (2002) Draft Mental Health Bill 2002. Cm 5538 –I, clause 78

Recommendation 57: The Commission recommends that Government should retain an equivalent of section 39 of the 1983 Act in new mental health legislation, whilst also considering identifying the chief executives of public authorities (whether commissioning authorities such as Primary Care Trusts or mental health service providers) as personally responsible for the identification and allocation of a bed within a specified timescale. This should be kept under review by the body responsible for monitoring the implementation of the new Act.

Use of Criminal Procedure (Insanity) Acts

13.9 On the 31 December 2001, there were 186 restricted patients detained in hospital under Schedule I to the Criminal Procedures (Insanity and Unfitness to Plead) Act 1991. Of these, 35 had been found by a jury to be 'not guilty by reason of insanity' under section 2 of the Trial of Lunatics Act 1883, as amended by the 1964 and 1991 Criminal Procedure (Insanity) Acts. The remaining 151 were found unfit to plead by a jury under section 4 of the 1964 Act, as amended by the 1991 Act. The population of resident patients detained under these powers shows a marked increase in recent years (Figure 41 below), as has the use of section 4 of the 1964 Act (Figure 42).

	1995	1996	1997	1998	1999	2000	2001
Unfit to plead	97	93	103	110	120	124	151
Not guilty by reason of insanity	24	25	23	25	23	28	35
Total	121	118	126	135	143	152	186

Figure 41: Resident patients detained under Criminal Procedure (Insanity and Unfitness to Plead) Act 1991, as of 31 December 1995–2001[383]

13.10 Once made, a hospital order under the Criminal Procedure (Insanity and Unfitness to Plead) Act 1991 is equivalent in law and practice to a hospital order under Part III of the Mental Health Act 1983[384]. As such, although it is arguable whether patients who have been hospitalised under the 1991 Act's powers fall within the Commission's remit, we do not exclude such patients from our attention on Commission visits.

Criminal Procedure (Insanity) Acts and fact-finding

13.11 One significant amendment introduced in the 1991 legislation to the Criminal Procedure (Insanity) Act 1964 was that, once a jury had determined an accused person unfit to plead, there must be forensic investigation before a jury of whether the accused did the act or made

---

[383] data source: Johnson,S, Taylor R (2002) *Statistics of mentally disordered offenders* 2001, National Statistics Bulletin 13/02, table 6

[384] Criminal Procedure (Insanity and Unfitness to Plead) Act 1991 Schedule 1, para 2(1)

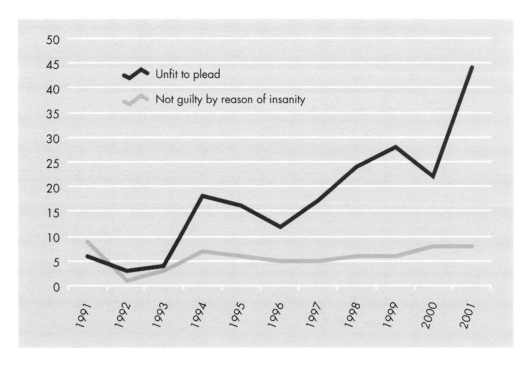

Fig 42: Admissions to hospital 1991–2001, England and Wales: Criminal Procedure (Insanity and Unfitness to Plead) Act 1991[385]

the omission charged against him or her. This change had been instigated by a case where a person had been detained for some time under the 1964 Act before it emerged that her confession of murder was false. In January 2003 the House of Lords determined that this fact-finding exercise of the court does not amount to a determination of a criminal charge for the purposes of ECHR Article 6[386]. Their Lordships' determination was brought about by a legal challenge to a finding under section 4A of the Criminal Procedure (Insanity) Act 1964 that a man accused of indecent assault (who was 13 years of age at the time of the alleged offence) 'did the act' but was unfit to stand trial. It had been argued before them that such a finding was to all intents and purposes a procedure to determine a criminal charge, but fell short of the guarantees of Article 6 in that the accused had already been found unfit to plead, give instruction or otherwise participate fully in his or her defence. Aside from the particular challenges relating to the case (including that indecent assault is by nature a crime of criminal intent, so that finding that the accused did the act is effectively to convict him of the offence, leading to stigma and requirements of registration under the Sex Offenders Act 1997), a general argument was placed before their Lordships to the effect that any detention subsequent to a finding of unfitness to plead should be under the civil powers of Part II of the Mental Health Act 1983.

13.12   The House of Lords' ruling rested on the question of whether section 4A of the CPIA 1964 involved the determination of a criminal charge. Their Lordships applied the tests established by *Engel v The Netherlands* (No 1) [1976]. In the first place, they found that domestic law does not classify the section 4A procedure as involving such a determination, given that the 1964 Act as amended expressly states that 'the trial' (meaning the criminal

---

[385] data source: as note 383, table 3

[386] *R v Secretary of State for the Home Department, ex parte H* [2003]

trial) shall not proceed after an accused is found unfit to plead. Secondly, their Lordships noted that the finding that a person 'did the act' could not be a conviction, as such a finding does not preclude subsequent trial for the offence at a future date if the accused person recovers the ability to plead. Thirdly, such a finding cannot culminate in any penalty, but may only culminate in acquittal or a hospital order. A hospital order is not a means punishing proscribed behaviour to deter, unlike sanctions provided by criminal law.

Criminal Procedure (Insanity) Acts and arrangements for hospital placements

13.13   A jury can only make either of the disposals discussed at 13.9 above on the written or oral evidence of two or more medical practitioners, subject to the requirements of medical evidence set out at section 54 of the Mental Health Act 1983. As such, for example, at least one medical recommendation must come from a doctor approved under section 12 of the 1983 Act. However, court disposals under the Criminal Procedure (Insanity) Acts differ from court orders under the Mental Health Act 1983 in that they are determined by the findings of a jury. There is, of course, no requirement on a jury that it must be satisfied regarding arrangements for a hospital place (as at section 37(4) of the 1983 Act) before determining that a person is unfit to plead or not guilty by reason of insanity. Once made, however, a court order under the Criminal Procedure (Insanity and Unfitness to Plead) Act 1991 must be implemented within two months.

13.14   The absence of a requirement equivalent to section 37(4) of the Mental Health Act 1983 (see 13.6 above) has not resolved dilemmas faced by courts in making disposals under the Criminal Procedure (Insanity and Unfitness to Plead) Act 1991. One case brought to the Commission's attention last year involved a patient with alcohol dependence, anxiety disorder and possibly other personality disorders. She was found unfit to plead under section 4 of the 1991 Act. Delays in locating an available bed and a doctor prepared to take responsibility for her treatment led to the judge threatening to have the case relisted for obstruction. For a time it appeared that the patient would be placed under the care of a consultant who believed compulsory hospital admission not in her interest and doubted that, had the patient been dealt with under the Mental Health Act 1983, she would meet the criteria for detention. This doctor was advised that he would have no choice but to take on the patient's care if the Home Office required him to do so. The situation was resolved by the identification of another doctor who was prepared to treat the patient within the hospital identified for her reception. It is clearly unsatisfactory that a patient may be ordered to accept treatment in hospital that is not deemed appropriate by the doctor administering such treatment, although we can see no mechanism to protect patients from this other than the discretion of authorities not to allow the situation to arise (see also Chapter 3.20-3 above on the limits of a doctor's duty as a public authority).

14

Prisons

14.1 The powers to provide compulsory treatment under the Mental Health Act 1983 are generally accepted to be not applicable inside prisons, where any treatment without consent must be justified under the common law[387]. The only power available under the Mental Health Act 1983 in respect of prisoners is that which allows their transfer from the prison environment to hospital facilities where compulsory care and treatment under the Act's powers are applicable[388]. The Commission's own remit with regard to prison healthcare is similarly circumscribed.

Transfers from Prison

14.2 There are often delays in the transfer process, particularly while a suitable bed is identified and made available, and we are pleased that the Prison Health Policy Unit now has a protocol for transfer delays of longer than three months[389]. The number of such delays during 2001/02 is shown in Figure 43 below.

2001/02 – monthly reporting				
	June 2001	Sept 2001	Dec 2001	March 2002
Number of prisoners assessed and accepted for mental health transfer by NHS	128	132	125	142
Number awaiting assessment/ acceptance but transfer pending	175	164	138	142
Number waiting longer than 3 months for transfer following acceptance	28	34	24	39

Fig 43: Transfer of prisoners, 2001/02: numbers waiting and delays over three months

data source: statistics from DOH, Prison Health Policy Unit, personal communication

---

[387] The Government view is stated in Department of Health (2002) *Seeking Consent: Working with People in Prison.* July 2002, para 1.4. A partially dissenting view, in relation to patients detained under section 3 at the time of imprisonment, may be found at para 1-283 of Jones R (2003) *Mental Health Act Manual*, eighth edition London:Sweet & Maxwell.

[388] Mental Health Act 1983, sections 47 – 53.

[389] Department of Health, HM Prison Service and the National Assembly for Wales (2001) *Changing the Outlook: A strategy for Developing and Modernising Mental Health Services in Prisons*, December 2001, para 3.20

14.3   The Prison Health Policy Unit during 2002/03 was refining data collection and some initial difficulties in definition and reporting have been addressed. From the 2002/3 data we know that, in the last quarter of the year (Jan-Mar 2003), 785 assessments were requested, 479 carried out and 221 prisoners transferred to hospital. Some of these activities will relate to prisoners whose assessments were requested or undertaken in earlier periods. At the end of the period, 33 prisoners had been waiting for longer than three months after their acceptance for transfer by the NHS.

> **Recommendation 58:** Data collected for future years should enable monitoring of the following aspects of prison transfers, and the time scales involved for each of these aspects:
>
> ✳ the number of requests for assessments from prisons;
>
> ✳ the total number of assessments carried out;
>
> ✳ the number of prisoners assessed and accepted for mental health transfer;
>
> ✳ the number of mental health transfers; and
>
> ✳ transfer delays of more than three months' duration.

14.4   At Figure 44 below we show the trends in transfer of sentenced prisoners to NHS facilities under section 47 over the lifetime of the 1983 Act. This data suggests a steady rise in the volume of transfers to medium and lower secure facilities up until 1993, when numbers have appear to have tailed off slightly. This apparent decrease *may* be no more than a reflection of a possible increase in the use of independent sector facilities, which are not counted in the chart, although figures available to the Commission are inconclusive on this[390]. The rate of transfers to High Security Hospitals has remained fairly constant. The numerical and proportionate increase in transfers to hospitals other than the High Security Hospitals has been explained by some commentators as a result of heightened awareness of the problems of mentally disordered prisoners and an increased willingness of prison medical officers to refer such patients to hospital[391]. There are a number of possible factors in the variation showed by transfers to facilities other than high secure units, including: availability of hospital beds; sentencing trends; the effectiveness of court-diversion schemes; or even rates of effective treatment within the prison system. We recommend this to the Prison Health Unit at the Department of Health and the National Institute for Mental Health England (NIMHE) as an area for further study.

14.5   Figure 45 below shows the transfer rates, since 1996, of unsentenced prisoners into NHS facilities under section 48 of the Act. There is a greater numerical use of section 48 than 47. This suggests that unsentenced prisoners are either more likely than sentenced prisoners to suffer from mental disorder, or at least to have such suffering recognised. Most unsentenced prisoners will be held on remand, although the section may also be applied to persons held under immigration legislation or other powers.

---

[390] Known transfers to private facilities under section 47 during this period are as follows:

87/8	88/9	89/90	90/91	91/92	92/93	93/94	94/95	95/96	96/97	97/98	98/99	99/00	00/01	01/02
0	1	2	5	15	7	18	23	16	5	7	17	24	18	17

Data source: DOH Stats Bulletins 1995/4; 1999/25 and 1999/26

[391] Huws R, Longson D, Reiss D and Larkin E (1997) *Prison transfers to Special Hospitals since the introduction of the Mental Health Act 1983* in Journal of Forensic Psychiatry Vol 8 No 1 May 1997 74-84, p82.

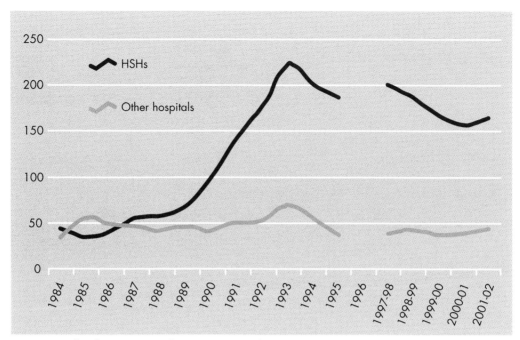

Fig 44: Transfers from prison under section 47, High Security Hospitals and other NHS facilities, 1984–2002[392]

14.6 A smaller proportion (average 5.5%) of transfers under section 48 are to High Security Hospitals than is evident over the equivalent period for transfers under section 47 (18% of all transfers under section 47 between 1996 and 2002 were to high secure care). The proportion of women prisoners to men prisoners transferred under sections 47 and 48 is, however, not dissimilar: women account for an average of 11% of sentenced prisoners and 13% of unsentenced prisoners transferred under sections 47 and 48 over this period.

14.7 As with patients remanded to hospital directly from the courts under section 35, section 48 patients may sometimes be subject to "dual detention", where a civil power of detention is exercised concurrently with the court or Home Office power. In the case of section 48, this may be considered if there is a likelihood of the patient suddenly ceasing to be a prisoner on remand (due to a case collapsing, or bail being granted, etc) whereby the powers of detention and treatment conferred by section 48 would immediately cease. We discuss dual detention at Chapter 13.1 above.

14.8 Around 140,000 people pass through the prison system annually, and the prison population at any one time is about half that number. Up to 90% of prisoners may have a diagnosable mental illness or substance misuse problem, or both[393]. Of those, we expect that only a small proportion will have a mental disorder of the nature or degree that warrants transfer under the 1983 Act, and indeed the above figures suggest a proportion of approximately one in 400

---

[392] data sources: 1984–1994 (calendar years): Huws R et al (1997) [see note 391 above], fig 1; 1996-2002 (financial years): data supplied by DoH Statistics Branch from KH15 and KP90 returns, see also table 4, DOH Statistical Bulletin 2002/26 . No data for 1996 was available in this format.

[393] Department of Health, HM Prison Service and the National Assembly for Wales (2001) *Changing the Outlook: A strategy for Developing and Modernising Mental Health Services in Prisons*, December 2001, Ministerial Foreword.

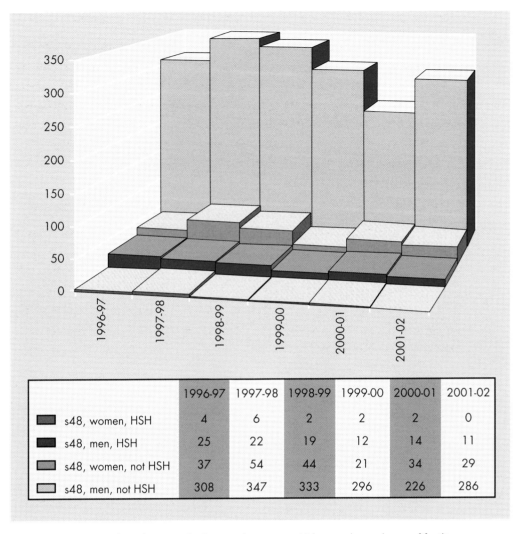

	1996-97	1997-98	1998-99	1999-00	2000-01	2001-02
s48, women, HSH	4	6	2	2	2	0
s48, men, HSH	25	22	19	12	14	11
s48, women, not HSH	37	54	44	21	34	29
s48, men, not HSH	308	347	333	296	226	286

Fig 45: Prisoners transferred to NHS facilities under section 48 by gender and type of facility, 1996–2002

data source: DoH Statistics Branch from KH15 and KP90 returns; see also see also table 4, DOH Statistical Bulletin 2002/26

prisoners overall are currently assessed as requiring transfer[394]. We suspect that the true proportion of prisoners who would meet the civil thresholds for detention is larger than this. It is likely that the threshold for admission under the 1983 Act is higher for prisoners than for other persons, given that prisoners are already in custody which may – rightly or wrongly – be considered as protective. The Reed Committee (1992) expressed concern at the often narrow interpretation of the requirement that treatment be "urgent" for section 48 powers to be used, and advised that section 48 "should be applied where a doctor would recommend inpatient treatment if a person were seen…in the community".[395] We doubt that this recommendation is observed in practice even today.

---

[394] i.e. transient prison population over one year (c.140,000) ÷ the average annual figure for Mental Health Act transfers 1996-2002 (c.350) ≈ 400. Therefore, approximately one in every 400 prisoners passing through the system will be transferred to psychiatric hospital under the 1983 Act. This suggests that prisoners may be about four times more likely to be detained under the 1983 Act than non-prisoners.

[395] Review of Health and Social Services for Mentally Disordered Offenders and others requiring similar services (1992) final summary report, HMSO para 9.6iv

Safeguards for mentally disordered prisoners awaiting transfer and treatment

14.9 In our response to the Draft Mental Health Bill of 2002[396], we suggested that consideration must be given to the Commission for Healthcare Audit and Inspection and any associate bodies' responsibilities in relation to prison healthcare services. We also urged the Government to consider whether prisoners who have been assessed as meeting the criteria for compulsion but who are waiting for transfer to mental health facilities should be considered as a specific group whose needs might be met by specific safeguards, such as the right to advocacy services or oversight by a healthcare inspectorate.

Developments in the prison service for mentally disordered prisoners.

14.10 The Department of Health report *Nursing in Prisons*[397] acknowledged that nurses and healthcare officers do their best within current arrangements, but concluded that "prison health care does not and can not provide" adequate secondary level mental health care. The report raised concerns about prisoners with mental health problems being kept alone in their cells for long periods of time, particularly at night. It compared this with practice in the NHS, where "seclusion is used only as a last resort under the direction of a psychiatrist following strict protocols"[398].

14.11 We acknowledge the work being undertaken to address the deficiencies in prison healthcare during our reporting period. The key shift over this time has been partnership of the Prison Service and the NHS. We recognise the achievements made towards implementing the NHS Plan and National Service Frameworks for Mental Health operative in England and Wales, all of which encompass the care of prisoners.

14.12 The basic principle underlying the changes in prison healthcare is that, allowing for the prison context, services should be provided as far as possible in the same way as they are in the wider community. Therefore, just as the focus of service development outside prisons is on community-based services, so the focus within prisons is on mental health promotion and "wing-based" mental health interventions. A key target over the next 3–5 years has been set as reducing the numbers of prisoners resident in prison-based health care centres, with resources re-deployed to day care and wing-based services[399].

14.13 One way of managing this, and perhaps the most dramatic change in service provision within prisons, will be the establishment of NHS managed "in-reach" teams in all prisons by 2006[400]. "In-reach" services for prisons are likely to play a broader role than their community-based "out-reach" counterparts. Whereas out-reach services' role is to help those with serious mental illness stay in contact with specialist services, "in-reach" services

---

[396] Mental Health Act Commission (2002) *Mental Health Act Commission Response to the Draft Mental Health Bill*, paras 6.19-20

[397] Department of Health (2000) *Nursing in Prisons: Report by the Working Group considering the development of prison nursing, with particular reference to health care officers.* Para 85.

[398] This may not, in fact, be an accurate account of NHS practice. See, for example, Chapters 11.17 & 12.30 above.

[399] Department of Health, HM Prison Service and the National Assembly for Wales (2001) *Changing the Outlook: A strategy for Developing and Modernising Mental Health Services in Prisons*, December 2001, paras 4.7, 10 and 4.8.

[400] Department of Health (2002) *Mental Health Bill consultation document*, Cmnd 5538-III, para 3.34.

will eventually be expected to provide general mental health services suited to all patients with mental health needs[401].

Extending compulsory powers into prison

14.14 It may be that the development of mental healthcare services within prisons can and should lead to fewer prisoners being transferred under sections 47, 48 or their equivalents in new legislation. It seems likely, for example, that in-reach services may provide the earlier intervention necessary to prevent less acute mental disorders from developing into crises. But we are concerned that the services currently under development within prisons may be expected to care for severely mentally disordered prisoners as an alternative to transferring patients to hospital facilities. In our view, unless and until prison facilities that are equivalent to hospital provision are available, the priority should be the transfer of severely mentally disordered prisoners to appropriate hospital facilities outside the prison walls. We share the Government's concern, however, that by implication many prisoners may be denied treatment or treated compulsorily without the safeguards of the Act, including the attentions of a monitoring body, whilst they are in prison.

14.15 We note with concern the suggestion that powers of compulsion could be extended to prison environments. The consultation document on the draft Mental Health Bill reasoned that, just as the draft Bill would provide a framework for the compulsory treatment in the community, thus severing the 1983 Act's link between compulsion and detention in hospital, so "there should be similar flexibility for patients to receive compulsory treatment in prison". Community treatment orders, in this model, would be allowed through the prison gates, so that prisoners could be made subject to them "just as if [they] were not in prison"[402].

14.16 Whilst Government accepts that the law would allow for compulsion only when appropriate services are in place and conditions are right[403], we question whether it has properly grasped what such service and conditions might be. We are concerned at the parallel drawn by Government between the use of compulsion in the community and prison, which suggests that in-reach or wing-based services may be expected to provide services under compulsion. We have argued instead that, for compulsory treatment within prisons to be legally or ethically justifiable, the level of service provision and support available to prisoner-patients should be at least equivalent to that which would be available elsewhere[404.] It is doubtful that in-reach services of any kind can provide the levels of service appropriate to provide compulsory mental health treatment. The prison "community" cannot offer any real equivalent to the support and care available outside prison, and any assumed equivalence between prison and the community outside greatly under-estimates the isolation and bullying of the mentally ill in prison, and the stigma of mental illness in such a situation.

---

[401] Department of Health, HM Prison Service and the National Assembly for Wales (2001) *Changing the Outlook: A strategy for Developing and Modernising Mental Health Services in Prisons*, December 2001 para 4.7

[402] Department of Health (2002) *Mental Health Bill consultation document*, Cmnd 5538-III, para 3.35-6.

[403] *ibid*, para 3.40.

[404] MHAC (2002) *MHAC Response to the Draft Mental Health Bill*, paras 6.1-6.21; see also Kinton M (2002) *Should we allow compulsory mental health treatment in prisons?* in Journal of Mental Health Law, Northumbria University Press December 2002 p304-307

14.17 This is not to say that the use of compulsion should not be contemplated within the prison environment, and the Commission has not taken a position that such compulsion could never be justified. There does seem to have been scant attention paid to the wider ethical implications of this, although we hope that the publication of responses to the draft Mental Health Bill proposals of 2002 may initiate a more considered dialogue. However, if appropriate treatment units were available within prisons, it could make sense to allow compulsory treatment there. We suggest that such units would have to be equivalent to in-patient units outside of prison. They would therefore be separate from the normal residential accommodation, staffed at all times with NHS professionals and able to provide the necessary treatment under the same quality-assurance arrangements (such as profes-sional regulation and inspection of services) as exist elsewhere in the NHS. We would also expect the same safeguards to be available to prisoner-patients as would be available to patients subject to compulsion outside prison, such as the oversight of a monitoring body, access to advocacy, ability to appeal against compulsion to a tribunal and to have tribunal oversight and safeguards applied to the treatment itself. Even if this infrastructure was in place, there should still be a requirement that transfer to an outside hospital should be considered if that would be in the prisoner-patient's best interests.

14.18 The Commission is deeply concerned at the current lack of monitoring, overview or general protection provided in relation to mental healthcare in prisons. In our view the potential for unrecognized or unchallenged coercive psychiatric treatment is extremely serious in a prison environment, where prisoners have far fewer residual freedoms than detained patients and may also feel that their compliance with psychiatric treatment may determine their assessment for release. It will not provide sufficient protection for prison healthcare to be monitored at the level of Primary Care Trust provision. Prisoners who are undergoing psychiatric treatment inside prison should be subject, at least, to similar visitorial safeguards as apply to psychiatric patients detained in healthcare establishments. Safeguards equivalent to those proposed in the draft Mental Health Bill of 2002 for incapacitated patients in healthcare establishments should extend to prison-based healthcare. This would provide mentally incapacitated prisoners who have not yet been transferred out of the prison system with the safeguard of a tribunal-style review and authorisation of their care plan.

Recommendation 59:

The Commission is opposed to the extension of powers of psychiatric compulsion under a Mental Health Act to the prison environment, especially whilst facilities available inside prison are not equivalent to those available on the outside.

If formal psychiatric compulsion is to be introduced to the prison environment at some future point, stringent safeguards at least equivalent to those available to non-prisoner patients outside the penal system must be in place, including Tribunal oversight and authorisation of care plans, appeal processes etc. There must also be appropriate and robust monitoring of the use of compulsion and inspection of facilities used by a suitably expert body.

Part 4

Diversity and Human Rights Practice

15

Equal opportunities and human rights

15.1 Article 14 of the European Convention of Human Rights provides that its rights and freedoms "shall be secured without discrimination on any ground such as sex, race, colour, language, religion, political or other opinion, national or social origin, association with a national minority, property, birth or status". This list is illustrative, not exhaustive[405]. It is therefore a fundamental requirement of all human rights-based practice that it is under-pinned with proactive and effective equal opportunities measures. We are encouraged by developments in this area since the passing of the Human Rights 1998 and Race Relations (Amendment) Act 2000, but do not underestimate the challenges faced by practitioners and policy-makers alike.

15.2 In the context of planned reorganisation of equality bodies for the UK (and therefore not specifically in the context of mental health services), the British Institute for Human Rights (BIHR) has suggested that the historic separation between equalities and human rights agendas that is peculiar to the UK has narrowed the focus of the equality agenda to a primary concern with individual redress for anti-discrimination[406]. This may be true of many points of mental health service delivery, but it is perhaps an overly harsh verdict in relation to service planning, particularly in relation to race equality where the Race Relations (Amendment) Act 2000 and non-statutory initiatives have emphasised authorities' positive duties to attend to equal opportunities at a structural level. However, we believe the BIHR charge is partly justified, in that there has been little attempt so far to make explicit the connection between anti-discrimination and human rights practice. For example, the necessity *under the Human Rights Act* of change in Black and ethnic minority patients' experiences of mental health services, and the role that human rights principles have had and will have in effecting this change, could have been emphasised in the report *Inside Outside: Improving Mental Health Services for Black and Minority Ethnic Communities*[407]. Such an emphasis could explain the

---

[405] In *R (on the application of T and S (a minor, by her next friend T) v Secretary of State for Health and Secretary of State for the Home Department* [2002], Sir Edwin Jowitt said that the word 'status' in Article 14 "is not to be considered narrowly but should be given a purposeful construction" [para 86]. As such Article 14 could encompass discrimination against any person on the basis of status, whether such status is a matter of self-identity or societal-imposition. 'Mental disorder' itself could be encompassed. In *R (on the application of Pretty) v Director of Public Prosecutions* [2001], Lord Hope held that Article 14 is capable of extending to discrimination on grounds of mental or physical capacity [para 105].

[406] British Institute for Human Rights (2002) *Something for Everyone: The impact of the Human Rights Act and the need for a Human Rights Commission*, British Institute for Human Rights, researched and written by Jenny Watson, page 16. (available from 020-7401 2712 or www.bihr.org).

[407] Department of Health (2003) *Inside Outside: Improving Mental Health Services for Black and Minority Ethnic Communities in England*. NIMHE. The Human Rights Act is mentioned only once in the main body of the report (as 'an additional imperative' to improve the experience of Black and minority ethnic patients, p7), and is not mentioned at all in the Ministerial Foreword to the document.

fundamental nature of the problems experienced by Black and minority ethnic patients and help to establish human rights awareness in a clear and forceful context.

15.3 We would like to see equal opportunities in the widest sense being acknowledged and promoted as a key component of human rights-based practice across all levels of service provision. The initiatives in relation to race equality could be a starting point for similar foci on women patients, older patients, children or patients with learning or physical disability.

Women Patients

15.4 The Commission was pleased to take part in last year's consultation over the strategic development of mental health care for women, organised around the Department of Health report *Women's Mental Health: Into the Mainstream*[408]. We recognise that the Department of Health has given women's services priority at a policy level[409] and we look forward to seeing the results of this in due course. A study commissioned by the Department of Health's Policy Research Programme and published in September 2002 concluded that while some services have improved so far, there is little indication of sustainable improvements in mainstream mental health service for women[410].

15.5 In our Ninth Biennial Report we noted some slow progress towards implementing NHS directives on safety, dignity and privacy in mixed environments[411]. Commissioners' reports suggest that the 95% implementation by the target date of 2002 of objectives relating to women's safety, privacy and dignity, which included establishing separate washing and toilet facilities and safe sleeping arrangements alongside more general organisational arrangements, has not been met in any meaningful sense, although we understand that this target is considered achieved by the Department of Health. Some hospital managers have informed the Commission that resource limitations have prevented them meeting basic accommodation standards. In some hospitals, however, excellent womens' services are being developed and implemented.

15.6 We have previously warned that some services may comply with the basic elements of the Government's objectives without in reality offering a quality service to women. The Commission has listed the following issues to be addressed by service commissioning bodies and providers in providing care to detained women patients (see Figure 46 below). In our Eighth Biennial Report (1999) we suggested to Government that services could also be required:

---

[408] Department of Health (2002) *Women's Mental Health: Into the Mainstream*. Strategic development of mental health care for women. London, October 2002. Summary document also available. The Mental Health Act Commission's response to this consultation document (December 2002) is published on our website www.mhac.trent.nhs.uk

[409] see also Department of Health (2003) *Secure Futures for Women: Making a Difference*; Department of Health (2003) Women-only and women-sensitive mental health services. Expert briefing. NIMHE, Summer 2003 www.nimhe.org.uk/expertbriefings.

[410] Barnes M, Davis A, Guru M, Lewis L and Rogers H (2002) *Women-only and women-sensitive mental health services: An Expert Paper* University of Birmingham Department of Social Policy and Social Work. This report is summarised in the NIMHE briefing referenced at 394 above, but is also downloadable from www.socialresearch.bham.ac.uk

[411] Mental Health Act Commission (2001) *Ninth Biennial Report 1999-2001*. London: Stationery Office. Chapter 6.33 *et seq*

* to have policies relating to women's safety available on every ward and reviewed every two years;

* to identify through risk-assessment women who are particularly vulnerable to sexual exploitation or harassment and also men who have a history of harassment or violence towards women;

* to monitor all incidents of sexual harassment to identify problems in service provision;

* to ensure staff are appropriately trained in gender awareness and the safety and special needs of women patients; and

* to appoint a designated officer with oversight for women's issues[412].

We continue to suggest such measures as elements of good practice in women's services.

Service commissioning bodies and service providers should agree and monitor services for women patients to ensure that such patients can:

* lock bedroom doors, using a system capable of being overridden by staff in an emergency;

* have a choice of a female key-worker;

* be in contact with other women;

* have the opportunity to take part in women-only therapy groups and social activities, but have the choice of taking part in mixed groups where appropriate;

* engage safely in a full range of such activities, even where their number is small compared to the hospital population;

* have physical health checks on admission;

* have access to a female doctor for medical care;

* have access to a female member of staff at all times; and

* be assured of adequate supervision at night.

Fig 46: Commission Practice Guidelines: service for women patients
(Recommendation 63, MHAC (2001) Ninth Biennial Report, Chapter 6.38)

15.7   We are concerned that the increasing physical segregation of sexes within acute services may have a deleterious effect on women's access to therapeutic and recreational activities, fresh air etc. We have found this to be the case even in the High Security Hospitals, where patient populations fluctuate less than other services and patients stay for longer periods to allow for more comprehensive individual care-planning (issues relating to women patients in the High Security Hospitals are discussed at Chapter 12. 52 *et seq* above).

15.8   In the coming two-year period the Commission intends to undertake a specific study of the nursing care and treatment of women detained under the 1983 Act, with a particular focus on the position of detained women patients who are in a minority in mixed-sex facilities.

Older patients

15.9   A primary concern of the Commission in relation to older patients is that such a large number of them fall outside of the scope of our operations. A great number of so-called

---

[412] Mental Health Act Commission (1999) *Eighth Biennial Report 1997-9.* London: Stationery Office. Chapter 10.72

"Bournewood" patients, who lack mental capacity to consent to their care and treatment but are nevertheless compliant with it (see Chapter 8.1 *et seq*), are likely to be older patients suffering from dementia or depressive illnesses. There is little overview of the general standards of care and treatment for this group of patients and no body with responsibility for considering the human rights aspects of *de facto* compulsion. It is acknowledged that such patients may be prescribed inappropriate neuroleptic medication in an attempt to treat behavioural complications of their disorders, with a number of adverse effects[413]. Although we welcomed guidance on implementing the medicines-related aspects of the NSF for older people in our last Biennial Report, we doubt that this guidance alone will even start to challenge practice:

> "These drugs [neuroleptics] should not be used for people with dementia, except in exceptional circumstances, and yet the use of them on old people is going up and up. It's a clear correlation it seems between lack of experience, lack of training and poor staffing… It's absolutely a violation. And it's covert, we picked up the issue of covert medication because of this issue…"[414]

Research on this issue by the Alzheimer's Society, commissioned by the Department of Health and carried out by a medical team, questioned the clinical appropriateness of the use of neuroleptics in 83% of nearly 1,000 care plans relating to older persons in care homes in the Thames region[415]. Although the inappropriate and covert use of psychiatric medication is one extreme example of malpractice that may be largely hidden from public view, but is now coming to the attention of Government, it is just one of possibly many other impositions on this group's human and legal rights that is not, at present, subject to any specifically focussed monitoring:

> "People in a care home with dementia who are there supposedly with their consent, don't have any rights or safeguards at the moment. If they were sectioned they would have much better safeguards… But it's a whole group that's completely ignored. And locked doors are quite common"[416].

15.10 The Commission has similar concerns over the care outside of statutory frameworks and regulation of learning disabled patients.

Recommendation 60: Future arrangements for monitoring of the use of compulsion should extend to mentally incapacitated patients receiving psychiatric care and treatment under all circumstances.

15.11 The progress report issued by Government in 2003 on the implementation of the National Service Framework for Older People provides few details of mental health services, as milestones for the mental health standards all fall in 2004[417]. The Audit Commission's 2002

---

[413] see Mental Health Act Commission (2001) *Ninth Biennial Report 1999-2001*, London: Stationery Office. Chapter 6.62.

[414] Julia Cream of the Alzheimer's Society, quoted in British Institute for Human Rights (2002) *Something for Everyone: The impact of the Human Rights Act and the need for a Human Rights Commission*, p52

[415] John Ezard *Nursing home patients given tranquilisers needlessly, research shows.* Guardian, 10 February 2003.

[416] *ibid*, note 414, p50.

[417] Department of Health (2003) *National Service Framework for Older People: a report of progress and future challenges*, 2003. www.doh.gov.uk/nsf/olderpeople.htm.

report *Forget Me Not* suggests that mental health services for Older People are "patchy", with a particular problem being gaps in service provision for early intervention and specialist nursing home provision. In particular, the Audit Commission found variations in the levels of dependency of patients with dementia in acute psychiatric beds, suggesting that thresholds for admission (not necessarily under the 1983 Act, but including such admissions) were being influenced by the availability of alternative services. Furthermore, three-fifths of acute psychiatric wards did not consistently offer separate nursing areas for elderly patients with dementia, elderly people with functional illnesses and younger people with functional illnesses[418]. Hospital provision is therefore not always ideally suited to treat older patients with dementia safely, and yet is used in the absence of alternatives. The Department of Health's own progress report also describes progress as "patchy"[419]. Nevertheless the Commission recognises the value of the NSF in raising awareness of the need for holistic services for elderly care, particularly in dementia services, and establishing standards for services.

Deaf Patients

15.12   The Commission raised a number of concerns in relation to deaf patients in our Ninth Biennial Report, including the likelihood that deaf patients are grossly over-represented in the patient population of mental hospitals as a result of poor diagnosis, miscommunication and misguided treatment plans. We also highlighted the limited specialist services available for the care and treatment of deaf patients with severe mental illness. These concerns were brought into focus by the inquiry into the care and treatment of Daniel Joseph, which recommended a nationally co-ordinated strategy for deaf people[420].

15.13   The Commission welcomes the publication of the Department of Health consultation document *A Sign of the Times: Modernising Mental Health Services For People who are Deaf* (2002), which accepts the Daniel Joseph Inquiry's recommendations and sets out proposals for service development[421]. We shall take a great interest in the results of this consultation.

15.14   It is still the case that detained deaf patients are particularly vulnerable to abuses of their ECHR Article 5(2) rights to be informed of the reasons for their deprivation of liberty in a language that they can understand. We continue to call on Government to provide information leaflets on the Act that will be accessible to persons whose first language is British Sign Language [422]. The Commission is reviewing its own information leaflets and will consider the communication needs of deaf patients in that review.

---

418 Audit Commission (2002) *Forget Me Not 2002.* London: Audit Commission Publications, February 2002, p 30.

419 Department of Health (2003) *National Service Framework for Older People: a report of progress and future challenges*, 2003. page 32.

420 *Report of the Independent Inquiry Team into the Care and Treatment of Daniel Joseph* (2000) Commissioned by Merton, Sutton & Wandsworth and Lambeth, Southwark and Lewisham health Authorities. April 2000. Daniel Joseph, who was profoundly deaf, was made subject to a hospital order with restrictions in 1998 having pleaded guilty to manslaughter with diminished responsibility and having another charge of attempted murder left on file.

421 Department of Health (2002) *A Sign of the Times: Modernising Mental Health Services For People who are Deaf.* London, stationery Office www.doh.gov.uk/mentalhealth/signofthetimes.htm

422 Mental Health Act Commission (2001) *Ninth Biennial Report 1999-01*, London: Stationery Office. Chapter 6.48, 6.54 & Recommendation 68

Black and Minority Ethnic Patients

16

16.1 In our Ninth Biennial Report, we wrote in some detail of the specific problems faced by Black and minority ethnic patients. We argued that mental health services as a whole suffered from insufficient understanding of the diverse religious and cultural needs of Black and minority ethnic patients and that this amounted to institutional racism, as defined by the 1999 Macpherson Report into the death of Stephen Lawrence:

> "…the collective failure of an organisation to provide an appropriate and professional service to people because of their colour, culture or ethnic origin".

We argued the need for all aspects of mental healthcare services to be subject to strategic equality programmes aimed at establishing clear policies, procedures and guidelines for service delivery together with robust monitoring, implementation and review procedures. Equality programmes should aim to address the proposals for implementation set out in the Home Office guide to the Race Relations (Amendment) Act 2000[423]. We also suggested outline programme headings, and suggested our own 'regional consultation exercises' as a potential model for services to adopt[424].

16.2 We are very pleased at the appointment of the Commission Chairman, Professor Kamlesh Patel OBE, as the National Institute for Mental Health in England's Acting National Strategic Director charged with implementing the Black and minority ethnic mental health programme. Alongside his work with the Centre for Ethnicity and Health at the University of Central Lancashire, Professor Patel was instrumental in ensuring that the Commission initiated its own ongoing equality programme in 1996.

16.3 The Commission's National Visit of 1999, operated in conjunction with the Centre for Ethnicity and Health and Sainsbury Centre for Mental Health, examined aspects of the care and treatment of detained patients from Black and minority ethnic communities[425]. The visit focussed on issues of ethnic monitoring; racial harassment; staff training in race equality

---

[423] Home Office (2001) *Race Relations (Amendment) Act 2000: New laws for a successful multi-racial Britain: proposals for implementation.* London, Home Office. Chapter 6.

[424] Mental Health Act Commission (2001) *Ninth Biennial Report 1999-01*, London: Stationery Office. Chapter 6.21-32 and Appendix D

[425] The preliminary report on the findings of this visit was published as Sainsbury Centre for Mental Health (2000) *National Visit 2. Improving Care for Detained Patients from Black and Ethnic Minority Communities, Preliminary Report.* London, Sainsbury Centre. The key findings and conclusions from that report are also summarised at Appendix C of the Commission's *Ninth Biennial Report* (2001).

and anti-discriminatory practice; and the use of interpreters. As a result of this work the Department of Health commissioned a report from the University of Central Lancashire Centre for Ethnicity and Health (supported by the Commission) to aid the development of policies in these areas. The report, *Engaging and Changing: Developing effective policy for the care and treatment of Black and minority ethnic detained patients*, published in October 2003[426]. Whilst we refer to and quote from the main recommendations from this publication in the remainder of this chapter, we hope that readers of this report will refer to it directly to ensure that it achieves wide dissemination and influence.

16.4   The Commission was also represented on the external reference group led by Professor Sashidharan, a member of the Mental Health Task Force and Medical Director of North Birmingham NHS Trust, whose report *Inside Outside; Improving Mental Health Services for Black and Minority Ethnic Communities in England*[427] set out proposals for the Department of Health as a result of consultations similar in methodology to the Commission's own 'regional consultation exercises', which we described in depth in our Ninth Biennial Report[428].

16.5   The coming into force of the Race Relations (Amendment) Act 2000 has created specific duties for public authorities to assess all policies and functions, to identify and remedy those which have an adverse effect on different racial groups. Implementation requirements of the 2000 Act include engaging with Black and minority ethnic communities to consult on service delivery. Services should find that the consultative model expounded in *Engaging and Changing*,[429] which builds in part upon the Commission's experience in its consultation exercises, provide a useful template for developing consultation with the scope and breadth of effective community engagement.

16.6   The Commission is pleased to see the spread of policy-level activity and enthusiasm for change in the delivery of a more equitable mental health service to patients from Black and minority ethnic backgrounds. From Government down through all levels of the service we believe that it is now beginning to be accepted that "if discrimination is to be identified and rooted out… there are few quick fixes and only long-term, whole systems approaches are likely to make a difference"[430] as we have held in past Biennial Reports[431]. In this area Government does seem to have now embraced a facilitative and leading role demonstrated by the October 2003 publication of *Delivering Race Equality – A Framework for Action*, a consultation document that has resulted from the Department's Race Relations (Amendment) Act impact assessment on mental health services. The consultation document is supported by a newly established Black and minority ethnic mental health programme within NIMHE, adopting a whole systems approach intended to help services identify problems they are facing in providing equitable services; support services in finding

---

[426]   Department of Health (2003) *Engaging and Changing: Developing effective policy for the care and treatment of Black and minority ethnic detained patients.* London: National Institute for Mental Health in England, UCLAN & MHAC October 2003

[427]   Department of Health (2003) *Inside Outside: Improving Mental Health Services for Black and Minority Ethnic Communities in England.* London. National Institute for Mental Health in England www.nimhe.org.uk

[428]   MHAC (2001) *Ninth Biennial Report 1999-01*, London: Stationery Office. Appendix D.

[429]   Department of Health (2003) *Engaging and Changing: Developing effective policy for the care and treatment of Black and minority ethnic detained patients,* Chapter 10.3.

[430]   Department of Health (2003) *Cases for Change: Introduction p7. National Institute for Mental Health.*

[431]   see, in particular, Mental Health Act Commission (2001) *Ninth Biennial Report 1999-01*, London: Stationery Office. Chapter 6.13.

solutions; and monitor services' progress in delivering those solutions. We hope that the improvements envisaged by this programme to mental health services in general will provide a real benefit to the service experience and outcome for Black and minority ethnic detained patients. We also hope that this will act as a precedent for similar engagement across a number of human rights issues pertaining to detained patients.

The diversity of black and minority ethnic communities

16.7   Underlying the term 'Black and minority ethnic patients' is a complex mosaic of people who categorise themselves in census classifications other than 'White British'. The largest subgroup (in terms of census classification) is the very heterogeneous "Other White" category, which encompasses people of at least three continents. Then, in descending order of numerical size according to the census, there are categories of Indian, Pakistani, Irish, Black Caribbean, Black African, mixed ethnic backgrounds, 'Other Asians', Chinese, 'Other Black' and 'Other Ethnic Group'. These subgroups obviously have a diverse range of religious beliefs, values, histories, cultures and socio-economic experience. In fact, what unites them for our purposes is precisely that they generally fare worse when it comes to access to mental health services, service experience and outcome in comparison with the white majority community.

The inequalities of service provision to Black and minority ethnic patients

16.8   The Commission raised issues of concern in relation to the experience of Black and minority ethnic patients in its First Biennial Report, which covered the years 1983–85. Three specific areas were identified:

(i)   The lack of recognition that the needs of Black and minority ethnic patients may be different to white patients. In particular, the Commission highlighted translation and interpretation issues, domestic issues such as dietary or clothing requirements, religious needs and isolation from other members of Black and minority ethnic communities.

(ii)   There were 'suspicions' in Black and minority ethnic communities that mental health laws may be "operated, at times… against their best interests" and that "cultural features are not always considered when diagnoses of mental illness are made".

(iii)   That originally no Commissioners had been appointed from the Black and minority ethnic communities themselves[432].

Twenty years on, we can report excellent progress in relation to issue (iii) above. Roughly one quarter of all Commissioners now come from Black and minority ethnic communities[433] and we strive continually to ensure that Commissioner membership reaches all sections of the community.

16.9   In relation to the concerns we raised over twenty years ago about mental health services and the operation of the Act, it would appear that there have been few significant overall improvements in Black and minority ethnic patients' experiences of mental health services under the Act. There are, of course, examples of excellent practice in relation to many areas

---

[432] see Mental Health Act Commission (1985) *First Biennial Report 1983-85*, London: Stationery Office, p 54

[433] As of May 2003, Commission membership stood at 176, of whom 22% were Black or from an ethnic minority group.

of mental health care for Black and minority ethnic patients, some of which we describe below. But the following highlighted issues show that there is still a long way to go before equity in service provision is achieved for Black and minority ethnic patients.

The overrepresentation of Black and minority ethnic patients amongst the detained population

16.10   There is continuing evidence of overrepresentation of many Black and minority ethnic groups in the detained patient population. There are, surprisingly, still no officially collated figures on the use of the Act by ethnic category, but the Commission's own figures in relation to the proportion of Black and minority ethnic patients made subject to detention continues to suggest over-representation of many categories (Figure 47). This is consistent with most research findings. A recent systematic review of published research suggested that the statistical odds on a Black and minority ethnic patient being detained under the Act, compared to a similarly unwell white patient, are at least 4:1[434]. Research undertaken for the Department of Health has suggested that Black and minority ethnic patients may be six times more likely to be detained than their white counterparts[435].

16.11   Statistics collated by the Commission using the census categories from 2001 are shown separately at Figure 48 below. Commission data is collated from voluntary returns provided to every hospital that we visit, but it remains substantially incomplete. Our ability to improve upon this is severely constrained by the resources available to us, but the Commission is currently planning a major census of Black and minority ethnic patients in 2004, in conjunction with NIMHE, so as to obtain once and for all a firm baseline of information and to encourage the establishment of robust ethnic record keeping and the production of key performance indicators for future monitoring purposes.

> **Recommendation 61:** Given the importance placed upon ethnic monitoring in health services, we hope that statistics on the use of the Mental Health Act by ethnic category will be collated in future by the Department of Health through existing arrangements to collate such data by gender, legal category etc, so that the expertise and resources of Departmental statisticians can be applied to this important task.

16.12   In a study published in 2001[436], the Social Services Inspectorate found that the percentage of people from Black and minority ethnic groups who were assessed for possible detention was generally disproportionate to the local estimates of local populations (Figure 49). These findings are supported by data from the University of Manchester Mental Health Social Work Research Unit, which is discussed at Chapter 8.70 *et seq* above. The SSI study found that detention rates from such assessments were similar for both White and Black and minority ethnic groups (63% and 69% respectively).

---

[434] Bhui, K; Stansfield, S; Hull, S, Priebe, S, Mole, F & Feder, G (2003) *Ethnic variations in pathways to and use of specialist mental health service in the UK; systematic review.* British Journal of Psychiatry 182:105-116

[435] Audinin, B & Leliott, P (2002) *Age, gender and ethnicity of those detained under Part II of the Mental Health Act 1983.* British Journal of Psychiatry 180:222-26.

[436] Social Services Inspectorate (2001) *Detained – inspection of compulsory mental health admissions.* February 2001.

Ethnic Group	Mental Health Act Admissions				
	1996/7 (n=29,426)[1] %	1997/8 (n=33,552)[2] %	1998/9 (n= 35,097)[3] %	1999/0 (n= 40,024)[4] %	2000/01 (n= 23,793)[5] %
White	84.0	83.3	85.0	88.2	87.7
Black Caribbean	5.4	6.2	5.2	3.6	3.1
Black African	2.7	2.5	2.4	1.7	1.4
Black other	1.8	2.0	1.5	1.1	0.9
Indian	1.7	1.6	1.4	1.5	1.4
Pakistani	1.3	1.0	1.4	1.2	1.3
Bangladeshi	0.4	0.6	0.4	0.4	0.3
Chinese	0.3	0.3	0.3	0.2	0.3
Other groups	2.4	2.5	2.4	2.1	3.6

1 ethnicity not known (1996/7) = 2,102 – not included in table
2 ethnicity not known (1997/8) = 1,505 – not included in table
3 ethnicity not known (1998/9) = 1,204 – not included in table
4 ethnicity not known (1999/0) = 5,029 - not included in table
5 ethnicity not known (2000/1) = 811 not included in table
(n.b. underreporting and ethnicity unknowns may have distorted residual analysis. See 16.11 for discussion)

Fig 47 : Mental Health Act admissions by ethnicity in England & Wales 1996-2001

Mental Health Act Admissions 2001-2002, % by ethnic category

Ethnic category	%	Ethnic category	%
British	84.4	Black African	1.1
Irish	0.5	Black Caribbean	2.5
Other White background	3.2	Other Black background	0.8
White & Black Caribbean	1.5	Indian	2.3
White & Black African	0.7	Pakistani	1.3
White & Asian	0.1	Bangladeshi	0.3
Other Mixed background	0.2	Other Asian background	0.5
Chinese	0.2	Other Ethnic background	0.9

Fig 48: Mental Health Act Admissions by ethnic categories, England & Wales, 1/4/01 – 31/3/02

Data collected by MHAC, n = 23,090

Percentage of minority ethnic groups in population and amongst those assessed under the MHA 1983

Local Council	% minority ethnic population local analysis	% minority ethnic MHA assessments n=998
Barking & Dagenham	7	17
Bolton	8	11
Cambridgeshire	5	7
Derby	10	16
Hackney	33	47
Nottingham	11	26
Rochdale	7	16
Southwark	18	38
Walsall	10	14
Warwickshire	3	3

Fig 49: Percentage of minority ethnic groups in population and amongst those assessed under the Mental Health Act 1983, 2001

Source: Social Services Inspectorate (2001) Detained – inspection of compulsory mental health admissions, table 1

16.13 We cannot be sure of the causes of this overrepresentation, and they are likely to be complex and varied. It is generally recognised that Black and minority ethnic communities tend to be concentrated in inner city areas characterised by social deprivation, including poverty, educational disadvantage and discrimination in the labour force. Black and minority ethnic communities may also show particular age, gender and marital status profiles in comparison to other groups, all of which may be factors in admission rates that confound straight comparisons of one ethnic group against another. However, even studies that adjust for these factors still report excess compulsory admissions among Black and minority ethnic patients[437]. It seems likely that amongst the causes of the overrepresentation of Black people in compulsory psychiatric care we should look at diagnostic and risk-assessment practice; patients' experience of inpatient care and how this effects the health outcome of admission; access to community-based services and attitudes towards seeking help at the early onset of illness.

16.14 Research by the Sainsbury Centre for Mental Health has suggested that many people with mental health problems from the Black African and Black Caribbean communities may be caught in a cycle of fear and prejudice. Negative experiences or perceptions of mainstream mental health services may dissuade people from accessing services until crisis point, at which point they face a number of additional risks, such as over and misdiagnosis, police intervention and the use of the Mental Health Act. These adverse pathways into care influence the nature and outcome of treatment and thus perpetuate the unwillingness of Black communities to engage with services at an earlier stage. The University of Central Lancashire's Centre for Ethnicity and Health has identified a similar pattern of accessing services only at times of fundamental breakdown or crisis amongst South Asian communities, although this is caused not so much by distrust of services as by lack of knowledge of them, and stigma of seeking help, with networks of family, friends or specialist South Asian Community-based staff taking on roles provided to other communities by primary care services[438]. Such reluctance to seek help early in the onset of mental health problems, and the concomitant experience of mental health services only at times of extreme crisis, may be one causative factor behind the high suicide rate amongst women from South Asian communities (and also amongst the Irish community in general).

16.15 The *Inside Outside* report has suggested national standards that:

* all services have access to crisis teams and 'crisis residential alternatives' to hospital; all patients on the enhanced Care Programme Approach have a crisis plan that specifically addresses how to minimise coercion; and that the pathways to care and the use of Mental Health Act in relation to ethnicity could then be audited, with an expectation of year-on-year reductions in variations by ethnicity.

* All assessments (including Mental Health Act assessments) should be carried out with the individual, carer or family members and if necessary with interpreter, translator or advocate support. Assessments should aim to establish a care plan that is mindful of individual religious, cultural and spiritual beliefs, and has a clear identification of recovery and outcome, so that Black experience of mental health services becomes less negative[439].

Such standards could prove challenging to practitioners using the Mental Health Act 1983 with current resources. We hope nevertheless that government will give consideration to these and other suggestions made by in the *Inside Outside* report.

---

[437] Bhui *et al* (2003) [see note 434 above] p113

[438] see, for example, Department of Health (2003) *Engaging and Changing: Developing effective policy for the care and treatment of Black and minority ethnic detained patients*, section 3.2

[439] Department of Health (2003) *Inside Outside: Improving Mental Health Services for Black and Minority Ethnic Communities in England.* NIMHE p26 - 27.

Ethnic monitoring

16.16   Ethnic monitoring has been mandatory for in-patient services since 1995, and yet many such services are still struggling to record and monitor patients' ethnicity. In many instances, staff appear to lack confidence to ask about a patient's ethnicity; in others they did not see the need. Monitoring may be seen as bureaucratic, intrusive and meaningless for staff who have not received adequate training in its purpose, or adequate training in cultural awareness, or who can see little use being made of the data collected in terms of service improvements. Yet effective ethnic monitoring can have a real impact on service development and the delivery of comprehensive, holistic care programmes[440]. We believe that the Department of Health could encourage better ethnic monitoring by collating national returns relating to the Mental Health Act and publishing the results alongside its existing statistical bulletins (see 16.10-1 and recommendation 61 above). In this way Government could ensure that services develop monitoring systems that can report at a national level and that data used to identify regional or national trends is accurate.

16.17   The Commission commends the *Engaging and Changing* recommendations for services on ethnic monitoring to all service managers. We summarise these recommendations at Figure 50 below.

Summary of *Engaging and Changing* recommendations to services relating to ethnic monitoring

∗   Board-level commitment to ethnic monitoring needs to be established, emphasising the importance of the work and committing to use systems that harmonise across services.

∗   Patients should self-assign their ethnicity using 2001 census categories (following CRE guidance on supplementary categories to take account of local need).

∗   Patients should receive information in accessible format on ethnic monitoring, explaining its purpose and assuring of confidentiality.

∗   Recording ethnicity should be an integral part of the admission procedure, with clear guidelines available to staff about how to request such information and what to do when it is not immediately forthcoming.

∗   Staff recording, analysing or monitoring ethnic data should be trained to do so.

∗   Secondary questions should be asked around language, dialect, religion, familial origins, diet etc.

∗   Information should be held at ward level, where it should be used to inform individual patients' care plans; and should be fed into a Trust / service wide system, where it should be used to monitor
   • the use of the Act;   • treatment regimes;
   • complaints;   • use of therapies and activities;
   • violent incidents;   • harassment incidents;
   • self-harm;   • deaths;
   • seclusion;   • control and restraint;
   • meetings with Commissioners on MHAC visits;   • MHRT outcomes; and
                                                         • requests for SOADs.

∗   Collected data should be analysed, disseminated and used to take positive action to reduce service inequalities.

Fig 50: Summary of *Engaging and Changing* recommendations to services relating to ethnic monitoring

---

[440]   see, for example, Department of Health (2003) *Engaging and Changing: Developing effective policy for the care and treatment of Black and minority ethnic detained patients.*

Racial harassment

16.18   A lack of racial harassment policies outlining how to deal with harassment between patients, as well as between staff and patients, continues to be a problem. The death of David Bennett starkly illustrates the need for effective policies in this area. David Bennett died in a medium secure unit having been restrained for 25 minutes, following an incident sparked by racial abuse directed at him. The coroner recognised that the lack of a racial harassment policy and procedure in the unit was a contributory factor in the events that led to his death[441]. Government has recognised generally that insufficient attention has been paid to ethnicity and gender and protection from abuse/harassment in acute mental health care[442] and has made it a minimum standard for Psychiatric Intensive Care Units and low secure units to operate "a clear policy on equal ops and racial harassment which all staff and patients are aware of…covering staff/patient and patient/patient harassment…signed up to by Trust Board & with monitoring of adherence"[443].

> **Recommendation 62:** The Commission recommends that services enhance minimum standards set by Department of Health guidance by adopting the recommendation from *Engaging and Changing* that, alongside an establishment's anti-bullying or general harassment policies, which should include racial harassment in their scope,
>
> > "…in a mental health setting, a separate section or stand alone policy aimed at protecting patients from racial harassment by other patients, by visitors or by staff should be established to acknowledge the special need for protection of these patients. A clear definition of racial harassment should appear on the policy, encompassing the continuum of behaviours… including forms of subtle racism…"
>
> Department of Health (2003) *Engaging and Changing: Developing effective policy for the care and treatment of Black and minority ethnic detained patients*, p5

Interpreting services

16.19   Patient records examined on the National Visit 2 showed that one in five patients from Black and minority ethnic communities did not have English as their first language. Even though a number of these patients may speak English, at times of stress or distress patients' abilities to understand or communicate in that language may be reduced and interpreting provision should be made. Interpreting the communications of patients with mental health problems, especially at times of crisis, is a skilled job and should not be undertaken by interpreters with no training in mental health issues. This will be particularly important in the establishment of specialist advocacy services (see Chapter 9.10 *et seq* above).

---

[441] Mental Health Act Commission (2001) *Ninth Biennial Report 1999-01*, London: Stationery Office. Chapter 6.26. At the time of writing the independent inquiry into Mr Bennett's death is preparing its report. The MHAC gave evidence to that enquiry, thus retaining its involvement and close interest in the case. See also Chapters 10.31 & 11.29-30 above.

[442] Department of Health (2002) *Mental Health Policy Implementation Guide: Adult Acute Inpatient Care Provision*

[443] Department of Health (2002) *Mental Health Policy Implementation Guide: National Minimum Standards for General Adult Services in Psychiatric Intensive Care Units (PICU) and Low Secure Units.* Para 9.2.1.

We summarise the recommendations of *Engaging and Changing* relating to interpreters at Figure 51 below.

16.21　Staff training on race equality issues, anti-discriminatory practice and the delivery of a culturally sensitive service is seen by many services as an 'extra' rather than a part of mainstream service delivery. This can particularly be a problem where there are small Black and minority ethnic communities, leading to a vicious circle of poor service delivery and poor awareness of how to make improvements.

Summary of *Engaging and Changing* recommendations to services relating to the use of interpreters

✳ Service policies should contain a clear statement of the duty and commitment to provide interpreting services in accordance with NSF and Mental Health Act Code of Practice requirements. Standards should be established for the use of interpreters on admission; at assessments during the formation of care plans; at significant clinical meetings; and when new interventions are introduced.

✳ Children under the age of 16 should never act as interpreters. Other family members, acquaintances and untrained staff should not act as interpreters for significant clinical events. In an emergency untrained interpreters should only be used to communicate the minimum information necessary until a trained interpreter can be found. Telephone interpreters should only be used in an emergency.

✳ Day-to-day communication needs may be met in part by befriending and advocacy organisations, and service engagement with such organisations in the community should be encouraged at policy level. Where bilingual staff are used as interpreters in any capacity, their training needs should be considered and care should be taken that the role does not compromise their professional engagement with the patient or role within the service

✳ Services should work in partnership and pool interpreters. The use of interpreters should be recorded, monitored and evaluated for quality and accessibility.

Fig 51: Summary of *Engaging and Changing* recommendations to services relating to the use of interpreters

16.22　*Engaging and Changing* includes detailed recommendations on training policies and practice which service managers should take up. The report recommends that:

✳ training should be practice-based and mandatory for all staff, regardless of their patient contact, provided at induction and as a part on an on-going programme of refresher courses;

✳ training may be supplemented with information packs to guide staff on elements relating to culture, faith and ethnicity. Such information must, however, not take the place of asking the patient and carers about the patients' preferences.

Providing culturally sensitive care

16.23　The above measures should establish the ground for the provision of services that are sensitive and appropriate to the cultural and religious requirements of diverse communities. Links into the community and meaningful consultation with Black and ethnic minority groups are central to developing such services, as service changes must be responsive to issues raised in such consultative processes. The *Engaging and Changing* report specifies some aspects of religious and cultural sensitivity in service provision that are not mentioned above, but which have been raised in past Biennial Reports of the Commission, such as:

* Ensuring that patients have access to worship space, faith leaders and religious/faith groups, and that staff are informed of and sensitive to religiously / culturally significant dates.

    The Commission was impressed by arrangements made at Rampton Hospital to inform staff and patients of the significance and observances of Ramadan. The hospital's information sheet included times of sunrise and sunset.

* Ensuring that culturally appropriate food is made available to patients.

    The *Engaging and Changing* report outlines an initiative undertaken by South London and Maudsley NHS Trust, which established a 'food group' to establish dietary needs and preferences of patients, including those from less well-established ethnic groups. Central to the exercise was the use of a food workbook through which patients could express concerns, ideas and solutions to catering issues.

* Ensuring that personal care requirements (such as hair or skincare products) are made available to patients.

    The *Engaging and Changing* report shows, for example, that some services are engaging specialist hairdressing services for their Black patients.

* Ensuring that patients can access culturally appropriate opportunities and materials for leisure and education.

    Engaging and Changing highlights that Ashworth Hospital has established a cultural forum to provide an opportunity for Black and minority ethnic patients to meet one another; access particular newspapers, magazines, films, food and music; and discuss and address issues relating to cultural needs.

16.24 Whilst we continue to look to services to engage with issues of anti-discriminatory practice and race equality on a holistic, service-wide level and not as a series of piecemeal and unconnected initiatives, the above examples may give an idea of how relatively modest initiatives can make a significant difference to Black and minority ethnic patients' care.

17

Children and Young People subject to the Mental Health Act

Admission of Children & Adolescents under the 1983 Act to adult facilities

17.1 The Commission's last three Biennial Reports have highlighted our concerns over the treatment of children and young people under mental health legislation[444]. In our Ninth Biennial Report (2001), we presented data to show that of 1,082 children and young people admitted to hospital under the Act during 1999-2001, 378 young men or boys and 246 young women or girls were admitted to adult wards. This represents 62% of total admissions under the Act for children and young people. It is clear that the Code of Practice guidance at Chapter 31.22, which states that placement of detained children and minors in adult environments should be 'exceptional', is not being met across mental health services.

17.2 Figure 52 below shows the number of children and adolescent admissions to adult facilities that we were informed of over this reporting period. The data prior to November 2002, when we introduced a standard form for services to return within 24 hours of admitting a detained child or adolescent to adult facilities, is likely to show considerable under-reporting, so the figures below do not necessarily show an increase in these inappropriate placements. The Commission introduced standardised reporting procedures in 2002/02, although there are still some problems in our data collection and retrieval regarding the identification of patient gender. Despite this we present the available data to give as accurate a picture of child and adolescent admission to adult facilities as is available at the present time (Figure 52).

	Children			Adolescents			Total
	Male	Female	N/S	Male	Female	N/S	
2001/02	5	8	12	32	24	57	138
2002/03	19	19	21	79	55	20	213

Fig 52: Children and adolescents admitted to adult wards, England and Wales 2001/02 & 2002/03

data source: MHAC

---

[444] see Mental Health Act Commission (1997) *Seventh Biennial Report 1995-7*, Chapter 10.9; MHAC (1999) *Eighth Biennial Report 1997-9*, Chapter 10.74-80; MHAC (2001) *Ninth Biennial Report 1999-2001*, Chapter 6.40-7. London, Stationery Office

Recommendation 63: Authorities should be placed under a mandatory requirement to inform a body such as the Mental Health Act Commission of the admission of children or adolescents to adult mental health facilities. Government might consider establishing such a requirement as part of a wider reporting duty for authorities that could encompass Mental Health Act, Children Act and informal admissions of children and adolescents to all types of mental health facility. Such a requirement could facilitate planning across authority boundaries based upon adequate knowledge.

17.3   The level of admissions of children and adolescents to adult facilities shown at Figure 52 above is despite the welcome strategies and guidance from Government, stemming from its 1997 response to the Health Committee on Services for Children and Young People[445], and 1998 commitment to improve the provision of appropriate, high-quality care and treatment for children and adolescents through building up locally based Child and Adolescent Mental Health Services (CAMHS)[446]. The latter included the aim that users of CAMHS services should be able to expect in-patient care in a specialist setting, appropriate to their age and clinical need. If, as in the Welsh Assembly Government's 2002 Policy Implementation Guidance, we should "take the term CAMHS to mean all services that impinge on the mental well-being, mental health problems and mental disorders of children or young people before their majority"[447], this aim is not being met. It is therefore of some concern that documentation relating to the National Service Framework for Children does not recognise this problem explicitly, and indeed suggests, erroneously in our experience, that the burden of care for children and adolescents undergoing acute psychiatric crisis normally rests with children's wards whilst appropriate arrangements are made[448].

17.4   During 2002/03 the Commission aimed to visit any minor admitted under the 1983 Act within two or three days of that admission. During the year the Commission was notified of 213 such admissions and undertook 166 visits. Although at first sight the number of admissions may seem high, the Commission's continued interest in these very vulnerable young people appears to be stimulating much earlier responses from mental health service providers, social services and commissioning agencies. It is becoming clear to everyone that this type of admission is inappropriate and every effort is made locally to get the minor moved to a more appropriate facility as soon as possible. The discrepancy in notifications and patients visited on adult wards is largely due to patients being transferred to more suitable facilities before such a visit could be arranged.

---

[445] Department of Health (1997) *Government Response to the Report of the Health Committee on Services for Children and Young People, Session 1996-97.* London, HMSO. See MHAC (1999) *Eighth Biennial Report,* para 10.74.

[446] Department of Health (1998) *Modernising Mental Health Services: National Priorities Guidance 1999/00 - 2001/02.* LAC(98)22.

[447] Welsh Assembly Government (2002) *Mental Health Policy Implementation Guidance for Child and Adolescent Mental Health Services : Commissioning the NHS-funded Component of Child and Adolescent Mental Health Services.* Cardiff, Welsh Assembly Government. para 1.5. CAMHS issues specific to Wales are discussed at Chapter 18.14 below.

[448] Department of Health (2003) *Getting the Right Start: National Service Framework for Children. Standard for Hospital Services.* London, Department of Health www.doh.gov.uk/nsf/children/gettingtherightstart para 4.27

17.5 Commissioners visiting minors detained in adult facilities are specifically chosen and trained for the task, and only visit singly if they have passed police vetting procedures. Commissioners check the patient's situation against guidance from the Code of Practice and find out whether the patient has their own room, whether they feel safe, have any concerns or require anything. We can also find out how long patients stay in hospital and in detention. After interviewing the patient in private, the Commissioners complete summaries of their visit, which will form the basis of for analysis and a short report to be prepared over the Winter period 2003/04 (see also Figure 54 below).

17.6 Because of the lack of available data, it is not possible to say whether the majority of minors admitted to adult wards are detained under the Mental Health Act or subject to other powers[449]. We are grateful to West London Mental Health NHS Trust for providing us with the breakdown of their admission figures for 2002/03 shown at Figure 53 below, which suggests that formal compulsion under mental health legislation is not necessarily the most prevalent route for the admission of minors. Because even the capable refusal of consent to admission or treatment by this group of patients may be overridden by parents or persons with parental responsibility, this also suggests that the compulsion of minors in hospital may, in fact, take many forms other than those provided by the 1983 Act. As this is the case, monitoring which has a focus only on the formally detained may be inappropriate with this group of patients.

17.7 The figures at Figure 53 above may not be typical, especially in that there is no recorded use of the Children Act over the year. We believe that all hospitals should be collecting this kind of data and that a central body should receive and collate it. In Chapter 20.26(c) below we suggest that a future monitoring body that succeeds from the Commission should receive routine notification of the use of powers of compulsion.

17.8 The National Service Framework for Children requires hospitals receiving and treating minors to have policies, liaison arrangements and protocols in place to ensure collaborative working methods within specialist areas of services and across different services[450]. In addition, the Climbié Inquiry[451] has highlighted, among other things, the need for careful documentation of observations and information sharing between professionals working in different organisations. We urge agencies responsible for children to review their policies and procedures for sharing information to ensure that these meet with Climbié Inquiry recommendations.

---

[449] see Mears, White, Banarjee, Worral, O'Herlihy, Jaffa. Hill, Brook & Leliott (2001) *An Evaluation of the use of the Children Act 1989 and the Mental Health Act 1983 in Children and Adolescents in Psychiatric Settings (CAMHA-CAPS)*. London, Royal College of Psychiatrists' Research Unit, for uses in CAMHS settings. The Commission is unaware of any similar-scale research study of admissions of minors to adult wards. Mears *et al* suggest that the Children Act is not much used for detention for mental health problems.

[450] Department of Health (2003) *Getting the Right Start: National Service Framework for Children. Standard for Hospital Services*, para 4.27, *Emerging Findings*, paras 7.7 - 7.8.

[451] Dept of Health & Home Office (2003) the *Victoria Climbié Inquiry: report of an inquiry by Lord Laming*. London, Stationery Office www.victoria-climbie-inquiry.org.uk. This report went to press in the week before the release of the Children's Green Paper. The Commission notes the intention to introduce a Children's Commissioner and ensure joined-up services, to build upon the echoes of Lord Laming's recommendations in the Children's NSF *Emerging Findings* (para 7.8). See also Department of Health (2003) *Safeguarding Children. What to do if you're worried a child is being abused. Children's services guidance.* May 2003. www.doh.gov.uk/safeguardingchildren

Minors admitted to adult wards 01/04/02 – 31/03/03, all legal categories, West London Mental Health NHS Trust (Ealing/Hammersmith & Fulham/Hounslow)				
Gender	Age on admission	Duration of admission (number of nights)	Legal status on admission	Change in legal status
M	16	1	s2	to informal
M	17	3	informal	-
M	17	13	s2	to informal
M	16	93	s2	to s3
F	17	48	informal	to s2 to s3 upon transfer
F	17	1	informal	-
F	16	3	informal	-
M	15	10	informal	-
M	17	11	s2	informal
F	17	22	informal	-
F	17	8	informal	-
M	16	120	s2	informal
M	17	269	informal	-
M	16	32	s2	informal
M	17	51	informal	-
F	17	74	informal	-
M	17	6	informal	s5(2) to informal
M	17	16	s2	informal
M	17	33	informal	s5(2) to s(2) to informal

Fig 53: Minors admitted to adult wards 01/04/02 – 31/03/03, West London Mental Health NHS Trust [452]

Recommendation 64: We hope, in due course, that Government will issue advice for authorities on requirements in relation to information sharing which takes account of the Climbié Inquiry recommendations and helps services fit them within the existing context of the demands and exclusions of the Data Protection Act and requirements of the Children Act.

17.9   We are pleased that Government has acknowledged the need for the development of protocols and liaison arrangements, having called in our Ninth Biennial Report (2001) for:

∗ all mental health services providing care to children and adolescents detained under the Act to have agreed working and referral arrangements with appropriate medical and psychiatric expertise in CAMHS (Ninth Biennial Report, recommendation 64)

∗ the Department of Health to consider the need for England to have standards and protocols for the care of mentally ill minors detained in adult units, as already exists in Wales (recommendation 66)

∗ all NSF local implementation strategies should identify the mental health care needs of children and adolescents and plan appropriate provision to meet those needs (recommendation 65)

∗ We hope that in the development of the Childrens' NSF, the Department of Health will also consider formats for its information leaflets on the Mental Health Act that will be accessible to children (recommendation 67).

---

[452] Data supplied courtesy of Kevin Towers, West London Mental Health NHS Trust.

17.10 In voluntary self-assessment returns reporting progress against the recommendations of the Ninth Biennial Report, even amongst the 72 hospitals that chose to submit assessments (representing approximately a quarter of all detaining hospital in England and Wales), only 32 (44%) could claim to have adequately implemented policies in relation to the admission of children and adolescents.

17.11 Figure 54 below shows data available for analysis collected from 56 visits to hospitals that had detained a minor on an adult ward during 2002/03. Considered alongside the self-assessment returns outlined in 17.10 above, these indicate that there may be a considerable way to go to provide adequate services to minors placed in adult facilities.

Findings from 56 Commission visits to adult wards following admission of a minor					
Question	Yes		No		N/S
Is there a hospital policy relating to the admission of minors ?	14	25%	32	57%	10
Are all staff who come into contact with the patient positively police vetted, including bank and agency staff ?	36	64%	14	25%	6
Are staff who deliver care to the patient specifically trained to do so, including bank and agency staff ?	3	5%	45	80%	8
Do staff have access to a child and adolescent psychiatrist ?	35	63%	9	16%	12
Have staffing levels been increased as a result of the admission of the patient	11	20%	34	61%	11
Was the admission... planned ?	10	18%	27	48%	19
An emergency ?	48	86%	1	2%	7
Are there plans to transfer the patient ?	23	41%	24	43%	9
Are appropriate plans in place for continuance with education ?	6	11%	30	54%	20
Is there a planned programme of activities relevant to ability/age ?	17	30%	29	52%	10
Is there an advocacy service available to the patient ?	36	64%	16	29%	4
...and are advocates specifically trained in dealing with minors ?	22	39%	23	41%	11
Does the patient have his/her own room ?	48	86%	6	11%	2
Does the unit have seclusion facilities	29	52%	21	38%	6
...if so, has the patient been secluded since admission ?	6	11%	23	-	-

Fig 54: Commission findings relating to 56 visits following admissions of minors to adult wards, 2002/03[453]

17.12 The Commission's particular concerns stemming from this exercise are that:

∗ In a quarter of adult wards detaining minors, *all* staff members involved in the care of minors, or who come into contact with such patients, had not been subject to appropriate police-checks. We recognise that delays in processing such checks that are beyond hospital managers' control may have contributed to this shortfall, but particular care needs to be taken to protect this very vulnerable group of patients.

∗ We have serious concerns for the safety and security of the one in ten minors who were not provided with their own room when housed on adult wards.

---

[455] Data source: CVQ returns from 2002/03 available from the MHAC database. See Chapter 19.11(c) for a description of the CVQ exercise

* Staff assigned to care for minors on adult wards rarely had any specific training to do so. Commissioners recorded that staff had no training in CAMHS in 80% of wards visited. Only two-thirds of wards visited even had *access* to a CAMHS psychiatrist. Although the Commission does not wish to condone the administration of medication to minors by practitioners who are not qualified to make safe and professional judgments on appropriate interventions, these facts suggest that widely-available guidelines should be produced on the use of medication and other treatments for young people with mental health problems. Such guidelines, which should perhaps be prepared by NICE, should certainly address the issue of rapid tranquilisation and in-patient services[454].

* In a fifth of wards visited staffing levels had been increased to meet the extra demands of caring for a minor. On the other wards, these extra demands would have been likely to have a detrimental effect on other patients' care, which is not only unfair to other patients, but could also foster resentment against the minor and increase his or her sense of isolation.

* Only 11% of wards visited had managed to make arrangements for educational needs for the minor. Further research is needed on the implications of this figure, taking account of the level of mental disturbance and the relatively short duration of stay of many of the patients concerned. However, that Commissioners did not positively identify a planned programme of ward activities appropriate to a minor on 70% of wards is a definite matter for concern that is less easily mitigated.

* One fifth of minors who were detained on wards with seclusion facilities have been secluded during their detention. Whilst minors who are admitted to adult wards may be very disturbed and difficult to manage, we suspect that the less than ideal circumstances under which they are cared for cannot but be a contributory factor in problem behaviour[455].

17.13 The Commission's concerns about the inappropriate care received by many children and adolescent patients on adult wards were highlighted by two cases that occurred in separate London hospitals just before this report went to press:

* a 16 year old patient nursed on an acute adult ward was offered illicit drugs for sale under threat by adult patients on the ward. It is understood that it is common on this ward for patients to be threatened if they do not buy illicit drugs when offered by other patients.

* a 17 year old patient with learning disability who was undergoing an acute psychotic episode was physically attacked on an adult ward by another patient. He required medical attention.

Both of these patients were on high-level observations at the time of the incidents.

17.14 It must be emphasised that on their visits to children, Commissioners meet with many dedicated and caring staff who share the Commission's concerns over the circumstances in which they have to provide care to children and minors. We also find some examples of exemplary practice, where good liaison arrangements with CAMHS services have been established; staff are empowered by training and adequate support; and thought has been given to the special requirements of this particular patient group and their families.

---

[454] Mears, White, Banarjee, Worral, O'Herlihy, Jaffa. Hill, Brook & Leliott (2001) *An Evaluation of the use of the Children Act 1989 and the Mental Health Act 1983 in Children and Adolescents in Psychiatric Settings (CAMHA-CAPS)*. London, Royal College of Psychiatrists' Research Unit. This recommendation is made at para 1.4.7.

[455] see *Mental Health Act Code of Practice*, Chapter 19.5.

17.15 The Commission therefore looks forward to the development of better services for children and adolescents under the policy lead of Government and with continuing facilitation through Strategic Health Authorities. As particular facilities are identified and developed to be links to specialist CAMHS services there is no reason why emerging good practice cannot spread.

Good practice example
Arrangements for minors on an adult ward in Herts

Commissioners visited a detained minor on St Julians' ward, St Albans City Hospital, (Hertfordshire Partnerships NHS Trust), in June 2003. This is an adult ward designated to admit minors. There were 24 patients on the ward on the day of the visit (eight of whom were detained under the Mental Health Act). The patient was being nursed in a single room with en- suite facilities and had access to all areas of the ward. The ward is spacious with facilities for some indoor games, access to fresh air and no seclusion facilities.

The following is a summary of the findings on that visit:

∗ There were procedures and operational guidelines in place for staff who have to care for minors on the adult ward.

∗ All the staff on the ward were positively police vetted. Arrangements were in progress for enhanced Criminal Record Bureau checks for all staff who have worked on the ward.

∗ Two nurses were designated to key work any minor admitted to the ward: a senior nurse (F Grade) who is specifically trained to deliver care to minors, and an E Grade staff nurse who had recently been seconded to the Child and Adolescent Mental Health Services (CAMHS) to undergo training in the care of minors.

∗ Ward staff have access to Child and Adolescent Psychiatrist and also a Community Psychiatric Nurse from CAMHS.

∗ The daily nursing and medical records indicated that the patient was being provided with a good standard of care. There was evidence of agreed care plans being implemented and reviewed.

∗ An outreach Occupational Therapist from the CAMHS had visited the ward to discuss programmes of activity for the minor detained and structured activity had been planned and implemented.

∗ The records indicated that the patient had had his rights explained to him. The patient confirmed at the private meeting that he understood what was explained to him. The records also indicated that the patient's mother has been informed of the patient's rights in accordance with Section 132 of the Act.

∗ The patient's mother had been allowed to stay on the ward for most of the time, including being able to sleep over at night.

∗ An advocate from the Power Advocacy Services had been provided to the patient

∗ The patient confirmed to the visiting Commissioner that he was happy with his care on the ward.

The Commission commended the standard of care provided to the patient.

Contact: Tina Kavanagh, MHA Manager, St Albans City Hospital, Waverly Road, St Albans, Herts AL3 5PN

Good Practice Example
Child & adolescent services in Warrington

A Community Health Homes Team established around the Five Boroughs Partnership NHS Trust and other agencies provides a range of services to persons aged between 11 and 17, covering mental health needs, developmental disorders, learning disabilities and the legacy of life events such as parental separation and divorce, moving house, bereavement, violence, etc.

The multidisciplinary health team includes speech and language therapist, who also co-ordinates the project, a music therapist, an art therapist, two RMNs, a child and adolescent psychiatrist, a team secretary and will include a clinical psychologist.

The cluster of secure and open facilities run by social services and a charity provide:

Briars Hey, Rainhill	8 secure beds for young women
Gladstone House, Liverpool	18 secure beds
Red Bank, Newton-le-Willows	28 secure beds and 10 open places
St Catherine's, Blackbrook	12 secure beds and 5 open

The Nugent Care Society also runs a residential school for those not convicted of an offence.

The young men and women arrive through secure remand, detention and training orders, or welfare routes. The Team receives approximately six new admissions each week, and offers assessment, intervention and then transfer.

This approach does not distinguish between the different difficulties that face young people – whether these are behavioural, mental health, or developmental. The service is geared towards the needs of young people, rather than being set up on the basis of an 'adult service' that has been transposed onto a group of younger people. The approach could have wider application, and when the service is running at full strength it is proposed to apply for NHS Beacon status, carry out a full evaluation and disseminate information about their service nationally.

Contact: Judy Debenham, Community Health Homes Team, Five Boroughs Partnership NHS Trust, Hollins Park House, Hollins Park, Hollins Lane, Warrington, WA2 8WA. Tel: 01925 664000

Children and adolescent patients under proposed Mental Health legislation

17.16   The consultation on the draft Mental Health Bill of 2002 invited views on proposals to provide young people with a greater say in consenting to hospital admission and treatment. The Commission's response concluded that:

∗   The Commission supports the proposal that parents should have authority for decision-making for no more than twenty-eight days before the Mental Health Tribunal is involved.

* The safeguards proposed for mentally incapacitated but compliant patients should extend to children, rather than exclude them as the draft Bill suggested.

* Whilst 16-17 year olds may be treated as adults in law, they should not necessarily be excluded from CAMHS.

* The passing of new legislation is an opportunity to improve service provisions and procedures for children and young people by, for instance:

  - ensuring that all children and young people have a thorough initial mental health assessment that does not automatically rely on hearsay or previous assessments;

  - providing a statutory duty on authorities to provide age-appropriate patient information and advocacy to children and young people;

  - ensuring that specific monitoring duties are created in relation to children and young people with serious mental disorders, whether in CAMHS or adult facilities, with a specific focus of aspects of compulsion. Such a duty might fall to the body responsible for monitoring the use of compulsion, perhaps with a duty to report to the Children's Rights Director created under the Health and Social Care Bill. Monitoring should extend beyond simple admission data of both formal and informal young patients, to encompass access to specialist services, quality standards etc.

Future monitoring arrangements for child and adolescent care under compulsion

17.17 Future monitoring proposals for health care are set out in the Health and Social Care (Community Health and Standards) Bill 2003. The Commission for Healthcare Audit and Inspection (CHAI) will cover both NHS and independent providers while the Commission for Social Care Inspection (CSCI) will cover social care and the welfare of children. We welcome the inclusion of a Children's Rights Director in the latter body.

17.18 Our general concerns over proposals to charge the newly created, generic inspectorates with monitoring the use of compulsion are discussed at Chapter 20 below. These general concerns do, of course, extend to the use of compulsion in the mental healthcare of children and adolescents. But we also recognise (and discuss at 17.6 above) that the compulsion of minors can take much wider and less precise forms than is the case with adults. Therefore, while we maintain that specialist monitoring of the use of mental health legislation as a framework for the care and treatment of minors will continue to be a pressing need under new legislation, we acknowledge that a broader focussed monitoring is also required to ensure the protection of child and adolescent patients and the appropriate use of services.

Recommendation 65: The Commission urges Government to give careful consideration to providing specific and complementary duties to CHAI, CSCI, and the Children's Rights Director in respect of children with serious mental disorders.

Part 5

The Mental Health Act in Wales

18

The Mental Health Act in Wales

18.1 The overall use of the Act in Wales is shown at Figure 55 below. The peak of usage in 1998/99 is likely to be due in large part to the Court of Appeal's judgment in *Bournewood*[456]. In December 1997 the Court ruled that psychiatric patients lacking mental capacity, even if they are compliant with admission, could not be admitted to hospital informally. This position was reversed by the House of Lords on the 25 June 1998[457].

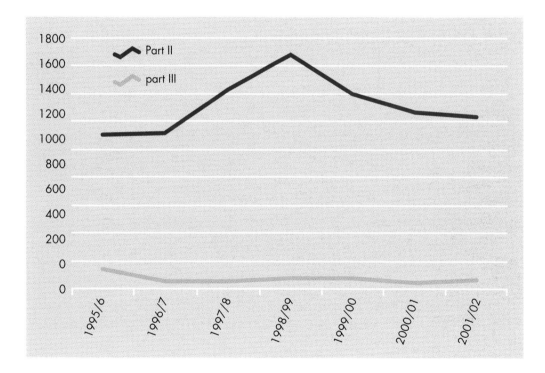

Fig 55: Admission by legal status, Wales, NHS facilities[458]

18.2 Overall uses the Act in have not returned to their pre-*Bournewood* level, with Part II usage having increased overall by about 10% from 1995/96. This rise in usage is most noticeable

---

[456] see Mental Health Act Commission (1999) *Eighth Biennial Report* para 1.31

[457] At the time of writing, the case had been considered further at the European Court of Human Rights but judgment had not yet been handed down. The Commission website (www.mhac.trent.nhs.uk) will provide up to date information. We discuss the general issues relating to incapable compliant patients at Chapter 8 above.

[458] data source: National Assembly for Wales, Health Statistics and Analysis Unit (2002) Admission of patients to mental health facilities in Wales 2001-02 (including patients detained under the MHA 1983) Report No: SDB 32/2002. 95% of all formal admissions in 2001/02 were to NHS facilities.

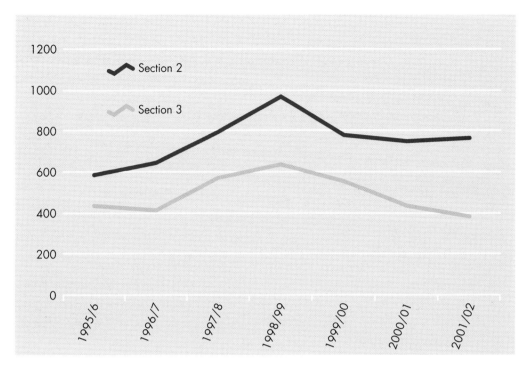

Fig 56: Use of section 2 & 3, Wales, NHS facilities[459]

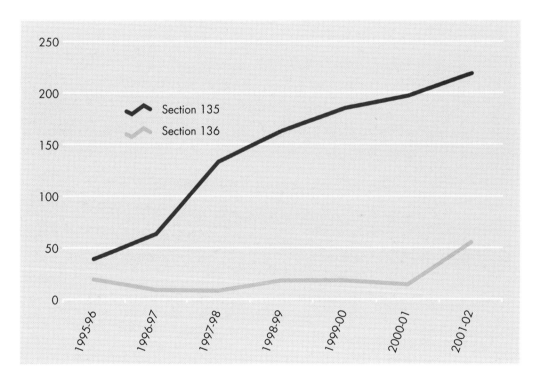

Fig 57: Use of sections 135 & 136, NHS facilities

in relation to the number of admissions for assessment and/or treatment under section 2 (Figure 56). The reasons for this overall increase are unlikely to be different to those discussed at Chapter 8.27 above.

---

[459] data source: as note 458 above

18.3 The most substantial rise in uses of the Act in Wales, according to the Welsh Assembly Government statistics, has occurred in place of safety detentions (Figure 57). However, it may well be that the apparent quadruple rise in such detentions actually reflects a positive change in mental health care provision. As places of safety are established in hospitals rather than police stations, as the Commission recommends, their uses will register in health statistics. No comparable figures of the use of places of safety in police stations or elsewhere are available to us to back up our supposition. We would welcome further research into this matter.

The detained patient population

18.4 In 2001-02, there were 16,723 formal and informal admissions to all mental health facilities in Wales, of which 1,378 admissions (8.2%) were under the Mental Health Act 1983 (excluding place of safety detentions) and other legislation. A similar proportion of formal patients were admitted during 2000-01 (7.8% – 1,372 formal admissions from a total of 17,631). In 1995/96 there were 1,242 formal admissions out of a total of 18,266 (6.8%) [460].

18.5 The increasing proportion of inpatients who are formally admitted appears more pronounced in snapshot figures of the patient populations over a longer timescale. At the 31 March 2002, 21% of mental health patients (464 patients) were detained under the Mental Health Act 1983 and other legislation, compared to 10% (295 patients) in 1992[461]. It may be that this increase in the proportion of detained patients is due in part to the increasing use of community-based out-patient treatment for informal care.

18.6 For the last five years, the proportion of women detained has been lower than for men, with a gap of 15% in 2002[462]. There are no nationally collated statistics on ethnicity and detention: we hope that this will be rectified in future collations (see Chapter 16 above for data collected across Wales and England on patients' ethnicity).

> **Recommendation 66:** Health Statistics Wales should collate data on patients' ethnicity for future publications of psychiatric hospital statistics.

The use of the Act in patients' hospital care in Wales

Staffing

18.7 Staffing continues to cause concern in relation to the standard of care of detained patients, particularly the difficulties in the recruitment of consultant psychiatrists and qualified nurses. Areas of concern include North Wales, Penbroke and Derwen, Cardiff, Pontypridd and Rhondda, Swansea and Bro Morgannwg. Trusts are keen to recruit, but the supply of

---

[460] National Assembly for Wales, Health Statistics and Analysis Unit (2002) *Admission of patients to mental health facilities in Wales (including patients detained under the Mental Health Act 1983)*, November 2002, SDR 58/2002, page 1.

[461] National Assembly for Wales, Health Statistics and Analysis Unit (2002) *Patients in psychiatric hospitals and units in Wales*, November 2002, SDR 59/2002, page 1.

[462] *ibid*, page 4. In 1996/97 marginally more women patients were detained than men

qualified staff is not adequate and competition is great. Commissioners have encouraged Trusts to provide resources for training health care assistants as qualified nurses. A policy to increase the number of ward clerks could also free nurses to have more patient contact. This would provide essential continuity of care for vulnerable patients who suffer from an over-use of locum doctors and bank nurses. Additionally, in some parts of Wales, there is a shortage of Section 12(2) appointed doctors. Commissioners were pleased to learn that Powys Local Health Board are being proactive in issuing personal invitations to general practitioners to become 12(2) approved.

18.8   The availability of occupational therapists is also patchy, which puts more pressure on nurses to provide therapeutic activities for patients. One of the most common criticisms by patients is a lack of meaningful activity during their period of detention. In some cases psychologists are not fully integrated into patient care teams.

Transfer delays

18.9   The Commission continues to be concerned at continuing delays in arranging patient transfers. In January 2003, for example, Cardiff and Vale NHS Trust reported 90 patients whose transfers to another level of care was delayed. Other particular areas of concern were North Glamorgan, Pontypridd and Rhondda, Powys and Pembroke and Derwen. In North East Wales it was reported that some patients had been waiting for over a year for suitable community places. Delays are caused in part by the conflicting priorities of health and social service organisations, and by a lack of available community resources. The closure of residential homes has had a great impact across Wales.

Low Secure facilities

18.10   There is a shortage of available low secure beds across Wales, although some gaps are filled by the extensive use of independent sector facilities. As a result, patients who would receive more appropriate care in a more restricted environment are nursed on acute wards for extended periods. This may be a causative factor behind the high levels of aggression and violence experienced by staff on acute wards. Aside from the obvious problems that this creates, it can also lead to patients being subject to special observations, taking nurses away from offering more therapeutic opportunities, and may lead to *de facto* detention for informal patients, due to wards being locked for extended periods. This is a particular concern in Cardiff. We suggest that the issue of low secure facilities is considered at a strategic level.

Examples Of Good Practice

18.11   Overall, Commissioners are pleased to record some general areas of practice improvement in the application of the Mental Health Act, largely due to the diligence of Mental Health Act Administrators. However, some aspects of Section 58 consent to treatment practice need improvement, in particular the proper recording of assessments of capacity to consent and the views of the patient (see Chapter 10.2 *et seq*).

18.12   Conwy and Denbighshire NHS Trust have created a very good system for recording patients' consent to treatment and for internal audit of issues around consent, highlighted at Chapter 10.21 above. They have also produced a questionnaire to patients who have been subject to control and restraint procedures about what could have been done in a more acceptable way.

18.13   Commissioners have been impressed with the arrangements made at Pontypridd and Rhondda NHS Trust to provide every patient with a structured plan of therapeutic care and activity and to allocate time with a qualified nurse, using a "tidal model of care". The Trust's engagement with users and carers is also encouraging, with user involvement extending to appointment committees.

Child and Adolescent Mental Health Services in Wales

18.14   In September 2001 the Minister for Health and Social Services launched the strategy for child and adolescent mental health services (CAMHS) in Wales[463]. The Commission commends the Assembly Government for the vigour with which it has followed up this strategy with mental health policy guidance[464].

18.15   Because of the shortage of inpatient facilities in or available to services in Wales, children and adolescents are often admitted to adult wards and, even when admissions are not emergency cases, available beds can be a long way from patients' homes. At Chapter 17 above we discuss at length the difficulties faced by children and adolescents admitted under the Act to adult facilities. These concerns are relevant to Welsh services, as is our concern that policy-level documents do not seem to explicitly acknowledge the problem. This may, in part, be a consequence of the Assembly's quite sensible inclusive definition of CAMHS to refer to all service that 'impinge' on children and minors' mental health care provision[465]. Whilst adult mental health inpatient facilities may therefore stand as CAMHS services by necessity, we hope that the Assembly will not lose sight of the largely inappropriate environments that such services offer for children and adolescent care. During 2002-03, the Commission was informed of 15 minors detained in adult wards in Wales, of whom Commissioners visited six. These were not confined to any particular Trust.

18.16   The Commission notes significant funding being invested in Pembroke and Derwen to provide flexible support for children and adolescents in the community and in West Wales hospital.

Services for women

18.17   Llanarth Court provides a forensic service for women with eight beds for acute patients and eight rehabilitation beds. It has very good facilities for occupational therapy, including a training kitchen, computer room, group therapy and relaxation. Classes include parenting and social skills; anger and anxiety management; and drug and alcohol awareness. This service could serve as a useful model for women's services in other parts of Wales and England.

---

[463] National Assembly for Wales (2001) *Everybody's Business – Child and Adolescent Mental Health Services Strategy Document.* Cardiff, National Assembly for Wales.

[464] i.e. Welsh Assembly Government (2002) *Mental Health Policy Implementation Guidance for Child and Adolescent Mental Health Services – Commissioning the NHS-funded Component of Child and Adolescent Mental Health Services.* Cardiff, Welsh Assembly Government

[465] *ibid*, para 1.5

Mental health strategy and policy in Wales

18.18 Mental health remains one of the Welsh Assembly Government's top three priorities for health improvement. Earlier strategies included *Mental Illness Services: A Strategy for Wales* (1989), *Child and Adolescent Mental Health Services for Wales* (2000, reissued in November 2002) and *Adult Mental Health Services for Wales: Equity, Empowerment, Effectiveness, Efficiency A Strategy for Adults of Working Age* (September 2001). These strategies are supported by an implementation plan, *A National Service Framework for Wales* (April 2002) and by *Commissioning Mental Health Services* (November 2002).

18.19 We welcome the commitment to principles of empowerment and social inclusion within the National Service Framework for Wales (NSFW). For example, authorities are required to meet the needs of specific vulnerable people who have a mental health problem and are already at risk of exclusion, such as individuals from ethnic minorities; individuals with disabilities; parents who have mental health problems; and homeless people[466].

18.20 The NSFW also requires authorities and agencies to develop arrangements relating to service user and carer empowerment, to ensure that service users and carers constructively participate in the development of plans to meet their individual needs. Specific requirements were placed upon authorities to provide have timely access to comprehensive, clear, appropriate and helpful information, in a range of appropriate formats and languages. This will include information in minority languages as well as English and Welsh, information on audio-tape and access to interpreters or people who can use British Sign Language if required.

18.21 Other Key Actions under the NSFW cover dedicated advocacy services, service user and carer involvement in service planning, design, delivery, monitoring and evaluation, carers' assessments, services for those with specific needs (such as physical disabilities).

18.22 At Chapter Six of this report we discussed the tools available to Government to promote and ensure the delivery of human rights-based mental health care services. We applaud the NSFW as even more robust in this respect than its English equivalent. We commend both National Service Frameworks, but especially those aspects of the NSFW highlighted above, as possible models for developing statutory requirements linked to the use of compulsion under the next Mental Health Act. It would provide a clear message to patients and professionals alike if such requirements were embedded and protected in primary legislation establishing powers of coercion.

> **Recommendation 67:** The UK Government should look to principles and requirements of the NSFW in determining statutory requirements upon services created under future mental health legislation.

---

[466] Welsh Assembly Government (2002) *Adult Mental Health Services: A National Service Framework for Wales.* Welsh Assembly Government, Cardiff . Key Actions for Standard 2

18.23   Other publications launched during the period include *Aspiration, Action Achievement: a Framework for realising the potential of mental health nursing in Wales*[467] and the Welsh Assembly Government formally launched its strategy for older people *When I'm 64… And More*[468] in January this year. This is to be followed by a supporting National Service Framework over the Summer of 2003. Services for older people with mental health problems are included in these documents.

18.24   The vision for partnership working in Wales is set out in another Welsh Assembly Government report: *Building Strong Bridges: Strengthening partnership working between the Voluntary Sector and the NHS in Wales*[469].

18.25   Together such strategies and the National Service Frameworks set out an ambitious agenda for modernising and improving mental health services in Wales, which we commend and look forward to seeing out into practice.

The Commission's activities in Wales

Visiting hospitals and detained patients

18.26   The Commission visited all units and wards with detained patients at least twice over 2001/02 – 2002/03. The Commission visiting team for Wales has three fluent Welsh speakers.

18.27   The main focus of Commission visits continues to be visiting and interviewing detained patients and monitoring the application of the Mental Health Act. In the past year, the Commission has established structured monitoring procedures to check on how well Trusts comply with the Code of Practice. There are examples of good practice, although hospital managers need to remain vigilant in their internal monitoring procedures. Commission Visit Reports should be received and reviewed by providers at Board level, with a Director at Board level taking lead responsibility for monitoring practice in relation to detention and treatment under the Act and the implementation of Commission recommendations.

> **Recommendation 68:** Providers should make it standard practice to give lead responsibility to a Director of their Board for monitoring the use of the Mental Health Act.

18.28   In future, Commissioners and the Team Manager will meet with chief executives of Trusts and Local Health Boards at least once during a two-year period, in addition to meetings with other levels of the service, and with the Welsh Assembly Government officers.

---

[467]   Welsh Assembly Government (2001) *Aspiration, Action Achievement: a Framework for realising the potential of mental health nursing in Wales.* Welsh Assembly Government, Cardiff. November 2001.

[468]   Welsh Assembly Government (2003) *When I'm 64…and more.* Welsh Assembly Government, Cardiff. January 2003.

[469]   Welsh Assembly Government (2002) *Building Strong Bridges: Strengthening partnership working between the Voluntary Sector and the NHS in Wales.* Welsh Assembly Government, Cardiff. October 2002.

The MHAC National Visit in Wales – focusing on specific communication needs

18.29 Detailed preparation for the Commission's first National Visit in Wales took place during 2002, with the visit itself taking place during early April 2003. Four teams of two people visited all eleven NHS Trusts and four of the independent providers who care for detained patients. They gathered information from 15 senior managers and 20 ward managers on the specific communication needs of detained patients and providers' policies and practice in seven areas of communication:

* Welsh Language;

* spoken languages other than Welsh or English;

* learning disabilities;

* visual impairments and blind people;

* hearing impairments and deaf people;

* physical disabilities; and

* low levels of literacy.

The teams then examined 43 patient records with the help of ward staff. Before the visit, providers had identified 46 patients as having specific communication needs, approximately 10% of all patients detained in Wales.

18.30 Findings were mixed. Many providers demonstrated excellent policies although these were rarely well known at ward level. Even so, many wards cited practice to support detained patients with specific communication needs.

18.31 An examination of patients' records suggested that while some providers can make arrangements to meet specific communication needs, these are not always routinely bedded into assessment and care planning.

18.32 While the sample was too small to make statistical inferences, it did appear that people with learning disabilities and low levels of literacy were likely to be reasonably well supported. In the north and west of Wales, Welsh-speaking patients were likely to be able to use Welsh, if they wished. Assumptions were often made that bilingual patients who spoke a language other than Welsh or English would find services in English adequate. People with sensory impairments and physical disabilities risked being poorly served, perhaps because few of the facilities visited catered specifically for people with this range of needs.

18.33 The full project report (*Empowerment and Understanding*) is due in winter 2003. The attention that this project gives to people with specific communication needs forms part of the Commission's equality programme, and is likely to be rolled out across England during the next reporting period.

18.34 The Commission appreciates the whole-hearted support that the Welsh Assembly Government has provided to this project.

18.35 As a result of its review of its Welsh Language Scheme, the Commission now requires providers, when they request the SOAD service, to identify the patient's preferred language.

The Commission will use this information to use this to deliver the SOAD service in the relevant language and upgrade its own information systems.

The Commission and the Welsh Assembly Government

18.36   The Commission met three times with colleagues from the Welsh Assembly Government during the period under review. Two of these meetings were our scheduled annual meetings, and the third was convened specifically to discuss more detailed issues related to the National Visit (see 18.18 above) and to routine visiting.

18.37   During summer 2002, the Welsh Assembly Government ran three broad-based stakeholder meetings, two of which Commissioners attended, and received many written responses as part of its consultation on the draft Mental Health Bill and on proposals for specialist advocacy. Assembly Members in plenary and in the Health and Social Services Committee also debated the draft Bill. Following these consultations and debates, the Minister for Health and Social Services, Jane Hutt, conveyed various concerns and comments raised to the Secretary of State for Health.

18.38   In Wales, as in England, discussions are taking place about the most effective way of monitoring both health and social care. At time of writing, proposals for future arrangements have not detailed. It is, however, anticipated that there may be a health inspection agency for Wales working alongside the Commission for Healthcare Audit and Inspection.

The Commission's Welsh Language Scheme

18.39   The Commission carried out a comprehensive review (2001-02) of its current practice with regard to Welsh and English language equality against the targets in its Welsh Language Scheme. The review drew on 23 Welsh Visit Reports for 2001-02, which covered 16 different service providers (11 NHS Wales Trusts and 5 independent providers), and assessed its own internal practice.

18.40   Reports showed a reduction in the number of patients requesting interviews in Welsh, from 22 in 2000-01 to nine for 2001-02. Commissioners carried out 180 interviews, nine (or 5%) of which were in Welsh. Most requests for interviews in Welsh were from North Wales. These interviews, carried out by Welsh-speaking Commissioners, provided a bilingual service to patients.

18.41   The Welsh Language Scheme sets out the various arrangements that the Commission will make to provide aspects of its services in both Welsh and English. Monitoring showed that there were no specific requests for correspondence or telephone calls in Welsh; for visit reports in Welsh (available to the general public in April 2002); or for a Welsh-speaking Commissioner to investigate complaints or attend inquests during the period. The Commission's response to this low demand is to recognise that it needs to be more proactive in promoting the fact that it offers a bilingual service

18.42   As a result of the review, the Commission has already improved its services to detained patients in Wales, some of whom are likely to prefer to use Welsh. For example:

* The Board has reaffirmed its responsibility for the Scheme;

* The pre-visit notification letter and request for information to Trusts and facilities in Wales now explicitly requests information about the language of choice of detained patients who wish to meet Commissioners. This will help the Commission to ensure either that a Welsh-speaking Commissioner is available for the interview or that interpreting services will be available; and

* Chairs of visits in Wales ask Mental Health Act Administrators or other liaison staff to remind patients that interviews are available in Welsh, ensure that Commissioners gather relevant information on Welsh Language use among patients and on the availability of our leaflets in Welsh and that they include their findings in reports relating to all visits in Wales.

18.43   The Review also identified several successes.

* All Commission leaflets are available in both Welsh and English, except that on neurosurgery which will be translated if the need arises.

* The publication of sections of the Commission's Ninth Biennial Report in Welsh;

* The Commission continues to promote its public identity in Wales in both Welsh and English; and

* The Commission's internal translation arrangements work well.

18.44   The Commission is arranging for web-based publication of a Welsh version of this chapter of our report, which will be expanded to include other parts of the report that are relevant to it.

18.45   As new monitoring arrangements become clear with the establishment of the Commission for Healthcare Audit and Inspection (CHAI) and any equivalent Welsh body, the Mental Health Act Commission will be revising its Scheme to fit with future arrangements and best practice in Welsh Language Schemes.

The future of Mental Health Act monitoring in Wales

18.46   Under emerging legislation and implementation arrangements, the Mental Health Act Commission is likely to merge with other bodies that monitor health services and become part of the Commission for Audit and Inspection (CHAI) – an Inspectorate covering all health services in England and Wales. In the meantime, the Welsh Government Assembly is considering what arrangements will best suit that nation. We are therefore working within this context of legal and organisational change and will ensure that our joint working and links with the emerging CHAI and any equivalent Welsh body will continue to deliver a service to detained patients in Wales.

6

The Work of the Commission and its Successor Bodies

19

The Commission's role and remit

The formal remit and powers of the Mental Health Act Commission

19.1   The Mental Health Act Commission was established by the Mental Health Amendment Act 1982 consolidated into the Mental Health Act 1983 (England and Wales). Scotland and Northern Ireland have separate legislation. Section 120(1) of the 1983 Act requires that the Secretary of State shall, for the protection of detained patients:

> '…keep under review the exercise of the powers and the discharge of the duties conferred or imposed by this Act so far as relating to the detention of patients or to patients liable to be detained under this Act and…make arrangements for persons authorised by him on that behalf…to visit and interview in private patients detained under this Act in hospitals…'.

Although the Commission necessarily undertakes a wide range of non-statutory activity in support of its formal remit, such as advice and guidance to mental health providers, the main function of ensuring the lawfulness of patient detention flows from the section 120 duty.

19.2   The Commission's remit and statutory functions as established by the 1983 Act and its delegated legislation are:

(i) Keeping under review the exercise of powers and duties contained within the Act in relation to detained patients.	MHA 1983 s120(1)(a), 121(2)(b)
(ii) Visiting and interviewing detained patients.	s120(1)(a), 121(2)(b)
(iii) Investigating complaints falling within our jurisdiction (this is a discretionary power).	s120(1)(b), 121(2)(b)
(iv) Appointing SOADs and s57 panels, and monitoring reports on treatment given to patients under their authority.	MHA 1983 s121(2)
(v) Reviewing on appeal decisions of High Security Hospital managers to withhold patients' mail. MHA 1983 s121(7)	MHA 1983 s121(7)

(vi)	Submitting proposals to the Secretary of State for the content and revision of the Code of Practice.	Statutory Instruments 1983: 894; 1995:2630
(vii)	Submitting proposals to the Secretary of State for treatments to which safeguards should apply.	Statutory Instruments 1983: 894; 1995:2630
(viii)	Publishing a Biennial Report.	MHA 1983 s121(10)

19.3   In pursuance of these aims, the Commission has unfettered powers of access to records concerning the detention of patients under the Act, including patient-identifiable information. As a Special Health Authority, we have appointed a Caldicott Guardian and comply with NHS requirements about the use of such information. Additionally the Commission Board has recently appointed a Freedom of Information champion who will oversee the implementation of the Commission's FoI publication scheme. We discuss rights of access to patients and patient records at 20.9 below.

19.4   A number of commentators have observed that the Commission's legal remit at (i) above technically encompasses monitoring the activity of the Mental Health Review Tribunal. This is discussed at 20.19 *et seq* below.

The activities of the Commission

19.5   Analysis and reports on the Commission's activities in pursuit of its remit are now published annually[470]. We have here restricted our reporting to a general overview, emphasising the purpose of activities to establish our discussion in the next chapter on the future arrangements that might be made to preserve their best aspects.

Visiting

19.6   The central aspect of the Commission's work in monitoring the exercise of powers and duties under the 1983 Act consists in visiting patients and healthcare establishments. In this reporting period we visited all hospitals that detained patients an average of three times and undertook around 19,000 patient related activities (e.g. checking records, interviewing patients)[471]. The purpose of visits as described in the Commission's visit policy is to:

*   meet with detained patients in private, particularly those who have asked to meet with members of the Commission. Meetings may be with individual patients or with groups of patients, including patient's councils;

*   observe the conditions in which patients are detained;

*   see how the provisions of the Act and the Code of Practice are being applied; and

*   offer advice and guidance on the implementation of the Act.

The highest priority is given to meeting with detained patients and to checking detention documents, although the Commission also produces reports for service providers on its findings from visits.

---

[470] Available from www.mhac.trent.nhs.uk

[471] Mental Health Act Commission (2003) *Annual Report 2002/03*, Table 2. Total patient-based activities 2001-2003 = 19,948. This is comparable with our last Biennial Reporting period: see *Ninth Biennial Report 1999-2001*, p100.

The Purpose of Commission Visits

The functions performed by the Commission's present visiting activity include:

* keeping a regular and detailed overview of specific establishments' services for detained patients;

* abstracting lessons from individual patients' or carers' experiences of local services under the Act;

* meeting with service users and carers, patients' councils, advocacy services and other voluntary organisations, and statutory organisations such as the police and ambulance services, to draw on their experiences of the operation of the Act;

* drawing together experiences of health and social services in the operation of the Act;

* identifying good and bad practice, sharing good practice and encouraging practice development;

* education concerning the application of mental health law and policy;

* providing expertise, information and/or advice to enable services to audit their own performance;

* scrutinising legal documents relating to the use of legal powers;

* identifying gaps or discrepancies between legal documents or formal care plans and the actual care being provided to patients;

* providing service managers with detailed reports on specialist aspects of their services, with recommendations for improvement;

* fostering relationships with service managers for the development of services through action-plans; and

* validating services' reported audit results.

extracted from the Mental Health Act Commission's response to the draft Mental Health Bill, September 2002.

Fig 58: The purpose of Commission visits

19.7   A more detailed account of the purpose of Commission visits was given in our response to the draft Mental Health Bill of 2002, extracted at Figure 58 above.

19.8   The Commission does not, however, visit only hospitals and nursing homes. In its meetings with Social Services Departments the Commission aims to encourage a co-ordinated approach to the operation of the Act and, in particular, to keep under review:

* the SSD's responses to the Act and the Code of Practice;

* the process of assessment, compulsory admission and detention under the Act, including the availability of ASWs and their communication with GPs, hospitals, Section 12 approved doctors and the emergency services;

* the planning and delivery of appropriate residential places, alternatives to detention and aftercare procedures and facilities; and

* the extent to which hospital and community services are able to integrate all aspects of a patient's detention from the initial assessment to the termination of aftercare.

19.9   The Commission also meets with representatives of the relevant commissioning bodies in order to encourage the latter to ensure that contractual arrangements adequately reflect the needs of detained patients, that the services provided meet such contractual requirements and to encourage commissioning bodies routinely to monitor services for detained patients. Its reports are copied to the relevant health commissioning body and NHSE regional office.

The Commission's review of its visiting practices

19.10 Over this reporting period we have been engaged in reviewing our visiting practice, completing this major piece of work in 2002/03. This is discussed in more detail in our annual report for 2002/03, although the following is an outline of its main features.

19.11 The review had four major focus areas:

(a) Visit planning

The visit programme has been adjusted to take account of the increasing numbers of large NHS Trusts (for which single visits are no longer practicable). We have reduced our demands upon services for visit planning information in recognition of the administrative burden placed upon services by inspectorates and visiting bodies. We also liaise with services regarding timing and focus of visits, to ensure compatibility with local arrangements and priorities where this is possible. A proportion of our visits remain unannounced to provide snapshot assessments of services.[472]

(b) Private meetings with patients

In this period the Commission has maintained its level of private meetings with patients, which are now backed up by new recording documentation that ensures appropriate follow-up of issues raised and will provide an evidence base for trend analysis and wider reporting. As part of a private meeting with a detained patient Commissioners will normally check:

* statutory documentation relating to detention;

* documentation relating to consent to treatment where the patient has been detained for three months or more; and

* documentation related to the queries and concerns raised by patients during a meeting.

Figure 59 below shows that new visit arrangements have resulted in a reduction of meetings between Commissioners and patients on an informal or group basis. This

Patient contacts/ document checks	1997–1999	1999–2001	% change	2001–2003	% change
Private meeting with document check	12,394	13,042	5.2%	13,188	1.1%
Informal meeting with patient	6,580	8,656	31.6%	6,543	-32.3%
Patients met in groups	742*	895	20.6%	217	-75.8%
Total direct patient contacts	19,716	22,593	14.6%	19,948	-11.7%
Documents checked with patient not seen	7,910	11,285	42.7%	14,804	31.2%
Total patient-related activity	27,626	33,878	22.6%	34,752	2.6%

Figure 59: Patient contacts 1997–2002

* data not collected in 1997/98, therefore estimated at 1998/99 activity levels.

---

[472] In 2001/02, 44% of visits were unannounced, although this was a unusually high proportion dictated in part by administrative practicality during reorganization of visiting practices. In 2000/01 14% of visits were unannounced, rising to 17% of visits in 2002/03.

reflects the Commission's need to use its limited resources where they will be most effective for patients' concerns and for the Commission's wider monitoring role. In this way the Commission is establishing a clear distinction between its role and that of advocacy services. This distinction cannot yet be put into practice rigorously, as patient advocacy is not yet available to all detained patients. We cannot change practices in anticipation of service proposals where this may disadvantage patients.

(c) Monitoring the implementation of the Act and Code of Practice

Figure 59 above also shows a significant increase in the number of patient documents checked where the patient is not seen on the visit. Over 5,000 of these document checks were undertaken as part of a revised procedure, introduced in 2002/03, for structured monitoring of issues relating to the use of the Act and compliance with the Code of Practice. This monitoring is undertaken using subject-specific Commission Visiting Questionnaires (CVQs), developed as a key element of the visiting review. Each CVQ collects data relating to local policies and practice and also examines in detail up to five patient records on each ward that is visited.

Figure 60 below shows the subjects covered by current and forthcoming CVQ questionnaires. The questionnaires themselves are available on the MHAC website or on request from the secretariat.

Commission Visit Questionnaires Subject Index

* Section 2
* Section 3
* Section 4
* Section 5(4)
* Section 5(2)
* Seclusion
* Control and management of aggressive and violent behaviour

* Section 17 leave
* Section 58 (consent)
* Section 62 (urgent treatment)
* Women's services
* Complaints
* Admission of minors to adult wards

Fig 60: CVQ subject index

(d) Reporting visits

A new visit report format was introduced by the review so that all Commission visit reports:

* set out overall conclusions against clearly stated objectives for each visit;

* are more concise, are exception based and include clear recommendations and action plans; and

* are issued in draft form to service providers for comment on factual inaccuracies before wider circulation.

Commission reports are issued to provider Chief Executives with the expectation that the recommendations will be considered at Board level. We have begun a series of biennial meetings with senior management teams of larger NHS Trusts and independent hospitals to take stock of reported issues, discuss progress and jointly agree priorities for future visits. We monitor progress against agreed targets between visits through a database incorporating all agreed action plans.

Once issued in final form Commission visit reports are public documents, available upon request from the Commission secretariat. At the time of writing, the Commission is considering other ways of making its reports available as a part of its Freedom of Information Act Publications Scheme.

The Commission's Investigation of Complaints

19.12 The Commission's complaints remit is set out in section 120(1)(b) of the 1983 Act, and states that the Commission may investigate:

(i) any complaint made by a person in respect of a matter that occurred while he or she was detained under this Act in a hospital or mental nursing home and which he or she considers has not been satisfactorily dealt with by the managers of the hospital or mental nursing home; and

(ii) any other complaint made as to the exercise of the powers or of the discharge of the duties conferred or imposed by this Act in respect of a person who is or has been so detained.

The first part of this remit enables the Commission to investigate any complaint from a patient who is or was detained under the Act. The second part, as interpreted by judicial review[473], enables the Commission to investigate complaints from third parties that are not only about those powers and duties explicitly mentioned in the Act but also issues that flow by implication from detention. The Commission is given the discretion not to investigate a complaint or to discontinue an investigation if it considers it appropriate to do so.

19.13 Since the introduction of the NHS Complaints Procedure in April 1996, our role in dealing with detained patients' complaints has changed a good deal. In the vast majority of cases the Commission's primary function is now one of monitoring complaints, advising and supporting detained patients through the NHS complaints procedure, advising them of their rights and corresponding with Trusts either on their behalf or in relation to perceived shortcomings in the way complaints are dealt with. We believe that, in general, hospital managers have developed better and more effective ways of dealing with complaints since the introduction of the NHS procedure. Most hospitals now employ staff whose main or sole job is to deal with complaints. The Commission, on behalf of the complainant, now places particular importance on the duration and rigour of the investigation and the quality of the final response sent to the complainant from the service. Consequently the Commission currently undertakes very few complaints investigations itself.

19.14 Complaints referred directly to the Commission, whether on visits or through the secretariat office, have remained at a constant level: on average at least one is received every working day[474]. Although many issues raised by patients on a visit are resolved locally, on occasion it is necessary for Commissioners to ensure that patients are aware of their rights

---

[473] *R v Mental Health Act Commission ex parte Smith* [1998].

[474] see Mental Health Act Commission (2003) Annual Report 2002/03, Table 2. Over 2001 – 03, the Commission received an average of 246 complaints each year.

to lodge a complaint through the NHS procedure and to offer assistance in this process. We also remind hospital managers of the need to ensure that patients are aware of the complaints procedure and how to use it. During 2002-03 there was an increase in the number of occasions where Commissioners helped patients raise concerns in this way. We have reviewed our practice during the reporting period to ensure a more pro-active approach. For example, where a complaint indicates a potential continuing risk to patients (e.g. where there are allegations of bullying and other abuse or when suicide is threatened) this is now referred to the visiting team for immediate action at the onset rather than waiting for the complaints process to be completed. Monitoring of complaints through the NHS procedure at the three High Security Hospitals was reviewed by the Commission in 2002 and resulted in a report comparing practice across the hospitals with a proposal to widen this approach to medium secure units[475].

Deaths of Detained Patients

19.15   For some years the Commission has, in furtherance of its general remit, asked service providers to notify it of any death of a detained patient, and a standard form for collecting this data was introduced in February 1997. Whilst the Commission records information on all deaths of detained patients, any unnatural death is the subject of a review. An important part of this process is attending the inquest, as this provides information relating to events that led up to the patient's death, the actions of staff and any pointers to whether established good practice was followed. The information obtained from the review process forms the basis of further work with the service to improve practice and is used to identify issues that require monitoring on future Commission visits. In this reporting period the Commission has also given evidence to the David Bennett Inquiry. During 2002-03 training was provided to ensure that a local representative of each visiting team is involved in the death review process to ensure that the information gathered can be disseminated more easily and used to inform the work of the Visiting Teams. In 1995, a review of the Commission's records on deaths of detained patients was published and a further report was issued in 2001 covering the period 1997 to 2000[476]. The Commission has submitted evidence based upon this report to the Joint Committee of Human Rights' inquiry into deaths in custody and human rights in September 2003.

Second Opinion Appointed Doctors (SOADs)

19.16   Under section 118, the Commission has a duty to appoint and remunerate SOADs, who are responsible for providing formal second opinions as set out in section 58[477]. The Commission arranges approximately 9,000 second opinions each year. Second opinion activity is discussed at Chapter 10.33 above.

---

[475] available at www.mhac.nhs.uk

[476] Bingley, Bannerjee & Murphy (1995) *Deaths of Detained Patients: A review of reports to the Mental Health Act Commission. A joint report of the Mental Health Act Commission and the Division of Psychiatry & Psychology, United Medical & Dental Schools of Guy's & St Thomas' Hospitals.* Published by the Mental Health Foundation; Mental Health Act Commission (2001) *Deaths of Patients in England and Wales; a report by the MHAC on information collected from 1 February 1997 to 31 January 2000.* Nottingham: MHAC.

[477] Section 58 provides that certain forms of treatment (ECT at any time and drug treatments after an initial three month period), shall not be given to a detained patient, unless the patient consents or an independent medical practitioner (SOAD) has certified that the treatment should be given notwithstanding the patient's refusal to consent or lack of capacity to do so.

19.17 The purpose of the Commission's role of appointing SOADs was described in the 1981 White Paper *Reform of Mental Health Legislation*:

> 'This will ensure that the opinions are independent and will enable the Commission both to monitor the use of the power to impose treatment and to offer advice on professional and ethical complexities…the Commission will build up considerable expertise in the care and treatment of detained patients and particularly on consent to treatment'.[478]

This conflation of the administration and monitoring of a system of safeguards, with both tasks allocated to the same body, creates a potential conflict of interest. This is most apparent when patients apply for judicial review of SOAD decisions or procedures, where the Commission has been a respondent to the action, ether directly or through our responsibilities for the indemnity of SOADs. It is also arguable that the Commission's overall monitoring of the effectiveness of the Second Opinion system cannot but have been influenced by its responsibilities for such a system. Whether or not this has actually had any practical effect, it is the case that the safeguards of section 57 and 58 have, in comparison with other aspects of the 1983 Act, been denied a truly independent overview. We also discuss this in relation to future legislative arrangements at Chapter 20.16 below.

Changing the Emphasis: the Commission's Work Programme 2003-05

19.18 Following significant investment in Information Technology systems during the reporting period the Commission is now in a much better position to analyse visit reports and to use the other data, such as notifications of deaths of detained patients, to provide a qualitative and quantitative picture of the operation of the Act and the implications for detained patients. As a result we are enhancing the work programme in 2003-04 (and possibly beyond[479]) in order to understand better the way in which patients are treated and to investigate and make recommendations in a number of areas of serious concern to Commissioners. For example, the seclusion practices of many providers require a closer and more focused scrutiny. We will undertake this enhanced programme in close co-operation with the Commission for Healthcare Audit and Inspection (CHAI), in part because these are matters of common and serious concern, but in part and importantly to prepare the ground for integration of visiting functions into the CHAI and the transfer of other functions to successor bodies.

19.19 The main areas in which enhancements are being considered are: extending notification requirements of the Commission to encompass a number of especially vulnerable patients, such as children and minors, and women detained on predominantly male wards; data analysis to support standards development in areas such as seclusion and consent; focussed visits and research projects including a National Visit on ethnicity and mental health and an investigation of CPA in relation to 'revolving door' detained patients; collaborative arrangements with the Commission for Health Improvement and National Care Standards Commission as a precursor to integration within CHAI; and additional relevant publications and guidance.

---

[478] Department of Health and Social Security, Home Office, Welsh Office, Lord Chancellor's Department (1981) *Reform of Mental Health Legislation*. HMSO, para 39

[479] subject to agreement with the CHAI, the progress of the Mental Health Bill and future arrangements for the MHAC establishment and funding.

20

Future monitoring of compulsory mental health care

Frequent attendance upon lunatic institutions can alone
give adequate idea of the difficulties of the service.

Phillippe Pinel, 1801[480]

The transition to new arrangements

20.1   In this final chapter we explore the future monitoring, inspection and regulatory arrangements that may apply under revised mental health legislation, and describe some of the
complexities in the transition of the Commission's functions to successor bodies. Much of
the discussion is necessarily speculative and requires a number of assumptions to be made,
especially about timescales. Undoubtedly many of these assumptions will change. In
developing a transition strategy we need to address a number of matters, including:

* ensuring that the Commission's statutory duties and functions continue to be
performed competently and properly during the transition period ;

* identifying the key statutory and other functions that need to be considered in any
transition arrangements;

* developing realistic and workable assumptions about successor bodies and timescales
for transfer, taking into account the legislative timescale for the Mental Health Bill; and

* ensuring that adequate plans are in place to manage the transfer of MHAC functions to
CHAI and successor bodies, requiring a transition strategy and risk management plan.

20.2   Where the State provides powers over mental health patients, there is also a reciprocal duty
to provide for independent review and monitoring of the use of those powers (see chapter
2.9 above). We were pleased to note the acknowledgement of this positive obligation to
protect against human rights breaches, and the Commission's role in meeting that
obligation, in the Secretary of State's Respondent Notice issued to the Court of Appeal in the
Munjaz case:

"the State has … discharged its positive obligations to provide effective protection
against…breaches [of the European Convention on Human Rights] because…
pursuant to sections 120 and 121 of the Mental Health Act 1983, the Secretary of State

---

[480] Pinel, Phillippe (1801) *A Treatise on Insanity*. First edition translated into English by D D Davis MD, 1806.
p.90n (Pinel's note). Facsimile edition published by Hafner, New York, 1962.

has made arrangements for the Mental Health Act Commission to visit and interview in private patients detained in hospitals under the MHA and for the Mental Health Act Commission to investigate complaints". [481]

The Court's judgment in *Munjaz* [2003] underlined this obligation, recognising that the State is under an obligation "to know enough about its ...patient to provide effective protection"[482]. In this chapter we examine the role of the Commission in providing this function, and how such a function might be preserved or enhanced in future monitoring arrangements.

The jurisdiction of the Commission

20.3   The requirement for monitoring discussed above can only be satisfied by a general healthcare inspection if it takes into account factors relating to compulsion and possible infringements of human rights. The proposal for the Commission's establishment in the 1981 White Paper Reform of *Mental Health Legislation* anticipated this in distinguishing the Commission's functions from those of inspectorial bodies:

> '...the Commission will not inspect and report on services in mental illness and mental handicap in hospitals and units in the way that the Health Advisory Service or the Development Team for the Mentally Handicapped do. The Commission's concern will be the particular problems that arise from detention of specific individuals in hospital rather than the general services that affect all mentally ill and mentally handicapped patients. The name "Mental Health Act Commission" has been chosen deliberately to emphasise its responsibilities for seeing that patients have full advantage of all the available legal safeguards under the Act...'[483].

20.4   The Commission's central remit as established by the 1983 Act is "to keep under review the exercise of powers and discharge of duties conferred or imposed by this Act"[484]. As we have discussed at Chapter 11, it is difficult to define exhaustively the 'powers and duties' conferred or imposed by the 1983 Act. Although there are explicitly stated powers and duties, there are also many other powers and duties *implied* by compulsion. This matter was considered in *R v Mental Health Act Commission ex parte Smith* [1998], which redrew and widened the Commission's previous understanding of its powers of complaint investigation and, by analogy, of its remit as a whole. The Court interpreted the exercise of powers and discharge of duties to pertain to "all those rights and duties which flow necessarily and by implication from a section 3 detention, and such other rights and duties that are expressly identified in the Act".

20.5   The broad definition of powers and duties established above, and the fact that the law does not (and probably cannot) provide explicit powers and duties covering all aspects of care and treatment under compulsion that may infringe patients' human rights, suggests that the

---

481 *R (on the application of Munjaz) v Mersey Care NHS Trust and two others; S v Airedale NHS Trust* [2003] Court of Appeal Respondent Notice issued by the Secretary of State, para 1.3

482 *R (on the application of Munjaz) v Mersey Care NHS Trust and two others; S v Airedale NHS Trust* [2003], para 58.

483 Department of Health and Social security, Home Office, Welsh Office, Lord Chancellor's Department (1981) *Reform of Mental Health Legislation.* HMSO, para 34

484 Mental Health Act 1983 Section 120(1)

new inspectorate must have a remit that is sufficiently broad and flexible to encompass wide-ranging issues of care, treatment and control, or else it could fail to meet the State's duties under human rights legislation.

20.6 During consultation on the Mental Health Bill in 2002, the Government acknowledged the importance of effective monitoring of the operation of the new Act once implemented. The consultation paper proposed that the remit of the new healthcare inspectorate to be established would include scrutiny of the proper application of the Act and that "[t]his role would be carried out by a specially established division of the inspectorate because the exercise of the function… will require special knowledge and expertise". The paper went on to say that the function should be focused on monitoring compliance with the law in decisions made under the Act about individual patients, by collecting information, visiting for cause, and associated activities[485]. Further, in relation to investigating and visiting, the consultation paper said that, following careful consideration, the Government proposed to supplement the role of advocacy with a special power to visit patients where there is cause for concern.

20.7 Effective monitoring and inspection of mental health services is essential, especially in relation to detained patients. Whilst we see many advantages and opportunities in the Government's proposals to integrate the Commission's monitoring functions into the CHAI and do not argue for a retention of a Mental Health Act Commission in its current form, the present role played by the Commission should not be diminished under the new arrangements. We believe that any new legislation must place a clear responsibility on the CHAI as an independent organisation to visit and review the needs of detained patients, as part of a general duty to promote high quality services for all mentally ill people. The Government has signaled that it does not want to diminish the monitoring safeguards provided to patients subject to compulsion under new legislation, but it is essential that such safeguards are not compromised unintentionally as a result of inadequacies in the legal provision or infrastructure.

20.8 In establishing the successor monitoring body to the Commission within a wider inspectorate, the challenge will be to preserve and enhance the specific focus on the legal and practice aspects of compulsion without placing artificial constraints on the jurisdiction of the body. Primary legislation could therefore allow that the remit of such a body extended to *any* matter pertaining to the compulsion of patients under mental health legislation, whilst specifying core duties as a statutory requirement. Any activity beyond such core statutory duties could then be determined by the body itself, through the governance of the healthcare inspectorate's Board, or defined further in secondary legislation or by Direction of the Secretary of State. Such a model could ensure that monitoring of mental health compulsion remains inclusive and flexible.

20.9 We believe that the duties on the Secretary of State to provide for independent and adequate monitoring of the powers and duties created by the next Mental Health Act must be stated on the face of that Act, and not relegated to secondary legislation or other Acts of Parliament. In this way the duty to monitor the use of powers is created by the same law that

---

[485] Department of Health (2002) *Draft Mental Health Bill – Consultation Document.* Cmnd 5538-III paras 3.1, 3.2

provides the powers, and cannot be separated from it. The Commission is empowered by the 1983 Act and by the Direction of the Secretary of State[486] to:

* visit and interview and, if the Commissioner is a registered medical practitioner, examine in private any patient detained under the Act.

* require the production of or inspect any records relating to the detention or treatment of any person who is or who has been detained under the Act.

The Commission recommends that the CHAI, or at least its Mental Health Act monitoring arm, should be empowered similarly in new mental health legislation. The right of access should also be extended to cover management documents, such as incident reports and general policies[487].

20.10   We have therefore suggested to the Department of Health that the next Mental Health Act should impose a duty on the Secretary of State that is equivalent to that imposed by section 120 of the Mental Health Act 1983. It would appear from the *Munjaz* judgment [2003] that human rights legislation makes such general oversight and monitoring of the use of compulsion an unavoidable duty of the State. Nevertheless, by enacting the duty in primary legislation Government could ensure that its intention is clear and protected from erosion or distortion as a result of any future political, organisational or other pressures, including any future changes to the organisation of the health service.

Recommendation 69: Any proposed mental health legislation that repeals the 1983 Act must retain, in some form, the duty on the Secretary of State to provide for the monitoring and review of powers and duties of that Act as they relate to the compulsion of psychiatric patients. Such a duty should be explicit and should establish core requirements of such monitoring, irrespective of the body that is charged with its undertaking.

The Commission's remit, *de facto* compulsion and community treatment

20.11   It is the Commission's view that the enactment of new legislation provides an opportunity to address its past requests that the monitoring remit should be extended to cover informal incapable patients subject to *de facto* detention[488] and to patients subject to community-based compulsion[489]. We trust any extension of statutory powers and duties to incapable informal patients and severance of the formal link between detention as a hospital inpatient and compulsory treatment in the next Mental Health Act will be reflected in the jurisdiction and resources of the body charged with its monitoring (i.e. the CHAI).

---

[486]   see MHA 1983 s120(4), and DHSS Circular HC(83)19, Appendix A.

[487]   *Report of the Committee of Inquiry into the Personality Disorder Unit, Ashworth Special Hospital* (1999) Vol 1 :1.30.4 . The Commission endorsed this suggestion in Mental Health Act Commission (1999) *Mental Health Act Commission Submission to the Mental Health Legislation Review Team.* Nottingham: MHAC. page 34

[488]   Mental Health Act Commission (1987) *Second Biennial Report*, 1985-87, London: Stationery Office. p50, see also subsequent Biennial Reports, as well as Chapter 8.10-11 and recommendation 17 above.

[489]   Government has not acceded to Commission requests that our remit be extended to patients subject to community-based powers under the 1983 Act. The MHAC requested that its remit be extended to Guardianship in 1991 (*Fourth Biennial Report* p45) and to Aftercare under Supervision in 1997 (*Seventh Biennial Report* p142). Neither request was granted.

Recommendation 70: Monitoring of compulsion under new legislation must be inclusive of all compulsion, including *de facto* detention (see recommendation 17) and compulsory treatment in the community.

The importance of visiting

20.12 Detained psychiatric patients remain one of the most vulnerable groups in society and, in our view, no general inspectorate role will compensate for the loss of a body whose primary task is to meet with and speak to such patients, and to focus specifically on the operation of powers and duties in relation to their care. Our contact with detained patients on our visits enables us not only to intervene directly in matters of concern to individual patients (which is a role that should increasingly be taken by emerging advocacy services), but also gives us a broad knowledge of the concerns expressed by such patients that we use to highlight more general issues of the care and treatment of detained patients. Advocacy organisations cannot be expected to fulfil this wider monitoring role, which might distract advocates from a disinterested representation of their clients' views.

20.13 Visiting practice must encompass:

(i) visiting on a regular basis all locations in which patients subject to compulsion may be required to reside or attend;

(ii) visiting particular locations and interviewing patients when there is general cause for concern through, for instance, analysis of information provided or general complaints;

(iii) visiting any individual patient where there is a reasonable cause for concern about their treatment or care under compulsory powers; and

(iv) unannounced visits at any time to any provider location where patients are subject to compulsion.

Some of these functions can be met without regular visiting of establishments, but many cannot. It may not be necessary to visit all establishments as frequently as at present. Some form of risk assessed visiting may be appropriate based on careful analysis of trends and other information available to the monitoring body. Regular visiting by the monitoring body of healthcare establishments where compulsion is used cannot and should not be replaced either by the presence of advocacy services within such establishments or by general visiting by the healthcare inspectorate.

20.14 We therefore believe strongly that successor arrangements to the Commission must include the particular activity of visiting patients detained in hospital. Such visits should continue to be undertaken by a spectrum of trained-for-purpose mental health professionals, service-users, advocates and carers. The visiting body must continue to have a gender-balanced membership with significant and meaningful representation from minority ethnic groups proportionate to those subject to compulsion under mental health legislation. We return to the question of visiting in our concluding comments to this chapter.

Sections 57 and 58

20.15   The administration of the consent to treatment safeguards of section 57 neurosurgery panels and section 58 Second Opinion appointments accounts for roughly a third of the Commission's present resources. This activity is discussed at Chapter 10.33 *et seq* above. We do not take the view that the administration of this system is a necessary part of monitoring the use of compulsion, and indeed we are aware that there may be good arguments to separate a monitoring body from this function to ensure no compromise of its objectivity. We discuss this further at Chapter 19.17 above.

20.16   Under proposals suggested in the draft Mental Health Bill of 2002, the administration of consent to treatment safeguards equivalent to the SOAD system under the 1983 Act will pass into the purview of Mental Health Tribunals. It is possible that the proposed arrangement would have its own problems of conflicting interests, given that the Tribunal may have provided authority for a patient's compulsion prior to its consideration of further imposition of treatment, but such difficulties are perhaps neither fundamental nor insurmountable.

Complaints

20.17   It could be argued that, as NHS complaints handling has improved markedly, largely as a result of the NHS Complaints Procedure, the Commission now has little practical role in investigating complaints. Furthermore, the advisory and supportive role that it now increasingly plays in seeing complaints through the NHS Procedure could conceivably be left to advocates and hospitals' complaints managers. However, removing the ability of either the Commission or its successor to investigate complaints from patients subject to detention (or other forms of compulsion) under mental health legislation would seriously weaken the statutory basis upon which such an organisation might intervene on behalf of those patients whose interests it should serve. Without the ability to take up investigations on behalf of patients, the Commission would have less to offer those patients that it meets with on its visits to hospitals and mental nursing homes, and would have less leverage with hospital managers when overseeing their handling of complaints. Thus the removal of the Commission's statutory authority to investigate patients' complaints would not only leave the organisation less able to intervene in cases where such intervention is warranted, but would also remove an important part of the organisation's statutory weight, with foreseeable consequences in its perceived image amongst mental health services. The Commission would want to see the complaints remit retained, with the discretionary element intact, in new legislation, and extended to complaints about community-based powers.

Advocacy and the monitoring body

20.18   The proposed special advocacy services could fulfil some of the general advocacy and complaints functions currently carried out by Mental Health Act Commissioners. In particular, they could ensure that patients are aware of their rights under the legislation and are able to interact positively with those responsible for their care. The Government should ensure that there is a statutory right to advocacy for all patients under compulsion and that the advocates concerned are properly funded, trained and managed. Advocacy services must remain separate from the monitoring body, and must not be expected to function also as visitors for the monitoring body or undertake similar activities that would compromise their proper advocacy role. The monitoring body could have a role in advising on standards in training for specialist mental health advocacy, as suggested in the consultation paper to the draft Mental Health Bill of 2002 (paragraph 3.4), but it probably should not be required to oversee the creation or accreditation of advocacy training programmes.

Monitoring of the Mental Health Review Tribunal

20.19   Because the Mental Health Review Tribunals come under the supervision of the Council of Tribunals and their hearings can be subject to legal appeal, the Commission has confined its observations about them over the years to the general. The Secretary of State has confirmed that it is not expected of the Commission to monitor the work of Tribunals under the present system. But under the proposed Mental Health Act, where the Mental Health Tribunal will have a much broader involvement in the exercise of powers and discharge of duties (including sanctioning compulsion and reviewing its own decision to do so when renewal of authority is required), this position may be less tenable for the Commission's successors . Whilst, of course, any arrangements for monitoring Tribunals would need to be kept distinct from any appeals process regarding Tribunal determinations, we believe that much important information on the use of powers and discharge of duties could be gained by a successor body from monitoring Tribunal activity, and the chance to influence practice (in, for example, the scope of care-planning) must not be lost to any monitoring body.

20.20   It is possible that difficult legal questions will arise as to responsibilities under the proposed Mental Health Act. In particular, where compulsion rests on the authority of a Tribunal order, it may be questionable whether the ultimate legal responsibility for that compulsion will rest with the health service provider or the Tribunal itself. Such questions could be particularly acute in situations where the Tribunal had reserved the right of discharge to itself, thus preventing a patient's clinical supervisor from ending compulsion on his or her own judgment and leading to delays in discharge. Even if the system works smoothly, there is bound to be an administrative delay whilst cases are referred back to the Tribunal for decisions during which time continued detention may be vulnerable to challenge under the ECHR[490].

20.21   But there may also be questions as to the ultimate legal responsibility in more general situations where a patient challenges treatment given under any care plan authorised by the Tribunal. It would seem, at the very least, that such challenges must be directed at both the healthcare provider and the Tribunal. Following the precedent set in *Wilkinson*, it would be possible that, where a dissenting medical opinion can be produced by a patient, all of the medical professionals involved, including medical advisers to the Tribunal as well as the patient's clinical supervisor, may be required to submit for cross-examination to the relevant judicial body. Where such dissenting opinions are produced at the time of the patient's initial 28-day Tribunal hearing, that hearing process itself is likely to satisfy the requirements if the ECHR, but this may not be the case in challenges to compulsion during the patient's subsequent treatment. We raise this matter so that consideration may be given

---

[490] see, for further discussion, Barber P (2002) *Ex parte KB: the road ahead* in <u>Bevan Ashford Mental Healthline</u> Winter 2002/Spring 2003

to assuring that patient's rights are respected whilst avoiding an intolerable burden on future tribunal or judicial systems.

The healthcare inspectorate and the monitoring body

20.22   The Government's approach to the rationalisation of regulatory bodies seems eminently sensible. There are potential advantages in the monitoring functions being administered in the context of a larger organisation charged with ensuring that the recommendations arising from an inspection/monitoring process are properly followed up and acted upon. Nevertheless it must be demonstrated that any "special division within a general healthcare inspectorate" as proposed in the Consultation Paper on the draft Mental Health Bill of 2002[491] will be sufficient to meet the requirement that "the State is under a particular obligation to protect the interests and human rights of those it places under compulsion for whatever reason, but especially when mental disorder may reduce a person's own ability to protect themselves"[492].

20.23   In the Commission's view it is essential that:

   (i)   patients subject to compulsion have a high enough priority within a general inspectorate (i.e. the CHAI) to ensure that their interests are properly safeguarded;

   (ii) inspectorate visits in relation to the monitoring of compulsion are of sufficient frequency to ensure that abuses and poor practice could not be overlooked;

   (iii) people with the necessary skills and expertise are available to monitor the implementation of mental health legislation and will be attracted to work in the CHAI; and

   (iv) responsibilities vested in the CHAI are deployed in collaboration with other inspection bodies (notably CSCI) so as to ensure that powers exercised in relation to patients subject to compulsion by social care providers are properly monitored. (The Mental Health Act Commission currently visits Social Service Departments and reviews social care for detained patients. In future the Commission for Social Care Inspection will have this role. It will be essential for CHAI and CSCI once established to work together closely on the needs of patients subject to compulsion). This will be particularly relevant in monitoring the use of non-residential treatment orders if established under the new Act.

Timetable for the new Act

20.24   At the time of writing the revised Mental Health Bill had not been published and thus it was not possible to predict the timetable for change with any certainty. The Bill is likely to provide for fundamental changes to many aspects of the detention process, including monitoring and regulation of the Act, and the way in which detention is sanctioned and reviewed by the revised Mental Health Tribunals (which in any event will be transferring to the Department of Constitutional Affairs). We expect that many aspects of these changes will require an implementation period of at least a year after the Act becomes law.

---

[491] Department of Health (2002) *Mental Health Bill Consultation Document.* Cm 5538-III (para 3.2)

[492] MHAC (2000) *A Successor to the Mental Health Act Commission. Response to the Green Paper Reform of the Mental Health Act.* MHAC Nottm. www.mhac.trent.nhs.uk/successorboby.pdf, para 5

Planning for the transfer of functions

20.25 Until the new Act comes into force and whilst any patient remains detained under the 1983 Act, we believe that it is essential for ensuring the lawfulness of such detention that the Commission continues to undertake its key visiting and Second Opinion functions as required by the 1983 Act. The revised Mental Health Tribunal arrangements may not be implemented until 2006 at the earliest (and possibly later) and thus there are likely to be many patients detained under the Mental Health Act 1983 for some considerable time. Any lapse in the monitoring of the powers and duties over detained patients may be open to judicial review challenges on either specific public duties established by the 1983 Act or general human rights principles. As the transition period may be quite lengthy we are concerned to ensure that planning for the implementation of the new Act includes consideration of a number of matters which at present have not been finalised.

20.26 Many of the points discussed at (a) to (g) below are necessarily speculative. Some may require resolution in any future legislation, statutory instruments and regulations, and some relate to the process of transition and the need to ensure all aspects of the legal protection of patients are carried through into new legislation.

(a) **Visiting for cause**

It is likely that future visiting programmes will be based on a risk assessment of provider performance and on an analysis of trends from information provided by all providers. Focused visiting to consider specific concerns (such as the use of seclusion and time-out) is likely to increase. There is no reason why the visiting function cannot be integrated administratively into the CHAI prior to the enactment of the new Mental Health Act, as long as the Commission's statutory duties can continue to be performed competently and properly. This implies no diminution of contact with patients and a continued focus on powers and duties of the 1983 legislation until the 1983 Act is repealed. Other aspects of the Commission's work (such as SOADs, or withheld mail reviews) are less likely to be appropriate for CHAI and may, for some time to come, continue to be managed separately from but linked to the new structures.

(b) **Complaints**

The Commission's role in relation to complaints is described at 20.17 above. Although the Commission does not investigate many complaints directly, it is involved in a large number of complaints indirectly through helping patients to make complaints and following up aspects of interest to it that have been raised through patients' complaints. As a by-product of the regular visiting programme, Commissioners are often in a position to intercede informally with patient concerns such that many do not become formal complaints. Although the Commission supports strongly the development of special advocacy, it is possible that such advocacy must remain reactive to specific patient complaints rather than proactive in the way the Commission is able to function at present. The CHAI's role in taking on the Commission's complaints functions will be complicated by its proposed designation as the second stage body for dealing with complaints that have not been resolved locally. Carefully designed protocols may be needed to regulate the interface between the monitoring and inspection functions (possibly fulfilled by some form of specialized mental health visiting function), the special advocacy service, and the second stage complaints process.

(c) Notifications

The Mental Health Act Commission requires notifications of all deaths of detained patients and in some cases attends inquests and reviews the reason for the death of the patient. The National Patient Safety Agency will in future have a role in relation to all adverse incidents and will receive non-attributable information about unnatural deaths of patients. We would like to see a process established whereby notifications of deaths and other critical incidents are sent to CHAI and a non-attributable subset of the core data is transmitted to NPSA. In this way the agencies involved can ensure they have consistent information about unnatural and unexpected deaths. The CHAI will then be in a position to enquire more fully into those deaths where there may be cause for concern; the NPSA will be able to encourage root cause analysis of such adverse incidents locally, provide overall statistical information on the level of incidents and collate information which may throw light on causation.

In addition, the establishment of the Mental Health Act monitoring function within the CHAI should allow an opportunity to provide routine notification of all uses of the Act to detain or compel patients, enabling the monitoring body to gather general statistics as a part of its monitoring and also track specific issues or cases as necessary. A system equivalent to that established under section 61 of the Act (providing progress reports on authorised treatment to the monitoring body) should be retained and enhanced by the adoption of routine notification (see Chapters 10.27-29 and 17.7 above)

(d) Code of Practice

The Department of Health is responsible for preparing, consulting on and publishing the Code of Practice under the Mental Health Act 1983. Under the draft Mental Health Bill of 2002 (Clause 1) it would retain this responsibility. The Commission agrees that responsibility for publishing Codes of Practice and other guidance should rest with the appropriate Minister, but it is vital that the independent monitoring body provides advice to the Minister on the contents of the Code of Practice and has a right to be consulted on it. The CHAI will need to provide evidence of the operation of the Mental Health Act to the Department of Health in order to amend the Code of Practice from time to time. This will require sufficient staff of appropriate expertise to be able to analyse the information received from mental health providers about the operation of the Act from Tribunal hearings, judicial reviews and other challenges to the operation of the Act, and to draw appropriate conclusions. Preparation and amendment of the Code of Practice is linked to the provision of advice and guidance to the field. At present the Commission offers informal advice on the operation of the Act, ensures that Commissioners are informed regularly of case law and policy changes, and in turn Commissioners are then able to ensure that providers are following the latest legal and policy advice. If in future providers are not to be visited on a regular basis by the equivalent of Mental Health Act Commissioners it may be necessary to have some other mechanism for ensuring that all providers are given up to date information on the operation of the Act.

(e) Considering appeals against withholding mail /monitoring telephone calls

At present the Commission functions as the appeals body for the withholding of mail to and from patients in High Security Hospitals under section 134 of the 1983 Act, and as an appeals body against the monitoring of phone calls made by 'high risk' patients in such hospitals by Ministerial Directive[493]. Although appeals in the former category are few in number (14 in this reporting period, 3 of which we upheld) and no formal appeals relating to telephone monitoring have yet been received, the process must continue until amended by new legislation, and some equivalent arrangement may be needed under new legislation.

(f) Mental Health Tribunals

Under the proposals in the draft Bill, Mental Health Tribunals will take on a role of approving the continued detention of patients after the first 28 days and reviewing that detention periodically. The Bill proposes that Tribunals will sanction the care plan provided for the patient by the RMO overseen and reviewed, we assume, by a representative of the proposed expert panel. At present it is unclear whether the expert panel will be part of the same organisation that manages the Tribunals (which in future will be part of the Department of Constitutional Affairs), or whether the expert panel will remain a separate function of the Department of Health. If the two are brought together in the same organisation there is a danger that 'legalism' and 'clinicalism' become too closely intertwined in a way that clinical care is 'trumped' by legal considerations at all times. Conversely, if the two are kept separate contestability between clinical and legal concerns will be assured, but at the possible cost of three way disputes between (i) the expert panel, (ii) the Tribunal and (iii) the constellation of RMO, patient and patient advocate that has drawn up the proposed care plan.

During the consultation process in 2002 many respondents noted that the procedures proposed in the draft Bill were likely to increase the number of Mental Health Tribunal hearings very significantly. Any significant delays in providing hearings for patients are likely to be challenged in the courts, leading to further expense and delay for patients. We believe that it will be essential to set clear performance targets for Tribunals and that patients must be able to obtain a Tribunal hearing within the time specified in the Act. It is unclear at present whether this aspect of the Tribunal's operation will be monitored by some external body (such as the CHAI) or whether that monitoring will be done internally within the Department of Constitutional Affairs.

It appears to be Government's intention that reviews concerning points of law in relation to Tribunal decisions or procedure will be dealt with at first instance by a separate appeals body (The Mental Health Appeal Tribunal) and then through the courts. We have argued that any monitoring body that is charged with keeping the operation of the new Act under review in a more general sense should extend its purview over Tribunal activity and decisions, and so gain a holistic view of the operation of the system of compulsion. The proposed Tribunal will have a wider role in such a system than its present counterpart, including sanctioning and providing the authority for compulsion

---

[493] The Safety and Security in Ashworth, Broadmoor and Rampton Hospitals Directions 2000, paragraph 29(2).

after 28 days. However the Mental Health Act Commission's statutory monitoring role may have been fettered by the directive that it should not include the present Mental Health Review Tribunal's workings from its monitoring scope, a similar fetter on its successor body will, potentially, have much more serious consequences (see Chapter 20.19 above).

(g) Second Opinions and Consent Arrangements

At present the Commission administers the system of statutory 'second opinion' authorisation of treatments falling within sections 57 and 58 of the 1983 Act. Under proposals set out in the draft Mental Health Bill of 2002 the process will pass the Tribunal administration, with doctors appointed to the Tribunal's Expert Panel taking a similar role to today's Second Opinion Appointed Doctors.

The Commission is keen to ensure that any benefits of current arrangements in relation to consent to treatment regulation be preserved under new legislation. For example, we argue at Chapter 10.25 above for the retention of some form of statutory documentation of a patient's consent status.

The authority to monitor the progress of treatments and the associated power to withdraw an authorisation and request that a further Second Opinion takes place in cases of concern (sections 61, 121) provides the Commission with a valuable tool, both to check the legality and appropriateness of treatments given after a SOAD's authorisation and to protect the interests of detained patients. The Commission would strongly support the retention and strengthening in new legislation of the requirement that RMOs should submit such reports, whether they do so to the monitoring body or to the Tribunal. Such strengthening measures could include the submission of reports for detained patients who consent to treatment as well as those who are incapable or refusing consent, and/or to extend the periods during which such reports are required to be submitted. This could be developed as a way for the Commission or its successor body to monitor the care and treatment of patients subject to compulsion throughout their psychiatric careers up to, or even following, discharge[494].

Concluding remarks

20.27   At the start of this chapter we quoted Phillipe Pinel's underlining, 200 years ago, of the fact that frequent visiting of hospitals alone can give "an adequate idea of the difficulties of the service". We believe that, whatever limitations the Mental Health Act Commission may have, its great strength over the last twenty years has been in the combined experience of its Commissioners of the problems and challenges faced within hospitals operating the 1983 Act, and faced by those who have come under its powers. Such experience comes partly from Commissioners' backgrounds as mental health professionals and service users, but it also comes through their visiting of services and meetings with patients and staff. It would be a matter of deep regret if successor arrangements fail to preserve a system of hospital visiting which retains this aspect of expertise coupled with a humane approach. We are confident, as were the Lunacy Commissioners of 1913 (see Chapter 1.10 above) that patients would wish to continue to receive the personal interest and attention of such a visitorial body.

---

[494] Mental Health Act Commission (1999) *Mental Health Act Commission Submission to the Mental Health Legislation Review Team.* MHAC, Nottingham. page 31

20.28   The Commission believes that there will be significant benefits to be had from amalgamation of healthcare monitoring and inspectoral bodies under the wing of the Commission for Healthcare Audit and Inspection. We wish to end our report, however, with a proposal that such amalgamation should make every effort to build on the expertise and personal attention fostered by the Mental Health Act Commission. We trust that the CHAI will seek to maintain specialist mental health visiting teams and that statutory duties will preserve the focus of such visiting teams on the use of powers of compulsion. Otherwise, it is possible that the attentions of inspectors may move onto less oppressive (and less difficult) areas of mental healthcare provision.

Psychiatric patients may sometimes break the law, become alarming or at any rate somewhat eerie to those around them. Something has to be done about them... in the interests of society such patients have to be made harmless. In the interests of the patients themselves some attempt must be made at cure. In many cases public safety demands the committal of the patient to hospital. He needs to be protected from doing violence. We want moreover to take him out of the public eye. We vary the form of segregation and try to make it humane so that relatives are satisfied and public conscience is appeased. Our own concept and interpretation of insanity involuntarily cause us to hide it away although it is one of the basic facts of human reality.

Karl Jaspers (1959) General Psychopathology, Seventh edition[495].

Seventeen years of labour and anxiety obtained for the Lunacy Bill in 1845, and five years' increased labour since that time have carried it into operation. It has effected, I know, prodigious relief ... and greatly multiplied inspection and care. Much – alas! – remains to be done, and much will remain; and that much will, in the estimation of the public, who know little and require less, overwhelm the good, the mighty good that has been the fruit.

Lord Shaftesbury, diary entry, 25 December 1850[496].

[495] Jaspers K (1959) *General Psychopathology*, Seventh edition. Translated by Hoenig, J and Hamilton, M W. Manchester University Press 1963, p 793 -794

496 quoted in Hodder E (1890) *The Life and Work of the Seventh Earl of Shaftesbury K G.* Cassell & Co, 1890 ed. p442

Appendix A

Table of cases cited

Case reference	Paragraph in this report where cited

U.K. Cases

A.R. (by her litigation friend J.T.) v Bronglais Hospital Pembrokeshire and Derwen NHS Trust [2001] EWHC Admin 792	8.65
Anderson, Reid and Doherty v the Scottish Ministers and the Advocate General for Scotland [2001] Court of Session x170/00	7.25
B v Barking, Havering and Brentwood Community Healthcare NHS Trust [1999] 1 F.L.R 106	9.50
B v Croydon [1995] 2 W.L.R 294	3.42, 11.66n
B v MHRT and Secretary of State for the Home Department [2002] EWHC 1553, QBD (Admin Ct)	3.13
Bolam v Friern Hospital Management Committee [1957] 1 WLR 582	3.35
Bolito v City & Hackney Health Authority [1988] AC232	3.35
Grindley v Barker [1798] 1 Bos & Pul, 875, 879	9.59
MP v Nottingham Healthcare NHS Trust (Secretary of State for Home Department and Secretary of State for Health intervening) [2003] EWHC 1782 (Admin)	3.21
Pountney v Griffiths [1976] Ac 314	11.6
Raymond v Honey [1982] 1 All ER 756 HL	11.6
R v Ashworth Hospital Authority ex p RH [2001] EWHC Admin 872	11.57
R v Ashworth Hospital Trust ex parte Munjaz [2000] M.H.L.R. 183	3.3
R v Bournewood Community & Mental Health NHS Trust ex parte L [1998] 2 W.L.R 764; 1 All ER 634	8.5
R v Broadmoor Special Hospital Authority and the Secretary of State for the Department of Health, ex p. S, H and D, February 5, 1998; C.O.D. 199	11.6, 11.49
R v Camden & Islington Health Authority, ex parte K [2001] EWCA Civ 240; [2001] M.H.L.R 24	3.19
R v Canons Park Mental Health Review Tribunal ex p. A [1994] All E.R.659	8.21
R v Doncaster Metropolitan Borough Council ex parte W [2003] High Court, 13 February EWHC Admin 192	3.19
R v East London & the City Mental Health NHS Trust ex parte Brandenburg [2001] EWCA Civ 239	8.38
R v Galfetti [2002] EWCA Crim 1916 CA (Crim Div)	13.5-6
R v Hallstrom, ex parte W (No2); R v Gardner, ex parte L [1986] Q.B. 1090; [1986] 2 W.L.R. 883; [1986] 2 All E.R. 306	4.1, 6.8, 9.48-9
R v Home Secretary ex parte D [2002] December 2002	3.24
R v Manchester City Council ex parte Stennett [2002] UKHL 34; [2002] 4 All E.R. 124	9.62
R v MHAC ex parte Smith [1998] 1 C.C.L. Rep 451; (1998) 43 B.M.L.R. 174	11.7, 20.4

Appendix B

Mental Health Act Commission Members 2001 – 2003

Ms M Agar*
Mr C Aggett*
Mr V Alexander
Dr H Allen
Dr T Ananthanarayanan*
Mr S Armson~
Ms S Bailey~
Mr A Backer-Holst ™
Ms C Bamber
Mr R Bamlett ™
Dr S Banerjee*
Mr M Beebe
Dr C Berry
Ms K Berry
Mr A Best
Mr A Bevan~
Mr J Blavo*
Ms L Bolter
Dr D Branford
Ms S Brindle~
Mr R Brown
Mr B Burke
Ms J Burton*
Mr M Cann~
Mrs S Campbell~
Ms M Casewell
Mrs B Chaffy~
Ms P Chann~
Mr H Chapman
Ns Noelle Chesworth
Miss M A Clayton*+Ch
Mr F Cofie
Mrs A Cooney
Ms S Cragg
Ms J Croton~
Mrs Ann Curno+ NED

Dr O Daniels*
Ms S Dare~
Dr C Davies
Mr H Davies w
Mr A Deery*
Mr Barry Delaney+
Mrs S Desai
Mr S Dharmabanahu~
Mr M Dodds w
Mrs M DosAnjos+w
Ms K Doeser~
Mr R Dosoo
Mrs P Douglas-Hall
Mrs G Downham
Mr A Drew
Mr R Earle
Mr T Eaton
Ms P Edwards*
Dr A El Khomy*
Mr H Field ™
Mr P Fisher*
Mr M Follows
Mr M Foolchand w
Ms A Flower~w
Miss D Frempong*
Ms E Frost
Mr S Gannon
Ms M Garner
Ms C Gilham
Mr M Golightly
Ms J Gossage
Dr H Griffiths*
Mrs C Grimshaw*
Ms A Hall~w
Mr G Halliday*
Mr N Hamilton~

Mr T Hanchen~
Miss C Harvey
Mrs S Harveyw
Mrs J Hassell~
Miss S Hayles
Mrs J Healey*
Mr S Hedges*
Ms K Herzberg~
Ms P Heslop
Ms C Hewitt
Mr D Hewitt
Mr D Hill
Mr M Hill*
Dr P Higson~w
Mr B Hoare
Dr J Holliday*
Mr D Holmes~
Mr W Horder
Mr J Horne*
Mrs B Howard
Mr P Howes
Mr C Inyama
Mr M Jamil
Ms D Jenkins+NED
Mr T Jerram*
Mr R Jones~
Dr O Junaid+
Dr A Kelly*
Mr N Khan
Mr S Klein™
Dr A Ananthakopan~
Dr S Knights
Mr G Lakes CB MC*
Ms A Lawrence
Ms S Ledwith
Mr P Lee

295

Appendix C

Second Opinion Appointed Doctors 2001-2003

Dr S W Ahmad
Dr M Al-Bacheri
Dr M Alexander
Dr M Alldrick
Dr S Ananthakopan
Dr T Ananthanarayanan
Dr R P Arya
Dr D Attapattu
Dr G Bagley
Dr D Battin
Dr C Berry
Dr J Besson
Dr M Bethall
Dr R Bloor
Dr J Bolton
Dr A Briggs
Dr A C Brown
Dr M Browne
Dr A Cade
Dr C Calvert
Dr W Charles
Dr A Chaudhary
Dr R Chitty
Dr J Colgan
Dr M Conway
Dr M Courtney
Dr C Cruickshank
Dr R Davenport
Dr I Davidson
Dr C Davies
Dr M Davies
Dr G Dawson
Dr V Deacon
Dr N Desai
Dr R Devine
Dr A Dick
Dr A Drummond
Dr G Dubourg
Dr K Dudleston
Dr D Dunleavy
Dr J Dunlop
Dr B Easby
Dr A Easton

Dr C Edwards
Dr H Edwards
Dr S Edwards
Dr A El-Komy
Dr G Feggetter
Dr S Fernando
Dr E Gallagher
Dr G Gallimore
Dr S Goh
Dr M Goonatilleke
Dr H Gordon
Dr G Grewal
Dr J Grimshaw
Dr K Gupta
Dr D Hambidge
Dr F Harrop
Dr G Hayes
Dr M Hession
Dr P Hettiaratchy
Dr S Hettiaratchy
Dr R Hill
Dr G Hughes
DR M Humphreys
Dr M Hussain
Dr G Ibrahimi
Dr S Iles
Dr J Jain
Dr H James
Dr S James
Dr P Jefferys
Dr J Jenkins
Dr B John
Dr D Jones
Dr S Joseph
Dr F Judelson
Dr S H Kamlana
Dr S Kanagaratnam
Dr G Kanakaratnam
Dr A Kellam
Dr J Kellett
Dr K Khan
Dr L Kremer
Dr N Lockhart

Dr M Loizou
Dr R Londhe
Dr B Lowe
Dr M Lowe
Dr E Lucas
Dr G Luyombya
Dr J Lyon
Dr P Madely
Dr S Malik
Dr B Mann
Dr H Markar
Dr E Mateu
Dr J Mathews
Dr H Matthew
Dr F Mckenzie
Dr D Mcvite
Dr P Meats
Dr G Mehta
Dr G Milner
Dr K Mosleh-Uddin
Dr N Murugananthan
Dr D Myers
Dr D Nabi
Dr G Nanyakkara
Dr C Narayana
Dr T Nelson
Dr H Nissenbaum
Dr M O'Brien
Dr A Okoko
Dr R Oliver
Dr R Orr
Dr D Pariente
Dr J Parker
Dr G Patel
Dr I Pennell
Dr A Perini
Dr J Phillips
Dr W Prothero
Dr E Quraishy
Dr D Rajapakse
Dr D Ramster
Dr S Rastogi
Dr M Razzaque

Dr E Richards
Dr J Rigby
Dr S Rowe
Dr J Rucinski
Dr R Sagovsky
Dr G Sarna
Dr G Shetty
Dr A Sheikh
Dr N Silvester
Dr S Singhal
Dr M Smith
Dr A Soliman
Dr C Staley

Dr N Suleman
Dr M Swan
Dr R Symonds
Dr A Talbot
Dr T Tennent
Dr R Thavasothy
Dr R Thaya-Paran
Dr R Toms
Dr N Tyre
Dr P Urwin
Dr H Verma
Dr N Verma
Dr N Wagner

Dr J Waite
Dr G Wallen
Dr A Walsh
Dr D Ward
Dr M Weller
Dr A Whitehouse
Dr Y Wiley
Dr A Wilson
Dr S Wood
Dr A Yonace
Dr A Zigmond

Appendix D

Mental Health Act Commission Publications

A full list of publications can be obtained from the MHAC Secretariat or through the MHAC website

Patient Information Leaflets

Leaflets are available in the following languages from the Commission:- Urdu, Bengali, Gujarati, Punjabi, French, German, Somali, Vietnamese, Cantonese, Mandarin, Tamil, Spanish, English, Welsh. Copies in English and Welsh can be downloaded from the Commission website (www.mhac.trent.nhs.uk). Bulk orders of any leaflet are £12 per 50 copies +£1.50 p&p from chiefexec@mhac.trent.nhs.uk or the Commission office.

Leaflet Number 1 – *Information for Detained Patients about the Mental Health Act Commission*

Leaflet number 2 – *Information for Detained Patients about Consent to Treatment (Medication)*

Leaflet Number 3 – *Information for Detained Patients about Consent to Treatment Electroconvulsive Therapy (ECT)*

Leaflet Number 4 – *Information for Detained Patients about How to Make a Complaint*

Leaflet Number 5 – *Information for Patients about Neurosurgery for Mental Disorder (Psychosurgery) and The Mental Health Act Commission*

Practice and Guidance Notes

Available on the MHAC website www.mhac.trent.nhs.uk, or individual copies can be requested free of charge from the Commission office.

Practice Note 1 – *Guidance on the administration of Clozapine and other treatments requiring blood tests* (issued June 1993, updated March 1999)

Practice Note 2 – *Nurses, the administration of medicine for mental disorder and the Mental Health Act 1983* (reissued March 2001)

Guidance Note 1 – *Guidance to health authorities: the Mental Health Act 1983* (issued December 1996, updated March 1999)

Guidance Note 3 – *Guidance on the treatment of anorexia nervosa under the Mental Health Act 1983* (issued August 1997, updated March 1999)

Guidance Note 2/98 – *Scrutinising and rectifying statutory forms under the Mental Health Act 1983* (issued November 1998, updated March 1999)

Guidance Note 1/99 – *Issues surrounding Sections 17, 18 and 19 of the Mental Health Act 1983* (issued August 1999)

Guidance Note 2/99 – *Issues relating to the administration of the Mental Health Act in Registered Mental Nursing Homes* (reissued December 1999)

Guidance Note 1/2000 – *General Practitioners and the Mental Health Act 1983.* (reissued May 2000)

Guidance Note 1/2001 – *Use of the Mental Health Act 1983 in general hospitals without a psychiatric unit* (issued August 2001)

Guidance Notes for RMOs & SOADs on R *(on the application of Wooder v Dr Fegetter & the MHAC.* (June 2002)

MHAC Response to the Mental Health Bill Consultation Document (September 2002)

The Mental Health Act Commission's FOI Publication Scheme, describing all information held by the MHAC that we make publicly available, is available on request or from the MHAC website (see Appendix F)

Appendix E

The Institute of Mental Health Act Practitioners' publications

Mental Health Act 1983 Statutory Forms Manual

produced in conjunction with Trecare NHS Trust
October 1999   £30

Mental Health Act 1983 Policy Compendium

produced in conjunction with the Mental Health Act Commission
May 2002   £40

A Guide to Mental Health Act Administration

produced in conjunction with the Mental Health Act Commission
May 2002   £70

Prices shown above include p&p.

IMHAP publications available from:
Frances Buckenham,
Gunfield Lodge,
Feock,
Truro,
Cornwall TR3 6SH.

Cheques made out to IMHAP should accompany orders.

A proforma invoice can be issued if required but manuals cannot be dispatched without prior payment.

Institute of Mental Health Act Practitioners
Yens Marsen-Luther (Chief Executive),
359 Norwich Road, Ipswich IP1 4HA .
Phone /fax 0845 2300105

Registered charity No 1081245

Appendix F

Contacting the Mental Health Act Commission

You can contact the Mental Health Act Commission at the following address:

Mental Health Act Commission
Maid Marion House
56 Hounds Gate
Nottingham
NG1 6BG

Tel: 0115 9437100

Fax:0115 9437101

E-mail: Chief.executive@mhac.trent.nhs.uk

Website: www.mhac.trent.nhs.uk

Index

The page numbers given in this index refer to the paragraphs. Graphs are indicated by the paragraph number immediately preceding the graph, and are italicised with the letter 'g'; notes by the italicised number and 'n'; recommendations by the italicised number and 'r'; and statistics by the italicised number and 's'.